Praise for
Pete Egoscue and the Pain-Free Method

"Extraordinary . . . I am thrilled to recommend it to anyone who's interested in dramatically increasing the quality of their physical health."
—Anthony Robbins, author of *Awaken the Giant Within* and *Unlimited Power*

"Pete Egoscue has totally changed my life. Never have I experienced such complete pain relief as I have by following the Egoscue Method." —Jack Nicklaus

"*Pain Free* is based on a very sound understanding of human physiology. It shows how we can break the circuit of pain and naturally heal one of the most significant disabilities of our times."
—Deepak Chopra, author of *The Path of Love* and *The Seven Spiritual Laws of Success*

"Whether you are in chronic pain or are a peak performance athlete, *Pain Free* can help you transform pain into power, and hurt into heart. Egoscue's methods will help you feel at home again in your body!" —Harold Bloomfield, M.D., author of *How to Heal Depression*

"*Pain Free for Women* answers the many questions I have about my health and my children's well-being. It has encouraged me to trust my instincts as a mom and to take charge of my family's health."
—Linda Lynch, former professional tennis player and mother of two

Also by Pete Egoscue with Roger Gittines

Pain Free
A Revolutionary Method for Stopping Chronic Pain

Pain Free at Your PC

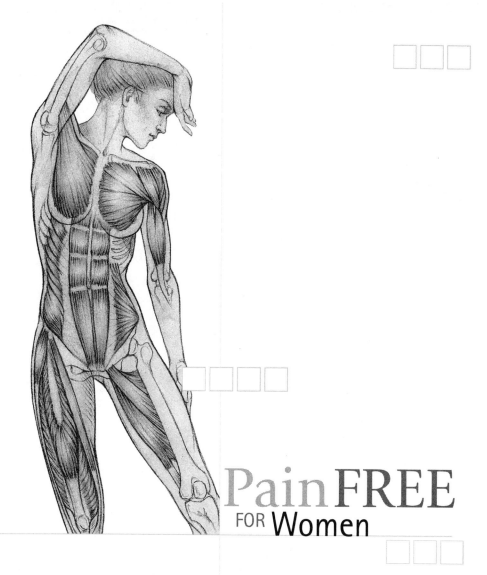

Pain FREE
FOR Women

Pete Egoscue
with Roger Gittines

BANTAM BOOKS

New York   Toronto   London   Sydney   Auckland

PAIN FREE FOR WOMEN
A Bantam Book

PUBLISHING HISTORY
Bantam hardcover edition published January 2002
Bantam trade paperback edition / July 2003

Published by
Bantam Dell
A Division of Random House, Inc.
New York, New York

Book design by Amanda Kavanagh, ARK Design, NY

Library of Congress Catalog Card Number: 200104398

ISBN 0-553-38049-4

Manufactured in the United States of America
Published simultaneously in Canada

BVG   10 9 8 7 6 5 4 3 2

Aristotle said, "In all things of nature there is something of the marvelous." This book is dedicated to all that is marvelous in women—their strength, resilience, beauty, and wisdom. The mother of all living.

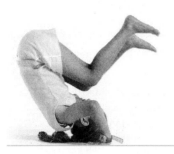

contents

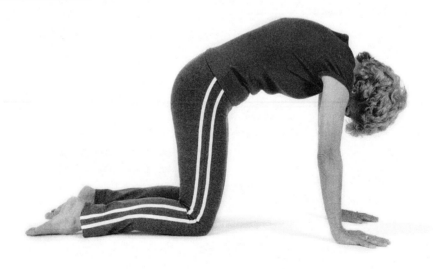

Disclaimer

For all of my books, I provide a disclaimer with a difference. The usual warning—"The following material is not intended as a substitute for the advice of a physician"—doesn't go far enough. Here's my take: This book is not intended as a substitute for the reader's independent judgment and personal responsibility. Health issues are too important to delegate to anyone else. It's always a good idea to seek information and counsel from as wide a variety of sources as possible, but in the end you make the decisions.

list of illustrations

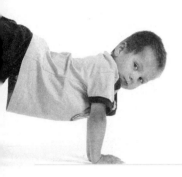

acknowledgments

If raising a child takes a village, producing a book like this one requires a small city of talented artisans, dedicated specialists, savvy advisors, and assorted invaluable friends.

First, I'd like to thank the "Magnificent Twenty," the models who literally embody the Egoscue Method in the pages ahead: Erica Bartnick, Lara Balderstone, Evelyn Carlson, Carolyne Jones, Chrissy Jones, Dottie Jones, Jack Jones, Sonia Jones, Alison Lewis, Jake Lynch, Linda Lynch, Mary Beth Mittleman, Kathy Mulherin, Cathy Murakami, Jennifer Park, Karolinka Placek, Liba Placek, Robin J. Wallace, Mathew Wezniak, and Donna Wood. Makeup artist CeCe Cantón did superb work. Illustrator Karen Kuchar and photographers Beth Bishoff and Nick Nacca demonstrated—to paraphrase Duke Ellington—images don't mean a thing if they ain't got that zing.

Without Troi Egoscue our photo shoots would have been fiascos. It took her organizational genius, eye for detail, endless patience, and boundless enthusiasm to make sure we got it right. Was I smart to marry her, or what?

Thanks to my co-author and friend Roger Gittines, my publisher and friend Irwyn Applebaum, and my editor and friend Robin Michaelson. Space is too limited to name everybody, but there are dozens of individuals who made a major contribution to this book by serving as volunteer sounding boards. They read early versions of the manuscript, offered comments, encouragement, and suggestions. Finally, I learned and keep learning something new and important each day from the staff of the Egoscue Method Clinic and from our many female clients. I'm a lucky and truly grateful author.

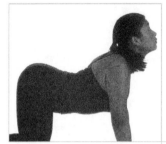

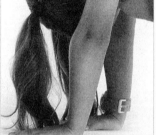

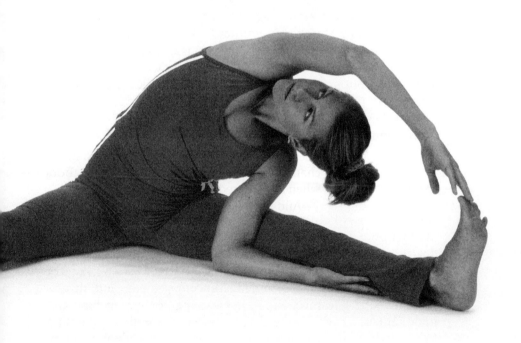

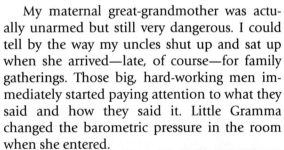

introduction

Women in Full

We were in love. I was about eight years old, and the lady in question—oh, she was seventy-five or so. Little Gramma. A tiny, wiry, fiery, tough, and talented woman who, as far as I was concerned, robbed stagecoaches by day and baked cookies for me by night. Never mind that fifty years ago even parched and dusty Oklahoma was a bit too civilized for stagecoaches, if not gunslinging great-grannies.

My maternal great-grandmother was actually unarmed but still very dangerous. I could tell by the way my uncles shut up and sat up when she arrived—late, of course—for family gatherings. Those big, hard-working men immediately started paying attention to what they said and how they said it. Little Gramma changed the barometric pressure in the room when she entered.

And when she departed, they gossiped about her. At that point Little Gramma had outlived her husband by about three decades and was doing just fine, thank you. She traveled across the country and around the world by herself and with friends. I knew her itinerary only by overhearing exasperated adults whisper, "She's in London—can you imagine?" Or, "I got a card from Paris—who does she think she is?"

But when Little Gramma came home, the idle chatter stopped, and she was back in charge, dispensing opinions and advice. Her recollections of what she had endured as a girl and young woman made that year's drought seem like a moist Irish springtime by comparison. She had a long memory as well as a hard head, a sharp tongue—and soft ways with little boys.

I'm thinking about her now because a friend asked me why I wanted to write a book about women's health. My answer: "Because of Little Gramma." To paraphrase the title of Tom Wolfe's novel, she was a woman in full. Not only did she embody the spirit of her time and her generation of women, Little Gramma represented women through time and across the generations. Her era spanned the buckboard and the boardroom. She could have taken the reins of either one.

She could hold her own, thanks—and so can you.

She possessed strength, stamina, and spirit—and so can you.

She could work and play as hard as any man—and so can you.

You, I assume based on the title of this book, are a woman. I'd like you and the rest of my readers to get to know Little Gramma because she hitches the past to the present. In today's world, where "You're so last week" is the ultimate put-down, it's too easy to lose track of where we've come from and, more importantly, from whom we've come. Consequently, we forget about all the Little Grammas of yesterday who held their own so that a long procession of kids, grandkids, great-grandkids, and more could hold their own too.

We need to refresh our memories and rediscover the source of their strength. Were they Steel Magnolias who never had a bad day? No, the secret was simple self-confidence. Not the Dale Carnegie kind, but a more fundamental, gut-level confidence. I'm convinced that it sprang from a complete and unshakable faith in the ability of their bodies to do what had to be done, and to finish what they started, no matter what, no matter how, no matter when. Little Gramma and her kind were smart because they were strong—and they knew it.

But what do *you* know? I'm serious. Do you know that your strength is the key to good health and long life? Do you know that the back pain or sore knees that perhaps motivated you to buy a book called *Pain Free for*

Women are not caused by your inherently fragile female bone structure or musculature? And do you know that lack of adequate motion—like lack of adequate food, water, air, and shelter—will make you sick and can even kill you?

Little Gramma knew without ever having to give these questions a second or even a first thought. Her knowledge was literally her strength. It made her tough, competent, happy, and beloved. While times have changed mightily, what she had is still available to every woman.

Hitting the Wall

This book is about women and their strength: how to recover it if it's lost, and how to keep it, build it, and pass it on to your daughters and sons, friends, and lovers.

My secondary purpose is to help you get rid of chronic musculoskeletal pain as well as the symptoms associated with conditions not usually linked with the musculoskeletal system (but they are), such as PMS, allergies, chronic fatigue, immune system weakness, eating disorders, depression, infertility, and breast cancer. It's a long list.

Since that *secondary* purpose sounds awfully primary in terms of magnitude, I'll explain. For more than thirty years I've been an anatomical functionalist, an alternative health care specialist concerned with optimalizing the human musculoskeletal system through proper alignment, posture, and muscular engagement. Using a unique, widely acclaimed form of exercise therapy that I developed, my Egoscue Method Clinic in Del Mar, California, helps more than twenty-five thousand people each year recover from sports injuries, backaches, joint pain, and other musculoskeletal disorders. During the course of this work, I've seen thousands of women of all ages and all walks of life improve their overall health using my programs that were primarily crafted to restore musculoskeletal strength, alignment, and function.

In short, I've observed a surprise dividend from these programs in the women I've worked with: they not only alleviated chronic musculoskeletal pain, but they also experienced vast improvements in other areas of their health that they had been led to believe could be addressed, if at all, only with drugs, surgery, or similarly invasive treatment regimens. The women received even elusive "macro" health benefits like higher energy, an enhanced sense of well-being, a revved-up immune system, and a hotter metabolic burn rate. I've studied this phenomenon carefully, and while I don't claim to be a scientist, I have observed direct correlations between improved strength and overall musculoskeletal health, on the one hand, and the ability to fight off various symptoms of disease, accidents, and aging on the other.

In a majority of cases, the women who came to the clinic in the last ten years reported that their significant nonmusculoskeletal health benefits accompanied measurable increases in strength, stamina, flexibility, and alignment. I'll share these findings with you, along with my thoughts on why this correlation exists, and how you can quickly and easily put the Egoscue Method to work on behalf of your own health.

In the pages ahead, you'll find menus of *E-cises*, a term I use to differentiate my Egoscue Method techniques for restoring strength, flexibility, and function from the more traditional heavy-duty exercise routines that measure results by the volume of sweat produced. By beginning this program, you're not enrolling in Marine boot camp—I can assure you of that. Think of E-cises as *easy-cises*. They are *easy* and *effective* because they reactivate the body's natural musculoskeletal functions and put them back to work, not only moving your muscles and joints without pain but properly energizing all the systems of the body. Being pain free starts with having the full use of your musculoskeletal system.

Although I'm addressing women in this book, I am not excluding men from my readership. Everyone's welcome. But there are two reasons for the slant that I'm taking. First, for many reasons (and we will get into them specifically later) the strange notion has taken hold that women don't need their full musculoskeletal system or don't have the physical resources to access it. That's simply not true, and a woman who buys into it puts her health in jeopardy.

Second, I've found that women are more receptive to addressing health issues because of their historical role as intimate, day-to-day caretakers of family and community well-being. Long before Hippocrates and his oath, there were Doctor Mom, Doctor Auntie, and Doctor Sis. She might have been a shaman or a shepherd, a nurse or a midwife, a good Samaritan, a good neighbor, or a grand lady. But she saw that the young were protected and nourished, so that they in turn would one day keep watch over their families and communities. Without her tender mercy and tough stewardship, I doubt humankind could have made it to the twenty-first century.

Today Doctor Mom is not necessarily a mother or a wife, but she most certainly is her mother's daughter. The mother-daughter continuum forms the main strand that ties together little girls, teenage girls, young women, women in their prime, and the wise women whom society too often dismissively labels as "elderly." The Irish may have saved civilization (as a best-selling book assured us a few years ago), but this female bond has saved humanity countless times and will do so again—I hope.

There's more than a trace of pessimism in my hopefulness, since it also contains doubts and misgivings. In the decades I've been an alternative health care practitioner, I've seen men go from perceiving themselves as nearly bullet-proof to accepting that their bodies are fragile and susceptible to all sorts of breakdowns and blow-ups. Until recently, I didn't see the same thing happening with women. Now I do, and it's profoundly disturbing.

Women's magazines, the news media, and the Internet are full of stories about "new epidemics" and new vulnerabilities, as well as new drugs and medical procedures to address them. The tenor and tone are alarming. It's as if women's health has hit the wall. Many women, particularly those in their teens, twenties, and thirties, seem to be losing contact with that bedrock self-confidence that I remember in Little Gramma.

To be sure, it's not all headlines and hype. Something is happening. The United States is not the world's largest market for over-the-counter and prescription painkillers for nothing. Men, women, and children are hurting in record numbers. But why?

You'll need to delve into this book for a comprehensive answer, but to summarize I'll just say three words: *lack of motion.* Modern life has drained away the full range of motion that shaped Little Gramma and her contemporaries. It's happened quietly and relatively quickly. We still move, but not as much and not in the myriad ways that we once commonly did. As a result, the musculoskeletal system is binding up and breaking down, taking the body's other systems down with it.

The Egoscue Method's E-cise menus can help you do something about this breakdown. Most of all, though, I want to help you remember. The poet Robert Frost suggested that one of the purposes and pleasures of a poem is to make the reader aware of something that she didn't know she knew. The memory of motion is the remembrance of good health.

Remember when you were eight and took your first solo bike ride?

Remember climbing the pine tree behind the house?

Remember marathon jump rope contests with your best friend?

Remember walking and running and skipping and dancing?

Take a moment to recall experiences such as these. Nothing? Don't worry, they're probably in there waiting.

Many women experience this kind of short-term memory lapse simply because they haven't been allowed the full and free use of their physical inheritance. Think of an heir and an heiress who both inherit a fortune. He gets to go on a spending spree, but she must live on a strict budget. As a result, his wealth is liquid, hers is frozen.

Likewise, the two sexes have lived with different standards when it comes to making use of their physical assets. Unlike men, women have had to battle for their sexual and reproductive rights, the right to develop the explicit strength and skills necessary to work at any occupation or play whatever game they choose, and the right to share equally the power and benefits of work and play. Not remembering experiences of strength is understandable. Memory is built on direct, firsthand experience, from great sex to a good workout. But a physical legacy that has never really been tasted and tested because it's walled off by cultural norms poses grave health consequences.

Luckily, you don't have to get involved in controversies about sex, reproduction, choice, and equality to rediscover what you knew all along: that your body's design is as tough and capable as any man's. It has the same overall number of muscles and bones, joints and tendons, ligaments and nerves. From head to toe exists vast potential strength, endurance, flexibility, and finesse. You're built to last eighty, ninety, a hundred years or more. Built to last without exotic drug therapy, high-tech gadgetry, and invasive surgery. Built to last without chronic pain, sickness, and frailty.

If you don't remember now, you will by the end of the book: *You are built to be strong and healthy.*

The Books Within the Book

Many health books use a problem/solution format, and this one is no exception. It's efficient and keeps the author from wandering off on side excursions. While I may take you on a few back roads, we'll always be moving toward the destination: practical ways to regain and maintain the strong, healthy musculoskeletal legacy that you were born with. It's *never* too late or too early.

I've organized the book along the chronological lines of physical development for several reasons. First, I hope you will see how your physical development unfolded from infancy to childhood, from adolescence to young adulthood, and on into middle age and the senior years; what I consider the *seasons* of a woman's life. It's important to gain perspective on the entire panorama. Second, by designating age categories, I'm able to create several books within the overall book. No matter what your age or situation, there is a place here for you. I've included information and insights on age-specific issues like the onset of puberty or menopause, together with simple, easy-to-perform E-cises to restore, maintain, and strengthen musculoskeletal wellness in the various seasons of life.

Does it surprise you that I consider puberty and menopause in relation to the musculoskeletal system? If there's one theme that my previous books have in common, it's that the motion-powered musculoskeletal system is the foundation and framework of human health and *all* the systems that support it. What you'll find in the pages ahead is the product of years of successful therapeutic applications based on that premise. When we move, we're not just going from here to there. Simple and complex movement underpins the efficacy of bone density creation, metabolism, visual acuity, balance, fertility, and many other fundamental processes and properties.

I believe there is a cause-and-effect link between musculoskeletal dysfunction and chronic disease, accidents, and aging. A growing body of evidence supports this belief, as we'll see, and it comes not a moment too soon. Mainstream medicine has recently discovered women in a big way. An amazing turnabout is taking place. In general, an absentminded indifference has characterized modern medicine's attitude toward women. Since science has been mostly a male-dominated enterprise, its preoccupations have tended to be those of the men who conducted or funded the research. I'll come back to this hot-button topic, but what needs to be said at this point is that because of the social progress women have made in recent years, medicine is taking unprecedented interest in their health. That would be unqualified good news—if it didn't coincide with the almost unconditional surrender to drug and surgical technology that's simultaneously occurring. These big high-tech guns are now being turned on women to treat their "special" needs, heretofore largely ignored.

I put quotation marks around "special" to suggest that you should be wary about this honor. Women do have special medical and health needs, and it's high time they are recognized. But if those special needs are seen primarily as abnormalities or flaws suitable only for the latest high-tech treatments, women's health will be subjected to a devastating onslaught. Menstruation, pregnancy, childbirth, and menopause—to name four "special" needs—are not abnormal, yet that is the tenor of much of the discussion they evoke, as well as the medical arms race mentality associated with the treatment options. We need to step back and cautiously examine this approach.

It deeply concerns me that women's transformation from forgotten patients to favorite patients is occurring at a time when aggressive measures disregard—and possibly undermine—the body's inherent strength and its built-in healing and wellness mechanisms. Women are vulnerable to these measures because their musculoskeletal systems are already compromised by cultural and social attitudes that suggest that women do not need strong muscles and bones. They certainly do need them—and not to buff up like weight lifters or bulk up like TV wrestlers, but for the sake of their health.

Therefore this book confronts two equally important problems: one, a modern lifestyle that increasingly confines women to an even narrower range and pattern of motion that causes chronic pain, premature aging, and poor health in general; and two, a dysfunctional musculoskeletal system (as a result of lack of motion) that is tempting medical technologists to intervene with ever more elaborate means to redesign and "improve" on what they regard as an inferior arrangement of muscles, bones, nerves, and other components.

These problems are big, especially in combination, but they're not insurmountable. My solution is to enable you to "improve" your musculoskeletal system *yourself* with a miracle drug that doesn't come as a pill or a potion. No drug company controls the patent. No hardware manufacturer can lease or license the process. It's called motion. Full, free, and spontaneous, it costs nothing and is easy to obtain and use. I'll show you how. The benefits are indeed miraculous.

A Beauty Secret

On any given day at the Egoscue Method Clinic, children as young as eight or nine will be happily engrossed in activities that are fun as well as therapeutic, while a few feet away an eighty-year-old great-grandmother does knee pillow squeezes or another routine from her menu of E-cises. Nearby a young mother might be enhancing the extension capability in her hips, while a teenage basketball star endeavors to strengthen her knees. The atmosphere is relaxed and supportive. We don't narrowly specialize in pediatric and geriatric—or thirtysomething-atric—therapy because, in the broadest sense, the musculoskeletal system of the young, the middle-aged, and the elderly is basically the same, once growth plates close in adolescence. (The precise timing depends on many variables.) The musculoskeletal system, no matter what its age, responds avidly to what I call *design motion* by increasing strength, agility, and stamina. For most of us, design motion has been supplanted by dysfunctional motion that puts tremendous wear and tear on our muscles and joints and undermines the musculoskeletal system's role as the solid foundation of our health.

The basis for that role and the basics of the musculoskeletal system will be presented in Part I. In case you knew it all along but didn't remember, the inner woman is an impressive work of art and biomechanical design. Four short chapters will explain all the anatomy you'll need in order to remember how utterly incorrect it is to say that "beauty is only skin deep." Beauty and health are *bone and muscle* deep.

In Part II, three chapters discuss infancy and early childhood, middle childhood, and adolescence. As I said earlier, it's important to know where we came from. The springtime of our youth has a profound effect on shaping our future health. We live every day with the musculoskeletal system that we built—or didn't build— as kids. Many clients who come to the Egoscue Method Clinic are stunned to discover that their joint problems, like bad backs or knees, have been brewing since childhood. Once they discover that, however, they understand how some of our deceptively simple E-cises quickly fill in these decades-old gaps. Chapter 5 will help readers with children understand a youngster's need for motion and learn what can be done to guarantee adequate amounts of it.

Women with children and women without children will have to cohabit the same space for a time. Meanwhile, I'll be addressing two different audiences simultaneously. Bear in mind that for a natural self-help solution to health problems to be truly effective, one must understand where the problem originated and why. *I had an accident* or *I'm getting old* don't cut it. I believe that self-confidence springs from self-knowledge.

At first, fixing five-year-old Jenny may not appear to be all that pertinent to fixing thirty-year-old Karen, who's never going to be five again. But as Jenny gets help, Karen's and Jenny's moms get the benefit of seeing the childhood origins of their own problems highlighted. It's a working self-knowledge that all of us need for the sake of motivation. I make no secret of it: the Egoscue Method requires time, effort, and commitment. The three chapters in Part II, with all their cross-talk, are here to help kids, to explain to moms what needs to happen, and to motivate all women to take action to stay strong and healthy. Menus of E-cises for children and teens are included in the Appendix.

In Part III, I'll introduce you to the Egoscue Method's principal tool: the E-cise. In Parts IV, V, and VI, we'll go deeper into the *seasons* of a woman's life, with separate chapters covering young adulthood, "prime time" (mid-thirties to menopause), and maturity (age fifty and beyond). Along with general E-cise menu programs to bolster alignment and strength, these parts offer targeted menus of E-cises to deal with childbirth, breast cancer, loss of balance, and metabolic weakness, with plenty of fix-it-now relevance.

As in Part II, some overlap among chapters occurs here because it is simply impossible to draw hard and fast demarcation lines between age groups. I won't be checking ID to see if you're old enough or young enough to visit a chapter, so come and go as you please in these timeless zones.

Part VI, which addresses what Keats called "the season of mists and mild fruitfulness," is a little more self-contained. Menopause does not follow a strict timetable, nor mean that the end of life's journey is close at hand.

Betty, a woman from Tennessee, came to the clinic a few years ago in her early eighties, suffering from hip and sciatic pain. After a week or so, as she was preparing to go home, Betty took me aside to thank me.

"The pain's gone for the first time in years," she said.

"Well, now it's up to you, Betty, to keep doing your program and stay healthy," I replied.

She nodded and lowered her voice a little, "And I'm not incontinent anymore."

"You didn't tell me about that."

"No, but I was—and now it's gone, that's what counts."

"You know why, don't you?"

"Yes, I know why."

Betty had restored her musculoskeletal system's strength, flexibility, and function. She was pain free and more—much more.

We helped her remember what she knew all along: at any age, health starts with a motion-fueled, functional, and strong musculoskeletal system. It's what Little Gramma, and all of our great-grandmothers, knew and remembered. It's what this book is all about.

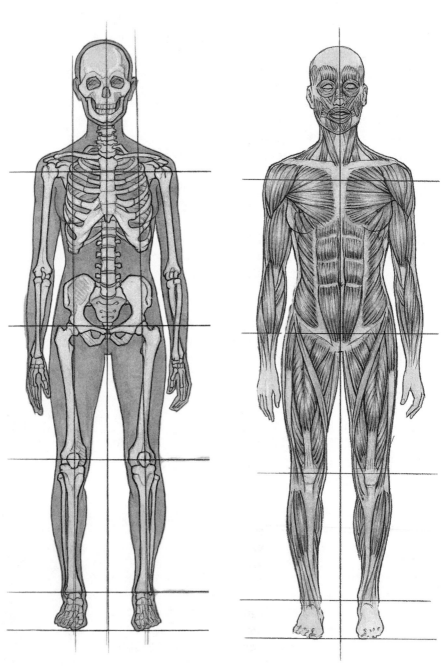

Fig.1-1   Fig.1-2

the basic woman

CHAPTER 1

structure and stricture

Look at the drawing of the human skeleton in Figure 1–1, and tell me whether it is male or female.

Take your time.

Give up?

It would require a lucky guess or specialized training to know you're looking at a female skeleton. Likewise, the drawing of the human musculature, in Figure 1–2, is also difficult to identify as female. I'll spare you a third illustration that makes the same point about the central nervous system.

What is my point? Muscles, bones, and nerves—the three major components of the musculoskeletal system—and the way they are assembled, are nearly identical for both men and women. The word *nearly* here isn't a loophole: it means we are roughly 99.99999999999 percent the same. Out of all our many bones, muscles, tendons, ligaments, joints, and neural axons, only two bones are slightly different in men and women: the pelvis and the femur.

The female pelvis is broader than the male's, with wider and deeper inlets and outlets, and it has relatively less overall bone mass. (Technically the pelvis comprises four bones, but I'm considering it as a single entity since these bones are fused in adults.) As for the femur (thighbone), its head end—the one that fits snugly into the socket of the hip joint to form the body's strongest joint—forms the connection at a more pronounced angle, giving the pelvis more leeway to tip into the birthing position. Because of the broader female pelvis, the female femur also has a slightly greater angle of incline as it descends to the knee.

That's it.

Anything else that you've heard or read about differences in joints, ligaments, and such is pure unproved conjecture. I won't even call it theory. I'm not knocking conjecture; I resort to it myself. But solid, undisputed evidence exists only for these two structural differences.*

As for the skeletal muscles, they have no gender-specific shapes, composition, or locomotor functions. An artist illustrating a medical text would probably have to include genitals or a profile to clue readers to whether they were examining a male or a female.

Gray's Anatomy, first published in the mid–nineteenth century, recognizes that the human musculoskeletal system is the same for both males and females. Most of the illustrations in the 1901 edition, for example, are genderless. Intricate black-and-white line drawings powerfully convey the ruggedness of the human biomechanical structures that are common to both sexes. Looking at them, you could be reading a blueprint for an immense and revolutionary machine possessing the sheer might and ingenuity to change the face of the world—and, in fact, you are.

Unfortunately, the *Gray's* example is not widely followed these days. The latest edition of a classic kinesiology handbook has only five or six illustrations using female models, compared with dozens showing men as examples of strength and overall function. The same is true of a thick human anatomy and physiology text that describes itself as intended for students in health, medicine, and biology programs. Perhaps those authors and publishers were chary about displaying the unclothed female torso; if so, we need to start growing up. I'd like to think that when Brandi Chastain exuberantly doffed her jersey to celebrate her team's 1999 World Cup soccer

*We'll discuss muscle and bone composition, and the effects of hormones, later in the book.

championship playoff victory, the gesture made the pages of anatomy texts safe for sports bras.

Farewell to Tarzan

The suggestion that men are the gold standard of musculoskeletal fitness and function does triple-barreled mischief. For starters, it helps mislead women to believe that no matter what they do, they'll never achieve strength and functional parity with men—or even come reasonably close. This leads to a "Boys are strong, girls are weak" mentality that reinforces stereotypes that help deny women access to their aspirations.

Second, the notion that a woman's body is substandard or abnormal invites pharmaceutical and technological means to come to her aid and to correct these shortcomings. One orthopedic clinic I know runs a newspaper ad that features an eye-catching illustration of a shapely, sexy leg—with the knee surrounded by construction scaffolding. The product is—what else?—reconstructive knee surgery for women. The ad even hints that beautiful knees are the work of a surgeon's scalpel. Inevitably, with more than 50 percent of the population as potential customers, the medical marketplace tries to provide a stream of new products to remedy the ever-widening circle of women's health problems and supposed design defects, like the "accident-prone" female knee.

The notion of female design defects leads to a self-fulfilling prophecy. If a woman is persuaded that her knees and muscles and bones are not designed to be strong and functional, the positive health benefits of having such strength and function will be lost to her. She will be frail, sick, and accident prone. No medical product ever devised can take the place of a healthy musculoskeletal system. But without a healthy system, there can only be a downward spiral of breakdown-intervention-breakdown-intervention. On that prediction, my crystal ball is absolutely clear.

The third piece of mischief is the supposition that men are stronger, fitter, and more functional than women. The male models in anatomy texts may seem that way, but their standard is a false one, because the vast majority of men have no material advantage. On average, men are somewhat larger (about 10 percent taller—big deal!), have less fat tissue (15 percent—how

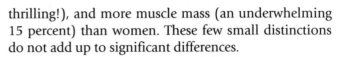

thrilling!), and more muscle mass (an underwhelming 15 percent) than women. These few small distinctions do not add up to significant differences.

A Curve That Keeps Us Straight

In Chapter 4 I'll explore more fully the differences—real and mythical—between men and women. In the meantime, we need to know more about the body's response to a force of nature that all humans must cope with: gravity. We tend to think of splitting the atom and landing on the moon as great feats of human genius. But they are nothing compared with our first conquest that took place about three million years ago, when Lucy knocked gravity on its butt.

Lucy is the name given to the fossil remains of our earliest known hominid ancestor to walk upright. She probably wasn't really the first, but with her demonstrated staying power, she can keep the gravity-buster trophy until someone with a better claim comes along.

Gravity is a useful service: it keeps animate and inanimate objects from whirling off into space. But it also creates a problem for the animate objects, which have to animate themselves. To accomplish the job, they have evolved intriguing skills such as crawling on the belly, swimming through the sea, and taking wing to fly. The one that most fascinates me, though, is the one that involves hoisting a heavy three-foot-long pod containing a couple of buckets of blood and gurgling tissue up onto a pair of jointed stilts that are secured to two small platforms that any novice engineer would see are too tiny to balance the weight. Performing this feat of animation would be quite a challenge in its own right. But contriving to lift and swing those platforms forward one at a time with a roundish eight- or nine-pound canister, the skull, riding precariously on top is truly astounding. Yet not only does this antigravity package stay upright and moving, it will shake its bootie and dance the Watusi (if it's old enough to remember 1960s dance crazes).

Truly, just standing up and walking is a biomechanical marvel that we take totally for granted. Try it. Stand up, walk across the room, and come back.

Savor the experience.

You've just used a vehicle that makes a Boeing 757 seem as primitive as a skateboard. The 757 can only taxi down a runway and fly. You can run, jump, stretch, bend over at the waist, punch with your left, jab with your right, tap a keyboard, throw a fastball, paint water lilies, or play a Chopin étude. You have these myriad abilities because you were born with the necessary equipment as well as the potential for using it.

The soul of this machine—its core—is the spine. Its characteristic S-curve is what defeats gravity. A backbone that was absolutely straight and rigid would likely have kept us on all fours, or left us stiffly upright, able to move forward but not back or to the sides; once we were knocked off our feet, it would be nearly impossible to rise. As you can see in Figure 1–3, the S-curve creates a center of gravity that runs on a straight line from the head through the rib cage to the hips and down to the knees and ankles. It brings all the skeleton's heaviest components into balance and links them together in a way that yields vertical stability and horizontal flexibility on three cardinal planes of motion.

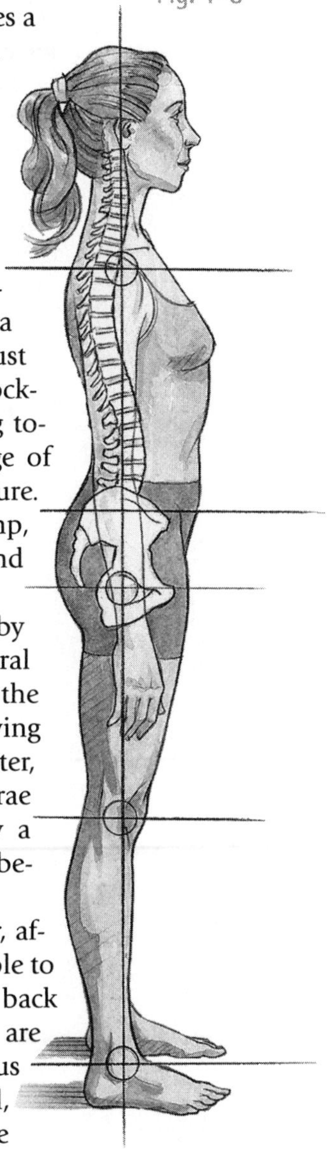

The spine and the pelvis are the musculoskeletal system's dream team. The spine rides on a pedestal formed by the pelvis's V-shaped sacrum, just above and around the bend from the hip-joint sockets. A head-to-toe connection is created. Working together, the pelvis and the spine allow us a range of motion that is unequaled by any other living creature. Without the spine we'd win the Olympic frog jump, but that's about it. Sans pelvis, we'd be second cousin to the rattlesnake.

The spine's S-curve configuration is produced by the shape and placement of the individual vertebral bones. Each is sized and molded to bring about the necessary overall angle to allow for a gentle flowing curve that's thicker and heavier at the base and lighter, tapered, and more flexible at the top. The vertebrae are stacked like poker chips, each separated by a small spongy pad, or disk, that acts as a cushion between them.

Although the bones of the spine hook together, after a fashion, what really keeps them united and able to hold the line of the S-curve is muscle power. The back has as many as five layers of muscles; the deepest are the spinal erectors, whose assignment is to keep us standing tall. But this assignment isn't easy to fulfill, given the persistence and power of gravity. The spine

Fig. 1–3

and its musculature need help from the rest of the musculoskeletal system.

That help comes mainly in the form of a superstructure that surrounds the spine on all four sides, like scaffolding. Stand up, and I will show you what I mean. Make sure that your feet are pointing straight ahead, parallel with each other, about twelve inches apart. Imagine a horizontal line running through your left shoulder joint and on through your right shoulder.

Imagine another horizontal line running through your left hip and on through your right hip. Imagine still another horizontal line running through your left knee on through your right knee.

Finally, imagine a fourth horizontal line running through your left ankle and on through your right ankle.

Fig. 1–4

Okay? Now imagine a vertical line coming straight up from your left ankle through your left knee and left hip, then passing to the inside of your left shoulder so that it bisects your left ear. Imagine the same thing on the right side.

What have you got?

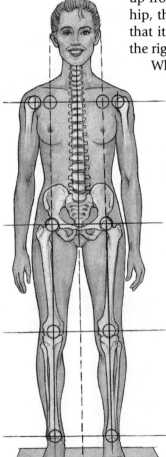

You've got a grid composed of horizontal and vertical lines that intersect at your principal load-bearing joints (Figure 1–4). The only ones that are slightly asymmetrical are the shoulders, because of the way we grow and how our shoulders work. Most people assume that the shoulder is the point where the clavicle attaches to the humerus (the upper-arm bone). And it is. But the shoulder is actually three points of articulation that constitute a joint complex spread out over enough real estate that the vertical lines of the grid cross it, even though not as obviously.

I'm running on about this because understanding the grid's role is fundamental to gaining an appreciation of how the musculoskeletal system moves smoothly and powerfully while staying erect. A grid consisting of exactly parallel horizontal and vertical lines is perfect for withstanding gravity's downward force. In the case of the musculoskeletal system, it uses the points of interaction—the ankles, knees, hips, and shoulders—to support, assist, and give the spine the structural integrity it needs without sacrificing flexibility.

This alignment of the joints allows us to shift our weight from side to side and front to back, so as to provide sequential four-point support when we walk and run—left front/right rear, right front/left rear, and so on. The hips and shoulders simultaneously rotate, rise, and fall in coordination. Meanwhile, the head, with its precious cargo of brains and eyes, stays level to look for danger and assess opportunities.

In the mechanical process that we call walking, roughly three and a half times your full body weight is projected downward onto one foot via the four load-bearing joints directly above, as the other foot is lifted off the ground and swung forward. The weight then transfers to the other side to repeat the loading of the foot, ankle, knee, hip, and shoulder. Individually, the joints aren't strong enough to handle that kind of a load. Not even the huge hip joint can take such a beating. But working together, it's a piece of cake.

The problem is that most of us ask our joints to go it alone. Our sedentary lifestyles have robbed us of our load-bearing alignment. The horizontal and vertical lines that I asked you to imagine are not parallel. The grid is askew; the scaffolding is tipped every which way. It's hardly an exaggeration to say that we are not walking so much as executing a controlled collapse. With each step, the scaffolding shudders and shakes forward, is caught just on the brink of falling, is steadied, and then is heaved forward again to bend and buckle. And away we go toward fatigue, stiffness, chronic pain, and increasing immobility.

Checking for Misalignment

The E-cises in this book are designed to correct and prevent musculoskeletal system misalignment. They are surprisingly effective and easy to do, because even though the body has undergone years of dysfunctional stress and strain, it never irretrievably loses its design.

When I first started out as an anatomical functionalist primarily helping people with back pain, I realized that every case—no matter how different the circumstances or the age of the individual—involved two things: observable skeletal misalignment and muscular weakness. What I developed was a method for strengthening key muscles and using them to restore and maintain alignment.

Over the years I've received many compliments and kind words about my work. But I don't deserve much credit—the human body is the real hero. If we pay attention, the body shows us what it needs in order to function properly. Once I realized that the starting point was always alignment—the grid, with its vertical and horizontal parallel lines—held in place by sufficient muscular strength to counteract the effects of gravity, I was able to see the misalignment and corresponding muscular weakness. When the grid is askew, there is dysfunction. Downward gravitational force guarantees it. The slumping structure stresses the joints and causes the spine to lose its S-curve. I can see it happening—and so can you.

Using a small carpenter's level, draw a vertical line from the top to the bottom of a full-length mirror. A crayon or lipstick will work fine. Then draw an intersecting horizontal line across the width of the mirror, at roughly chin height. Make sure the bubble on the level lines up in the middle of the capsule both times when you do this.

Now face the mirror, and stand at a distance that allows you to see your head-to-foot reflection. Take your time, and compare the horizontal line to the reflection of your shoulders. Relax. Let your posture settle into its normal configuration. Try to see whether the line on the mirror parallels a line that would pass horizontally across your shoulders. (Assume that your shoulder joint is formed where your upper arm connects with the clavicle of your shoulder.) Draw another horizontal line on the mirror to actually delineate your shoulders.

Compare it to the original horizontal baseline. Is the right end of the new shoulder line lower or higher than the left? In other words, do your shoulders slope away from the horizontal baseline? If so, your musculoskeletal system grid is lower on that one side, and each of the three remaining horizontals—the hips, knees, and ankles—are probably lower as well. Draw lines to mark them. The disparity will vary: one may slope to the right, while the others slope to the left. The more pronounced the variation, the more the musculoskeletal system is compromised.

To check yourself against the vertical line, turn sideways, and put your thumb on the hipbone nearest the mirror (the bony knob that's roughly at navel height). By edging forward or back, align yourself with the vertical line you drew so that it passes through the hipbone's reflection. Take a moment to relax, and look straight ahead, not sideways at the mirror. Get comfortable. Now turn your head slightly toward the mirror, just enough to see the reflection without changing the position of your torso. (Don't swing your head all the way around.) Where are your head, shoulders, knees, and ankles located in relationship to the vertical line? If your musculoskeletal grid is properly aligned, they'll be aligned with the hipbone. In other words, the vertical line will bisect the load-bearing joints and head exactly. But for most people that won't be the case. It varies from individual to individual, but a typical arrangement is for the ankle to be behind the line, the knee in front, and the head and shoulder in front too. Furthermore, if you switch sides, the line will fall differently.

If you wiggle around a little, you might be able to get your joints to line up better: by pulling your shoulders back, for instance, or straightening your neck. But that won't last long. Your muscles have lost their ability to automatically hold you in an aligned posture. They'll soon snap back into misalignment. That's what the E-cises in this book are going to fix.

Chronic Pain

Why bother? *Everybody's posture is different,* I hear the skeptics saying. And they're right—but they're also wrong. The grid is the standard template for the human musculoskeletal system. Everybody's posture is different because everybody's lifestyle is different, and individual lifestyle determines to what degree our posture matches or diverges from the template. But for most of us in the United States and the developed world, our lifestyle simply doesn't strengthen the right muscles enough to hold the musculoskeletal system grid in alignment as we move.

Human joints are a lot like hinges (and ball-and-socket couplings). If you've ever had a fender bender with your car, you may have experienced a problem opening the door because of the twisted frame. The hinges bind each time they operate. It's the same with a joint on a misaligned human frame. There's extra friction in the joint, and since our joints move hundreds and perhaps thousands of times a day, the stress does enormous damage in the long run.

Not only is it subjected to this extra friction, the misaligned musculoskeletal system can also no longer do an adequate job of assisting the spine. Here gravity makes a comeback. If, for instance, your head and shoulders are in front of the vertical line you drew on the mirror, the force of gravity is pressing down the top of your spine to transform the S-curve into a C-curve (Figure 1–5). All the carefully crafted bits and pieces of the spine that worked so well in the S configuration now must function under far different circumstances. Like binding hinges, the vertebrae start to drag against one another. Their cushioning disks flatten and protrude, the erector muscles are overtaxed, and the spine loses flexibility and strength.

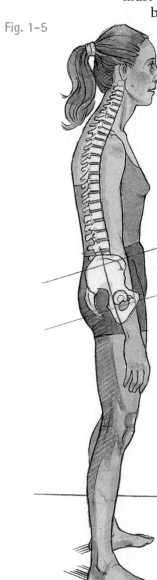

Fig. 1–5

Whenever I hear the phrase *Everybody has different posture*, I have to bite my tongue to keep from asking, "If everybody has different posture, why do they look so much alike?" On your next visit downtown, check it out. Bring those imaginary parallel vertical and horizontal lines along to hang in space, and you'll see a whole array of rounded backs, drooping shoulders and heads, hips that are tipped and rotated, crooked knees, and splayed feet. Those posture problems are symptoms, and they explain why more than 35 million Americans suffer chronic back pain. We're experiencing an epidemic of chronic pain and chronic disease because our musculoskeletal differences add up to the same thing—musculoskeletal dysfunction.

I could end this chapter by ticking off the evils of musculoskeletal system dysfunction, but instead I'll list the benefits of full, readily obtainable function, because that's where the book is headed:

- Higher energy
- More strength
- Better balance
- Increased resilience
- Greater flexibility
- A pumped-up immune system
- Improved metabolic efficiency

- Enhanced athletic performance
- Effective weight management
- Peace of mind and tranquillity
- Heightened sex drive
- Anti-aging. And—I almost forgot:
- Pain-free living, working, and playing.

I'd better stop here before I'm accused of overselling musculoskeletal system function. But I believe passionately in its benefits, and I genuinely doubt that it can be oversold.

I've seen all these benefits happen to women who were willing to trust their own instincts and turn away from the notion that full, functional musculoskeletal system health—including all of its dividends—is just a "guy thing."

Take it from Lucy, the woman with her two feet on the ground, the lady who knocked gravity on its butt.

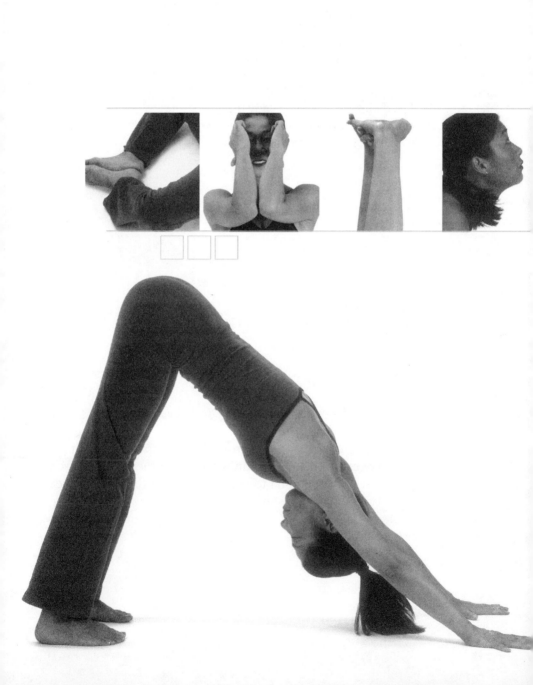

muscle and motion

The French philosopher René Descartes said, "I think, therefore I am." My take on the nature of being is slightly different: *I move, therefore I am*. Without movement, the *I*, in the sense of a living human presence and an accompanying conscious thought process, would not exist.

Where Descartes was plumbing the metaphysical depths, I am paddling in the shallow end of the gene pool, where basic functions like breathing, blood circulation, and metabolism take place. These functions are muscle-driven, as directly and decisively so as heavy lifting, trudging up a steep flight of stairs, and heaving a bulky carry-on bag into an airplane overhead bin. Muscle power is as elemental to every function of the human body as electrical power is to a refrigerator. If the wattage going to the fridge is insufficient, the ice melts and the vegetables spoil. Likewise, if muscle power is inadequate, the consequences from head to foot, inside and out, are drastic.

By the end of this chapter, I hope you'll have a new appreciation of exactly what your muscles do for you and what you do for your muscles. My purpose is to remove the "dumb and dumber" label that somehow got slapped onto muscles and persuaded many people to regard them as being of trivial importance except for athletes and stevedores. Three pounds of brain tissue are going nowhere without the musculoskeletal system.

By standing Cartesian logic on its feet—not its head—we can guarantee the mastery of the mind through the ministry of the muscles. We move, therefore we are.

Cut to the Bone

Our bones are sturdy. If I said that your femur (thighbone) is as solid as a rock, I'd be demeaning its true quality. A femur makes a rock look like—well, a rock: clumsy, brittle, and lifeless. Human bones are incredibly tough, flexible, and alive. Not only do they provide support for the body, they are a source of red blood cells and a reservoir of vital minerals that are central to our fundamental biochemical processes.

Even so, bones taken alone, or even bones strapped together with ligaments, don't amount to anything more than a formless heap of collagen and calcium. One reason that those skeletal models in classrooms and clinics—whether made of bone or plastic—hang from a stand and are loosely wired at the joints is that they would be too fragile and tipsy if glued together and propped up on two feet. What's missing is musculature.

Whether it is working individually or collectively, a skeletal muscle's first test of strength is its ability to give the skeleton the strength it needs to maintain structural integrity while bearing its own weight in an upright posture. Skeletal misalignment—the situation in which the horizontal and vertical lines of the grid are not parallel—is conclusive evidence of muscular dysfunction. The muscles are simply not doing their job.

But why not? Is it age? Disease? Accident? Individual variation? The answer is—none of the above.

The signature postures of musculoskeletal system dysfunction that we see all around us—and inside the frame of your own mirror—are primarily caused by lack of motion. I said that already in Chapter 1, and I'll be saying it many more times, so brace yourself. I'm out to *motionalize* your life.

Muscles operate on a use-it-or-lose-it principle. Anyone who has been bedridden with an illness for more than a few days knows this, as do those who drop out of an exercise class and rejoin a few weeks later. In both instances, there is a noticeable decline in muscular strength.

For a quick practical demonstration, sit on the front edge of a chair with your back straight and your arms at your sides. Bring your shoulders straight back, as if you were trying to squeeze your shoulder blades together. Hold this position for about ten seconds. Now relax. You probably haven't used those muscles for several days or even longer. Thus, the muscles that helped you draw your shoulders back are probably relatively weak. To verify that, notice that your shoulders have already returned to a slumped forward position. They are not strong enough to keep your shoulders square without an overt, conscious effort.

If you have time, do that same exercise again, holding your shoulders back for ten seconds, relaxing for ten, and then holding for another ten. Do a total of six sets. Notice that after each set, as your shoulders relax, their forward slump diminishes. At the end your shoulders will be straighter and closer to vertical alignment with your head, hips, knees, and ankles. What's happening is that relatively dormant muscles are being engaged, put to work, and strengthened. As they strengthen, the muscles automatically resume their task of supporting the musculoskeletal system grid.

It didn't take long, did it? The fact is that muscles are motion sponges. They soak up motion and expand accordingly. (But in a motion drought, they dry up.) They are gorging on the energy distilled by extra helpings of oxygen-laden red blood cells that are being pumped to them to support their increased activity levels. The body is fairly ruthless. It treats muscles like ancient galley slaves: no work, no food. The system is based on rewards and punishments. Fortunately, the rewards are readily available. As you just demonstrated, the simple act of repeatedly flexing and relaxing the shoulder muscles provides enough motion to activate this feeding and strengthening process. The payoff is immediate.

Later in this chapter, you'll see that some muscles work and eat more than other muscles, and that this inequity leads to trouble. First, though, I want to spend a bit more time on muscle mechanics, since I'm a firm believer in the old mangled maxim "What you don't know will hurt you."

No Pushing

Muscles seem so deceptively simple. They only have one card trick in their magic act—they contract. Or, even more banal, they twitch. When zapped by a neural pulse of bioelectrical energy, a bundle of muscle fibers shortens in length. This bundle is part of a larger muscle structure that is anchored at one end to a relatively stationary bone and at the other end to a bone that is more mobile, so the shortening of the fibers pulls the bones closer together. Other bundles get zapped—twitch!—and the bones are pulled back. Whether it's a laborer digging a hole with a shovel or Julia Child whipping up a soufflé, what's happening is basically the same: zap, twitch, zap, twitch.

To make use of the energy generated by the alternating zapping and twitching, the skeletal muscles tend to be paired off. One muscle flexes (pulls the bones toward one another), while the other extends (pulls the bones apart). Remember this concept, because *flexion* and *extension* are important terms in this book.

Flex and extend, flex and extend: it's a tug-of-war between muscles designed to be equals in terms of strength and function. Some muscles (including several that also flex *or* extend, depending on the joint) perform a third role: they stabilize joints or other components of the musculoskeletal system to allow them to smoothly open and close.

Moving the human body—I'm talking basics, like going from point A to point B, not anything fancy like ballet—requires coordination and teamwork on the part of the muscles. The team is made up of every skeletal muscle, not just the ones closest to the action. To walk a few steps, you shift your weight to one side—let's say the left—by stabilizing your left hip and knee, as you flex the muscles of the right thigh and knee. To lift the foot, you extend the muscles of the right hip. To swing it forward, the right side's knee and thigh muscles extend (move bones away from each other). As weight shifts back to the right side, the right hip muscles flex, the foot lands, and the hip and knee are stabilized for the impact. Meanwhile, the back and shoulder muscles are engaged in a similar process of flexion, extension, and stabilization. All the load-bearing joints—shoulders, hips, knees, and ankles—and their attendant muscles are involved.

This kind of teamwork is predicated on each team member having the strength and functional capability to carry out the assigned role. But as your mirror has shown us, even before the first step is taken, the musculoskeletal grid is misaligned. It's sagging under the weight of gravity. Key muscles lack the strength and functional capability to hold the vertical and horizontal lines parallel, let alone execute flexion, extension, and dynamic stabilization of the joints as they move.

A Disease Known as Progress

In sports or business it's relatively easy to improve a team's performance: you get rid of the duds. With the body, it can be done even more readily: you make every member a star by serving them the real "breakfast of champions"—motion.

Dysfunctional muscles are generally not diseased, aging, or broken. They are starved of motion. When I asked you to try the exercise with your shoulders, I said that some of those muscles probably hadn't moved for days or weeks. I wasn't kidding. We assume that because we lead busy and active lives, our musculoskeletal system is also busy and active. It is, but only in a piecemeal fashion. The conveniences of modern life—tools, furniture, appliances, cars—as well as architectural design and the routine tasks that we perform have bypassed parts of the body that people once relied on to meet their basic needs.

It's called progress. If your grandmother loved to garden or if she lived on a farm, she was probably pretty handy with a hoe to keep weeds under control. Just imagine, for a moment, using a hoe. This movement is pretty basic, but it engages all the load-bearing joints, plus the back, the arms (including wrists and hands), and the shoulders. Flexion, extension, and stabilization are under way throughout. Now here comes progress. A modern woman combats weeds by squirting herbicide out of a spray bottle. Most of her effort involves pointing the bottle, squeezing the trigger, and walking back and forth.

Yes, this is a lot easier than hoeing, but there's also a lot less muscular engagement and stimulation going on. I'm not saying that backbreaking physical labor is the only way to achieve a fully functional musculoskeletal system. But I want to show how our motion—even with weeding—is conscribed. Our muscles respond, but we have to ask them to. We have to find effective ways and means to stimulate our muscles to keep them functional—otherwise more and more muscles will opt out. And as that happens, misalignment increases along with stiffness, chronic pain, and disability. That's really not progress at all—it's pain and poor health.

Notice that I said that "we have to find" ways and means. That's a major change. In the past, motion found us. The environment kept our earliest ancestors in motion. From dawn till dusk, they were on their feet hunting, foraging, fishing, and herding. Along the way, they forged the powerful musculoskeletal system that is ours today. We are equipped both to walk vast distances and to run fast in short spurts, both to trot for miles and to crawl on our hands and knees. We have the apparatus to lift heavy objects off the ground and to hoist burdens overhead, to carry babies in our arms and the sick on our backs, and to climb hand over hand, to stretch, to bend, to throw, to push, to pull, to point the way. These muscles and bones tell a story that's more wondrous than any fairy tale and more startling than science fiction. And to examine the fossil remains of an ancient woman is to come face to face with the Queen of Motion.

The royal dynasty endures today, because her musculoskeletal system is yours. But you live in a different world, a different environment—one that was changed, ironically, by humankind's own motion-generated capacity for hard work, abstract thought, and ingenuity. The muscles and bones that support all of the physical attributes that I've listed above are still present, but the stimulation to engage them is not. We can do something about that without having to re-create the harsh and hostile environment of our earliest ancestors. What we need, rather than danger or hardship, is variety.

Anthropological evidence indicates that until about ten thousand years ago, men and women were engaged in pretty much the same daily activities: they hunted and foraged. While men occasionally worked together to bag big game and engage in warfare against rival bands, those occurrences were probably far from routine. Survival meant going out and filling one's belly with whatever was digestible, just as it did for any self-respecting squirrel, rabbit, or crow. It wasn't glamorous work, and everyone participated. They walked mile after mile, they stooped over to pick up seed pods, they climbed trees for fruits and birds' eggs, they pried rocks loose and turned over logs in search of grubs and insects, and they ran away from angry bees protecting hives full of honey. The more they roamed, the more they prospered, in body and mind. Eventually, someone picked up a stone or a stick and threw it. From then on, armed and dangerous, those puny two-legged creatures had a decisive advantage. While people certainly are what they eat, they are also what they *do* in order to eat. Our ancestors did a little bit of everything. They were complete generalists.

Today most of what we do with our arms is restricted to a small area directly in front of us, roughly from midthigh to midchest. Technology, usually in the form of a keyboard, a desk, or a steering wheel, brings work precisely into this zone, which I call "the box."

Do you rake the leaves in your yard or blow them? Do you beat your carpets or vacuum them? Do you chop vegetables with a knife or use a food processor? These relatively minor chores once routinely engaged muscles that are now not being engaged in the same way at all.

Yes, it takes muscle to flick a switch, but it takes roughly only one contraction. (To be exact, it takes a smooth and seamless series of contractions that blend into what feels like a single act of flexion or extension.) But the effort of raking, carpet beating, and chopping causes the contractions to take place again and again. These tasks gave muscles the wherewithal necessary to maintain their strength and functional capability. Without them, our range of motion has been steadily shrinking.

Basic yoga and simple stretching exercises feel so good because they rescue us from the box. When was the last time you got out of it? Think about it. If it was more than a half hour ago, it's time to escape. Try this (if you're not experiencing back or shoulder pain). Stand up with your feet parallel, about hip-width apart. Arch your back, and square your shoulders. Interlace your fingers as if you were about to pray. Raise your arms over your head, with your fingers still locked together, palms facing down, arms straight. Look at your palms, and roll them so they face the ceiling with the fingers still interlaced. Arch your back. Let your stomach muscles relax, and breathe deeply. Pull your arms back so they extend straight past your ears. Hold this position for a count of thirty.

Congratulations! You escaped from the box. How did it feel? I hope you noticed that your head, neck, arms, shoulders, spine, and hips formed one unit. When I do this E-cise—called a Standing Overhead Extension—I get a rush of energy and pleasure. As we move through the book, I'll introduce you to several more E-cises that you can use for quick and easy escapes from the box.

The Human Hummer

I cautioned you about doing the Standing Overhead Extension if you are experiencing back or shoulder pain because that pain indicates that dysfunction and compensating motion have taken a toll.*

Pain is a message. Aside from traumatic injuries that suddenly break, tear, or rupture musculoskeletal system components, pain is a way to slow us down before there's serious damage. It's the body's technique for letting us know that it's time to stop what we're doing and focus on correcting the underlying musculoskeletal problem. But correcting the problem doesn't mean just "killing" or deadening the pain with drugs or surgery. Pain, while uncomfortable and frightening, is rarely the main problem. It's a symptom of the problem. Too often, painkilling drugs and surgery only eliminate this symptom. They temporarily remove the pain, but its cause remains and will eventually start making trouble again. Health care problem-solving is all about cause and effect. If my back hurts, I want to find the cause so I can remove it. Pain is usually the effect, not the cause, so we need to be extremely skeptical of treatment regimens that make pain relief the primary objective.

Often when there is musculoskeletal pain, the chief culprit is compensating motion, or motion in which the

---

*Please consult my book *Pain Free: A Revolutionary Method for Stopping Chronic Pain* (New York: Bantam, 1998) to find special E-cise menus that address chronic musculoskeletal pain for specific parts of the body.

body functions—after a fashion—in violation of its own design. Here's how compensating motion works.

Motion is so important that the body rarely refuses to move. It can improvise a response to almost any stimulus. Humans are natural contortionists and acrobats. One of the chief reasons is that we are bifunctional—that is, the musculoskeletal functions that are on the right side of the body are the same as those on the left. Basically we have two of everything, and no matter what side they are on, these muscles, bones, and joints have an identical design. Neither right nor left has an advantage. Paradoxically, this equality also means we can do *different* things on each side at the same time. Walking again is a good example. While one leg flexes, the other extends. Or we can do the same thing on both sides at the same time, like rowing a boat with oars or bouncing up and down on a pogo stick.

Walking also illustrates how we are bifunctional front and back. Our muscles are mostly positioned (anchored) on either the front or back of the skeletal structure. The posterior (back) muscles tend to handle extension, while the anterior (front) ones manage flexion.

Neither side, right or left, is fully autonomous, because they share one crucial component—the spine. Caught in the middle, the spine depends on a balance of power between the two sides to keep it upright. But no built-in mechanism exists to prevent one side from overwhelming the other. For more than three million years such a mechanism was unnecessary: a motion-rich environment kept both sides equal, because each received an equal share of stimulus.

Bifunctionalism allows for hyperflexibility and spontaneity, so that we can handle a wide range of motion coming from any direction. But because of the spine's central location, we are also designed to operate symmetrically. The two sides interact equally as a single unit to support the spine, allow us to stand upright and stationary, or provide a smooth and flowing gait-pattern when we walk. In an environment that generates random motion demands, even temporarily asymmetrical stimulation will eventually be distributed to each side symmetrically. A person who walked uphill for an hour, for example, is likely to spend another hour walking back downhill.

However, our present-day environment doesn't generate many random motion demands—at least, not on a regular basis. Technology has eliminated both spontaneity and variety of motion. Today's patterns of motion are repetitive and limited. Consequently, some muscles and joints receive more stimulation than others. The functional equality between the two sides, and within them, is disrupted. Some muscles become strong, and others weak. Certain joints are condemned to hard labor, while others are on permanent vacation. This inequality drastically alters the balance of power between the two sides. Yet weak muscles still have work to do, like opening and closing joints, so those functions become compromised. For instance, the left knee may bear a disproportionate share of the body's weight, while the right knee, failing to fully open and close smoothly, twists laterally.

To get the job done in whatever haphazard fashion it can contrive, the body borrows muscles from other assignments. These conscripts are usually secondary muscles that handle stabilization duties, as well as rotation, adduction, and abduction. (I'll explain these terms in a moment.) They are closer to the surface than the prime movers and big posture muscles, which are attached to the bone for the sake of maximum leverage. Despite their disadvantages, however, the compensating muscles assume more and more power and responsibility. As they take over, dysfunction spirals downward. The less the big posture muscles and prime movers engage, the less capacity they have to engage at all. Weakness and dysfunction breed ever more weakness and dysfunction.

Once the compensating muscles come into play, the body enters a defensive phase, gradually sacrificing various individual functions in the interest of keeping the body semi-upright and semi-mobile. The paramount danger, the body knows, would be complete immobility; to avoid this catastrophe, the compensating muscles, as they struggle to keep us moving, allow the musculoskeletal system grid to slump. This dysfunctional posture generates a further sequence of dysfunctions: a stiff neck, a torn rotator cuff in the shoulder, herniated disks in the spine, sciatic pain, cartilage loss in the hip, and so on.

The Art of Improv

I promised to explain rotation, abduction, and adduction. I'll start by illustrating them. Figure 2–1 (a, b, and c) depicts a woman performing a jumping jack, that old standby of calisthenics classes. To move from position a to position b, she is abducting. Her *abductor* muscles, primarily in the hips and shoulders, are moving her bones away from the median plane that divides her body from front to back. To go from position b to position c, other muscles, called *adductors*, draw the bones inward, toward the same median plane.

Fig. 2–1

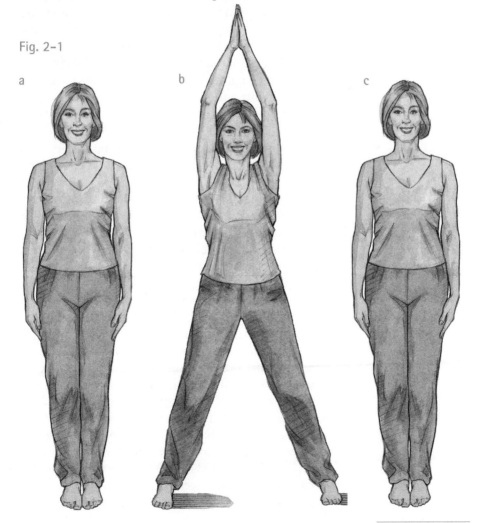

a   b   c

When the posture and prime mover muscles become dysfunctional, the abductors and adductors take over their work. Only they're not very good at it. During walking, the crisp heel-to-toe gait-pattern of the foot that's normally carried out by alternating flexion and extension becomes muddled, because abductors and adductors are designed to move bones sideways, not from front to back. Ingeniously, the body gets around this problem by sacrificing the design gait-pattern and substituting a destructive side-to-side waddle that's accomplished by rotation.

Rotation? For maximal flexibility and stability, most of our joints can rotate, so as to perform a limited amount of lateral movement; without rotation, we'd be as inflexible as the Tin Woodsman of *Wizard of Oz* fame. The compensating adductor and abductor muscles use this rotation capability to convert side-to-side movement into a series of angular tacking maneuvers, much as a sailboat solves its inability to point its bow straight into the wind by tacking. In effect, the abductor needs only a little knee flexion and hip extension to get the foot off the ground; then it can move the leg sideways with sufficient momentum to fake the leg's functional extension. The body supports this maneuver by toppling forward enough to swing the leg in an arc, and the hip stabilizer muscles go into rotation to bring the leg around to catch the weight transfer. It's a masterpiece of improvisation!

But it comes at a high price. The ability of the hips, knees, and ankles to improvise reflects the body's acrobatic genius. When the body is surprised by an unusual situation, its joints can respond in an unconventional way—they're tough enough to handle occasional stress. But the hips, knees, and ankles aren't designed to work that way all the time. When the stress becomes routine, damage begins to accumulate.

In this case, extra rotation in the hip socket is likely to strain the stabilizer muscles that are being pressed into service as ersatz extensors and flexors. In the process, these muscles lose their ability to help with the smooth operation of the joint. Cartilage may begin to scrape away. As for the knee, rotation of the femur (thighbone) has replaced flexion and extension. Instead of moving forward and back, the bone is twisting in the joint capsule—grinding, really, at the point where it joins the tibia and fibula, like a mortar and pestle (on the other end at the hip too). Below, the carefully balanced structure of the ankle starts wobbling, and the foot, which is designed to bear weight with carefully arranged traverse and latitudinal arches, flattens under the gyrating load that's bearing down from above.

For the Pleasure of It

Studies show that a majority of Americans do not exercise regularly, even though the health benefits are irrefutable, and it's no wonder. Burdened with a dysfunctional musculoskeletal system, it's hard enough for us to move just to accomplish the necessities of life, let alone for the fun of it—or the health of it. For many of us, moving is getting increasingly difficult and increasingly painful.

I hope I don't sound cynical, but I believe people do what makes them feel good. We are primarily motivated by pleasure. Ultimately, even the fact that we work hard confirms this rule because it yields us tangible rewards like money and comfort, as well as producing intangible compensation like prestige and feelings of accomplishment.

The same is true for movement. Marathon runners pursue the sport because it's challenging, fun, and—for all the blisters and sore muscles—pleasurable. A stroll through the park has similar appeal. Duty isn't much of a motivating factor.

Pleasure has many definitions and sources, but "lack of movement" is usually not among them. Even the early indicators of dysfunction, like poor balance, fatigue, and stiffness, can rob movement of just enough pleasure to make it easier for us to curtail our motion activities and to make excuses—"I'm not as young as I used to be," "I'm bored with biking," "Jogging is bad for my knees." Eventually, when the symptoms escalate into pain, the motivational equation will be fatefully reversed: since movement hurts, lack of movement avoids pain and therefore brings pleasure.

The linkage between pleasure and lack of movement scares me. As we've seen, once the stimulus of motion becomes scarce, an unavoidable undertow of dysfunction results. When moving ceases being a pleasure, pain is inevitable, along with an ever-escalating reliance on painkilling drugs, surgical procedures, and other high-tech products with dicey side effects.

In just a few generations, we've become bound to our cars and our desks, bound to our TVs and our computers, bound to convenience, consumer medicine, and the couch. Educators proudly announce cutbacks in physical education and athletic programs. From coast to coast, schoolyards and suburban backyards that once teemed with energetic children are now mostly empty. "Have bike will travel"—which could easily have served as a motto for American kids a generation ago—has been replaced with "Have minivan (with Mom at the wheel) will travel."

This trend will continue and probably intensify. We're going to have to learn how to deliberately supplement our body's minimum daily requirement of motion. Taking motion for granted—assuming that it just happens on its own—is a thing of the past. Many of us will have to rediscover and reforge the link between motion and pleasure. Some will find it easy to do and almost instantaneous; just a bit of topping off is all that's necessary. They're the lucky ones, with lifestyles that provide almost enough motion to stay fully functional. Others will have to work harder, endure a little drudgery at first, and overcome pain. Eventually, though, the pleasure principle will kick in again, guaranteeing that we'll want to stay in motion for no other reason than that it feels good—very good.

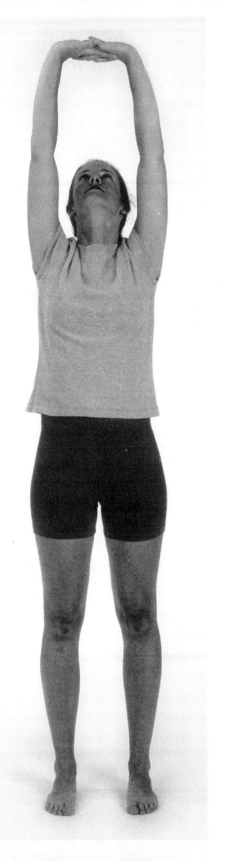

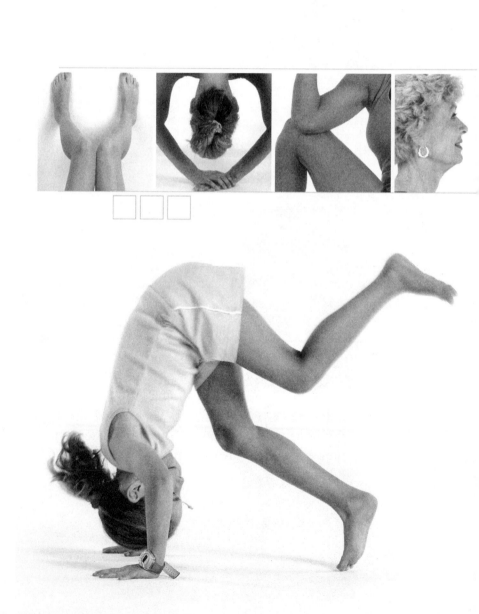

CHAPTER 3

living tissue and the river of renewal

Not long ago, Randy and Arlene, a married couple in their mid-fifties, came to the Egoscue Method Clinic after Arlene fell and fractured her radius, one of the forearm's two long bones. It had mended well, but the accident had convinced Arlene it was time—she was *getting older*, after all—to take some preventive measures. Randy was clearly of the opinion that the fracture was age-related and therefore whatever happened in the clinic wasn't going to have much effect.

□□□□

As we examined an X-ray of her forearm, I pointed to the radius and asked one of my favorite questions: "How old is this bone, do you suppose?" There was a moment of hesitation, as happens when a dumb question arises. Randy spoke first.

"Fifty-four. That's how old Arlene is. All her bones are the same age." I looked at Arlene, who nodded in agreement.

"Okay. See that line where the break occurred? It's lighter, like new putty or mortar. How old is that?"

There was another moment of hesitation, but this time Arlene answered. "It's new. Maybe six weeks old."

E-cises: Preview of Coming Attractions

In the Egoscue Method Clinic, we use E-cises to promote renewal and regeneration. These simple routines, many of them second cousins to stretching exercises and yoga moves, correct musculoskeletal system imbalances by strengthening and reengaging lost functions that cause damage. In Arlene's case, Standing at Wall let her feel her dysfunctional shoulder position (and feel the proper design position in contrast). By using a short menu of other E-cises, among them Cats and Dogs and Triangle, Arlene brought her hips and shoulders back into proper alignment, and strengthened the muscles to maintain the proper posture. Check them out. Page numbers for the instructions are in the index.

"So does that mean your radius is mostly fifty-four with a smidgen of six weeks where the break occurred?"

"Yeah—" Randy was ready, but Arlene cut him off: "No, that doesn't make sense. The process must be working on the entire bone, probably all the bones."

Randy didn't get it, but Arlene did. Bones are not static. Growth and regeneration are under way constantly—if we allow it to take place.

In Arlene's case, a cast and a sling were enough to allow regeneration. Her arm had been immobilized for nearly six weeks. Bone fractures don't allow for many other options. Even if a drug company could invent a powerful enough painkiller, using a broken arm and leg is usually impossible structurally. The loose ends of the bone have to have a chance to knit.

For most people, a broken bone is a once- or twice-in-a-lifetime event, but when needed, the regeneration mechanism still operates. In fact, it happens everywhere in the body. Whenever cells are used up, they're replaced. But in places where musculoskeletal misalignment and dysfunction have set in, regeneration is counteracted by excessive wear and tear. A cellular deficit becomes a tissue deficit and then a structural deficit.

Randy's readiness to blame Arlene's accident on her age, and his assumption that age would affect her healing prognosis as well, opens the door to a common self-fulfilling prophecy: "I'm getting older, so I'll have to live with this stiffness and pain." But what's really happening is that you're getting used to the symptoms of dysfunctional wear and tear, which are preventing full tissue regeneration in the joints. Without new growth and renewal, lo and behold—there's more stiffness and pain, confirmation that you're getting older and had better start acting your age. Actually, you're acting not your age but your dysfunctional posture and skeletal misalignment.

If she followed the conventional wisdom, Arlene would probably give up tennis, a sport she loves and does well. After all, her elbow hurt. And if she eliminated tennis, her elbow might indeed stop hurting for a while. But her musculoskeletal system dysfunction, which had its origins in her shoulder, would continue unabated, because her shoulder and elbow were still being used for other purposes. Consequently both joints—and their cartilage—would remain under stress. Months or years later, a skeptic who doubted that cartilage regenerates could use Arlene's sore shoulder and elbow as a prime example. "The cartilage is gone," they'd insist. "Cartilage doesn't regenerate itself. When it's gone, it's gone."*

Regeneration Versus Degeneration

Thirty years ago, when I started out as an anatomical functionalist, tissue regeneration as a subject received fairly little attention. Mainstream science had decided that, with the exception of a few mostly minor examples—the growth of hair and fingernails, the healing of skin abrasions, the knitting together of broken bones, and some other occurrences—human tissue did not regenerate in meaningful ways once it was used up or destroyed. While routine cell division did take place to a greater or lesser degree, depending on the nature and function of the tissue, the prevailing opinion was that for the most part the human body was a net consumer of nonrenewable resources.

Why are hair, nails, skin, and bones any different from other tissue? I wondered. Why would regeneration, a seemingly invaluable attribute, be wasted on mostly secondary characteristics? Bones, I understood—but nails and hair? Furthermore, I was puzzled by children: What is so special about youth that explosive tissue regeneration, in the form of growth, takes place from birth to the age of eighteen or nineteen? Does this astonishing capacity for nearly constant change really just stop of its own accord?

My musings weren't just idle speculation. The issue of tissue regeneration probably won't be featured on the front cover of *People* anytime soon, but it's extremely relevant to fixing the musculoskeletal system when it seems to be broken. Once upon a time, it was holy writ that joint cartilage would not and could not renew itself. That was strange, I thought. Back then I knew a sixty-five-year-old librarian who was an avid gardener; her next-door neighbor, also sixty-five, was an accountant and a devoted collector of antique silver teaspoons. Both women were approximately the same height and

*Arlene's right shoulder was hinged forward and more or less locked in that position, which shifted the flexion and extension work to her elbow. It contributed to the broken arm as well, since the shoulder joint was unable to cushion the impact of her fall.

weight; neither had ever banged up her knees in an accident. But the librarian's knees were pain free, while the accountant's were swollen and stiff. Could it be that the librarian's gardening was helping to renew her knee cartilage, I wondered, while silver spoon collecting did not make the same contribution to the number-cruncher's knees? If cartilage is finite, why didn't Mikhail Baryshnikov, the famous Russian ballet dancer, run out of it when he was twenty-five?

Every year at the Egoscue Method Clinic, I see dozens of people who have been assured by physicians that their joint pain was caused by cartilage loss. Yet after a couple of months of doing E-cises to restore function and strengthen the appropriate muscles, they're pain free. What happened to the lost cartilage?

In my first book, written more than ten years ago, I stated flatly that cartilage will regenerate itself if and when damaging joint stress caused by musculoskeletal misalignment is eliminated and function is restored. That statement drew a barrage of criticism from doctors, researchers, and physical therapists. When cartilage is gone, they scolded me, it's gone, and nothing short of a miracle will bring it back. But since then, cartilage has, in fact, been deliberately regenerated, first in a Swedish laboratory and then elsewhere in Europe and Asia. Pharmaceutical products and surgical procedures are now being marketed that supposedly enhance cartilage regeneration as an alternative to joint replacement surgery. It's not a miracle. If we just let the body do what it has always done, we will have plenty of cartilage to last a lifetime.

The same discovery has been made for tissue regeneration in general. We now know that the lining of the intestinal tract is sloughed off and replaced *every day.* Likewise, the liver can restore itself after losing *80 percent* of its tissue mass. As for blood, the body routinely creates enough new red blood cells for a pint of fresh blood each week, and far more in an emergency, by destroying and recycling old, used-up red blood cells. And researchers at Princeton University have recently shown that even brain cells, long thought to be finite in number in adults, arrive in the cerebral cortex by the thousands every day as bouncing, newborn neurons. In these examples and many others, the cells and tissues that are most active, and most subject to irritation and stimulation, are those with the greatest propensity to repair damage and renew themselves. Even at the cellular level, it pays to keep moving.

In that respect, muscle offers a working paradigm for all tissue: use it or lose it. All tissue thrives on stimulation and languishes in stagnation. The brain is no exception, and that's why the breakthrough Princeton research I just mentioned was so startling when first reported in the November 1999 issue of *Science*. Hardly a month later I personally may have seen it in action. Over the holidays I went to visit my eighty-five-year-old father at his home in rural Utah. He was fairly listless and unfocused. One day we ran out of things to do, and rather than hang around the house, we went on an expedition to the college where he had studied as an undergraduate. It was a long drive, but as the day wore on Dad got stronger, more alert, and more active. He was having a fine time and seemed to be getting younger by the hour. And maybe he was. Is it so far-fetched to believe that the stimulation was renewing his tissue, including his oxygen-carrying red blood cells, heart muscle tissue, and brain cells?

I can already hear the howls of protest: heart muscle tissue does not regenerate! True, there's no clinical evidence—yet. But the research on brain cell regeneration suggests that it's only a matter of time. The belief that adult brain cells could not replicate themselves was once sacrosanct. How else could we explain aging? It was so easy to blame it on tissue that just up and died because—the theory went—it was too specialized to regenerate. But now we know our highly specialized brain cells are renewable. So why wouldn't the same apply to all tissue, including heart muscle tissue? And if it does, then in cases of heart disease, we need to know what prevents the regeneration mechanism from working. What is interfering with it? In my father's case, a rut of sitting around at home, not moving much, and not being stimulated by new demands and experiences was enough to adversely affect his energy levels, metabolism, and mental acuity. Was tissue degeneration actually taking place? It's unclear, as is the question of universal tissue regeneration. But it's undeniable that an observable change for the better took place.

I've always wondered why negative health outcomes

are regarded as proof that the body is weak and flawed, yet positive outcomes are considered just a lucky fluke.

In his book *Spontaneous Healing*, Dr. Andrew Weil recalls that when he was in medical school, arteriosclerosis was considered to be irreversible. Once for the university newspaper Weil interviewed an expert on rivers, who observed that even what seemed to be hopelessly polluted rivers cleansed themselves if people stopped dumping toxic waste into them. Once the contamination levels dropped, he said, there were enough oxygen, sunlight, and beneficial organisms to allow a healing mechanism to kick in. Weil asked himself: "Why shouldn't arterial systems behave the same way? In fact, we have clear evidence that arteriosclerosis is reversible, if you simply stop putting into your body the substances that cause it (mainly saturated fat) and stop obstructing the healing system with your mind (by cultivating anger and emotional isolation, for example)."

A river of renewal runs through us all. Gradually, the view that the body is in a state of degeneration once adulthood is reached, is giving way to recognition that it constantly seeks regeneration and self-healing. This change in perception and attitude is deeply significant. Medical treatment that enhances self-healing and works in harmony with the body's own processes and logic is far more desirable than techniques that assume that the body is an accident waiting to happen. What may be

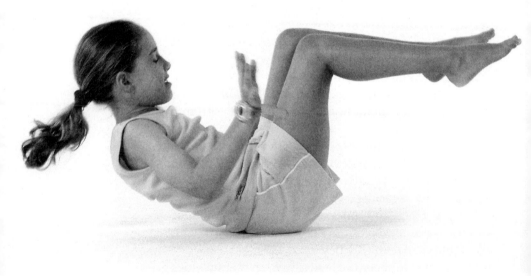

waiting to happen is health—if we let it. To understand and accept that the body's first priority is to keep itself alive—and that it endeavors to do that at all times—means we must learn to look beyond the symptoms to the causes of ill health.

In a polluted river like Weil's, the stench of dying fish is a symptom, not the cause. Introducing replacement fish and spraying billions of gallons of air freshener won't clean it up. There's nothing wrong with the river itself; what's wrong is what's being done to it. Likewise, in a person with arteriosclerosis, there's nothing wrong with the arterial system other than what is done to it. Yet we bomb it with drugs and ream it out with angioplasty. We attack the symptoms. Ironically, the attack on the symptoms leads only to the use of heavier medical artillery, because the patient never seems to make real progress. But there's no progress as long as we target the symptoms. The river that runs through us remains polluted.

Name That Tune

Amazingly and mysteriously, the body knows whether the river is pure and renewing or polluted and harmful. To illustrate this powerful trait, I need to abruptly switch metaphors from rivers to music and the body's *soundtrack*.

As a woman, you already know from your own experience of the monthly cycle that the body has its own inner logic and rhythm. It's neither accidental nor incidental. It's true not only for your reproductive system but for all the other systems of the body as well. Some of these cycles are harder to detect—or easier to ignore—than others. But each chord, each grace note and downbeat, resonates to produce that complex symphony we experience as an individual life. If we can learn to pay attention to the music, it will tell us what we need to know about our health.

Unfortunately, having a tin ear—or no ear at all (like Arlene's husband, Randy)—is a common condition. Some people think that listening to the music—paying attention to one's health—smacks of hypochondria or self-obsession. Others are afraid of what they might hear and learn if they listen, a fear that grows out of the fact that we're all mortal and cannot postpone death forever. But listening and learning can prolong life, because if we know what the music of good health sounds like, we can more easily keep the dial set to that frequency. If you don't know the tune that hums "All is well," what are you to make of silence? What about the odd notes that stop short of pain that seem to be conveying an important message nonetheless?

Psychologists often refer to the "tape" that people listen to in their heads, the soundtrack we carry within us. It's a medley of hope and fear, doubts and dreams. The optimist may be listening to "I can, I can, I can . . ." The pessimist hears "I can't, I can't, I can't . . ." My work has convinced me that before that track is laid down, our health lays down another one that establishes the beat and sets the tape's tone and content. In other words, the pessimist who hears "I can't, I can't, I can't" is experiencing not only a state of mind but a state of body. *The negative content is emanating from the body's own reading of its capabilities:* I can't (concentrate), I can't (summon the energy), I can't (control my tools).

Barbara is a perfect example. She loves to run along the bridle paths of Rock Creek Park in Washington, D.C. One weekend she was jogging with her friend Yolanda, who would have preferred to be inline-skating on the bike path. As they ran down a long hill, Barbara saw a stream ahead, with a natural bridge of stepping stones passing from one side to the other.

"I just pumped right along, pulling in front of Yolanda because the path was narrow," she recalled. "I hit the bank and kept on running, using the rocks without breaking stride. I looked over my shoulder. Yolanda was gone. I stopped to look, and she was back there on the other side of the stream, just mustering up the courage to jump to the first rock." She paused. "Yolanda is a gutsy woman. Those rocks were steady. It was no big deal!"

"Did you ask what the problem was?" I inquired.

"Yes. Yolanda said that when she first saw the stream up the hill, she was fine. But as she got closer and closer, her doubts started to rise. She wondered if the rocks were steady and whether the first one was too narrow—that kind of thing. By the time she got to the bank, she said there was no way she could make herself keep running."

I asked a few questions about Yolanda's posture. Barbara had noticed that her friend's left foot pointed straight ahead but the right flared outward when she ran. "She's got a hip disparity, Barb," I explained. "The left one is doing more work than the right, and that undermines her balance. At first, her mind was saying, 'No sweat—four steps and I'm on the other side.' But as she got closer, her body, processing the incoming visual data, was saying, 'You're going to have trouble landing on the right leg and transferring the weight smoothly into the left hip in order to extend the left leg for the second rock.' "

"Really?"

Really. Mentally, Yolanda started off ready to ford the stream. But her body wasn't ready and soon let her know it. Our muscles and joints have neural receptors that monitor their functions and report back to the brain through the central nervous system. The mechanism that produced Yolanda's mental tape—one track saying "I can, I can," the other warning "I can't, I can't"—knew all about her musculoskeletal system dysfunctions, and at the last minute it wouldn't allow the "I can" to overrule the "I can't." Why? Because she really couldn't. Off balance, Yolanda would have fallen into the stream.

Had it happened, Yolanda would have immediately said, "I knew it!" And she did know it. One of the first questions I ask any client who has injured herself is "Why do you think this happened?" I'm not looking for a specific anatomical answer, but a general sense of cause and effect: "Just before my knee popped, the right hip was really tight," or "My wrist hurts when I type, although when I pull my shoulder back, it feels better. I think it's a shoulder problem."

I tell my therapists at the clinic to go on red alert when a client says, "It may not be important, but . . ." Believe me, it will be important. The inner tape is rolling. One way to trigger a data download is to ask, "When your shoulder [or whatever] started to hurt last night, what did you do?"

"I got out of bed and sat in my reclining chair. You know, I put my feet up on the rest and leaned back. Eventually the pain eased and I fell asleep."

Here again, the system's internal monitor is reporting in, and instinctively this person knew what to do about it. By getting into the recliner, she put both hips into the same position—and her shoulders stopped hurting.

Many physicians discourage this kind of self-diagnosis because the information doesn't seem relevant. They're trying to treat a blown knee or a sore wrist, and the patient is yammering on about her hip and shoulder, or a night spent in the recliner. But sparking such an analysis is the equivalent of downloading data directly from the patient's neural receptors. The knee knows when there's a problem in the hip, and the wrist is equally aware of what's going on in the shoulder. Yolanda might not be able to tell me that she has a hip disparity, but I wouldn't be surprised to hear her say, "My right side feels weaker than my left, and I was afraid that I'd slip when my right foot went down on the first rock on that side." Or it may be even more basic: "I didn't think I could make it." If Yolanda's musculoskeletal system has determined that she doesn't have the functional wherewithal to cross the stream, no pep talk is going to get her across.

This checking or braking feature is particularly pronounced whenever our feet are off the ground. Balance is crucial to bipedal locomotion, so much so that two-thirds of our neural receptors are involved with balance. On the ground, if our balance is compromised by our position or skeletal alignment, there are a variety of ways our body can compensate. In the air, it doesn't have much to work with, and once our feet leave the ground, the monitoring system takes a dim view of any and all detectable dysfunctions that could interfere with keeping the body balanced and stable. That's why Yolanda got shut down.

The interactions and interplay that occur within the body are so extraordinarily complex that human life as we know it could not exist without our internal monitoring system. The "tape" that we may be aware of to some degree is just a surface manifestation of a far deeper process of stimulation, reaction, and response taking place among all cells, tissues, structures, and systems. There's no dark side of the moon in the body. We are totally wired, and this wiring, as Dr. Sherwin B. Nuland notes in his book *The Wisdom of the Body*, is our most precious gift:

> Like all communities of cells throughout the body, nervous tissue adapts to circumstances it encounters. But because it is uniquely equipped, qualitatively and quantitatively, to exchange information with its fellows, it has much more potential to do its adapting by coordinating itself with the re-

quirements of other parts of the body. It is the integration of parts of the brain with its other parts and its ability to act (at a tremendous rate of speed) on the basis from signals from every other tissue of the body that are the basis of the mind, of abstract thinking, and of much that has gone into the creation of a dazzling array of faculties that I have called the human spirit.

The "tape" and the rest of the monitoring system do become fouled up sometimes. Here's how. A stimulation always begets a reaction and a response, whether we are overtly aware of them or not. In Yolanda's case, the stimulation was the upcoming demand on her dysfunctional right hip to ford the stream. She reacted, and her response was to stop in her tracks rather than risk tumbling into the water. Stimulation-reaction-response. In other words, stimulation said Go!—while her tape said Whoa!

Ideally, Yolanda knew why her body responded this way because the information that she has a hip problem is on her "tape." But like the rest of us, Yolanda had another tape playing, one produced by a culture heavily invested in the notion that while the spirit is willing, the body is weak.

We have two tapes? I'm afraid so. Yolanda's first tape produced the original sequence of stimulation-reaction-response, and she stopped. Then she responded again, this time to tape number two, by lying to herself about why she stopped.

The Body Blame Game

Maybe *lying* is too strong a word. I'll put it another way. Modern science has set itself the task of definitively answering all questions, including Why do we live? and Why do we die? Death is such a disturbing thought that the easy move is not to answer it at all but to blame something for it. So we blame our worn-out, broken, malfunctioning bodies. The scientific quest, therefore, is to build a better body. This assumption of physical frailty provides the underlying theme that we hear on the second tape, the one produced by our culture. Yolanda heard and responded to this one during her run in Rock Creek Park. More often than not, the second tape drowns out the first one, which is the one we

The E-cise Alternative

E-cises work with the body's design to restore function. There's nothing wrong with the design of Yolanda's hips. Their function, however, has been disrupted by misalignment. E-cises work to realign the body's structure rather than redesign it through surgery or drug therapy. By avoiding redesign, E-cises preserve and enhance the body's internal systems—including the immune and metabolic systems—that depend on motion and proper musculoskeletal system function.

should be hearing in order to get an accurate readout of the body's internal monitoring mechanism.

Instead of accepting that her right hip was dysfunctional and doing something about it, Yolanda received an easier and more plausible message: "You're getting older" or "Women don't have the knee strength to bound across streams." Both messages are nonsense, and both come from the belief that individual physical shortcomings are the result of general design weakness in the body, fluky accidents, or gender-specific defects. This message is generated by our culture. Loud and pervasive, it induces us either to passively accept our seeming limitations, or to aggressively pursue technological remedies. Hearing the message, Yolanda might decide to give up running (since she prefers inline skating anyway) or to put orthotics in her shoes, use a knee brace, and eventually, once hip pain sets in, agree to undergo joint replacement surgery.

The last thing she'll think of doing is restoring hip function. I'm out to make it the first thing.

This progression from passive to aggressive responses is the usual pattern because it parallels the body's increasing disability and its pain of growing severity. Our stiffness and pain persuade us that the body is weak with age or prone to accidents. "Do something" becomes the imperative. When the arsenal is stocked with heavy weaponry, we pull the trigger. Increasingly drastic remedies seem entirely justified. But because they are aimed at the wrong targets, they don't work, beyond providing short-term relief for symptoms.

Meantime, the monitoring system is still reporting faithfully on the state of the body's health. But the warnings are now considerably more ominous, since it detects a far bigger mess: the original problems, their direct and spreading effects, and the impact of an excessive and misdirected treatment program. It's little wonder that many personal tapes are broadcasting "I can't, I can't, I can't." What's the bottom line when we've allowed a fixable musculoskeletal problem to worsen and added to it the calamity of needless powerful drugs and surgery? *Can't* is the bottom line.

Posture and Metabolism

Let's stay with the image of a tape recorder for the moment. As the reels slowly turn, they convey the important information in the first tape, the soundtrack. I hope you are listening to it, but even if you are not, something else is. I'm thinking of every organ system of the body. There are twelve of them: skeletal, muscular, nervous, integumentary (skin), circulatory, respiratory, reproductive, digestive, urinary, lymphatic, endocrine (hormones), and immune. Each of them is subject to stimulation-reaction-response.

Musculoskeletal dysfunction triggers (stimulates) a reaction and response in each of the eleven other systems. When the tape broadcasts the news that something is happening, it's not a warning as such—stimulus is initially regarded as neither good nor bad. But the news that important major muscle groups are not engaging needs to be known by all systems because, for starters, it's going to affect the metabolic process.

Yes, metabolism. One of the body's most complex biochemical operations, metabolism is the way the body provides fuel to its cells. Muscles play an important role in at least three ways. First, by creating heat from the friction of contracting and relaxing. The heat helps to essentially cook the food, oxygen, and water that we consume until they break down and recombine into substances that can be converted by the cells into usable energy. The more work the muscles do, the more fuel is available to the cells. And the reverse is true: the less work the muscles do, the less fuel for the cells. The second metabolic role for the muscles is that of being a major metabolic consumer. Large, active muscles have many muscle cells to fuel. This appetite serves to create an expanded metabolic capacity in order to meet muscular demand. But the metabolic supply isn't exclusively used by the muscles, though. When we rest or sleep, our muscles are relatively (and temporarily) inactive, and the fuel that's not needed by the muscles is diverted to other tissue and organs.

That's why poor posture—slumping, misaligned dysfunctional posture—indicates a metabolic dysfunction. Notice that I didn't call it a *symptom*. Poor posture is actually a *cause* of metabolic dysfunction. Once the deep muscles—the ones closest to the bones and joints—disengage, the metabolism backs off because the body's monitoring system tells it there are fewer cellular mouths to feed and reduced means to do the feeding. The other eleven organ systems immediately lose

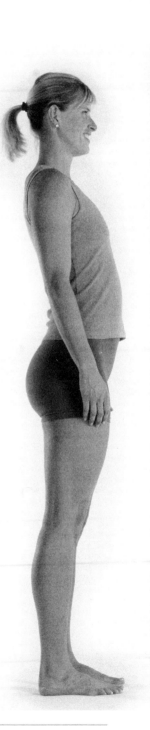

the benefit of a revved up, efficient, fully functional metabolism. The energy they need to carry out basic functions is no longer as abundant. It puts a strain on every organ in the body and the roughly 75 trillion metabolically dependent individual cells.

The third important metabolic role played by the muscles is this: reduced muscular engagement means reduced oxygen intake and distribution. Oxygen is the combustion agent that the metabolic process uses to refine the fuel (primarily glucose, amino acids, and enzymes) needed for the operation of the body's cells. Disengaged and dysfunctional major muscle groups mean that the primary vehicle for getting oxygen into and around the body isn't in optimal condition. But suppose circumstances require optimal metabolism. A sudden demand for physical exertion, the effects of stress, or severe illness all call for extra energy to support extra work from the body's organ systems. They depend on the support of a fully functional metabolic process. Since muscular action is involved with drawing oxygen into the lungs and assisting the heart and circulatory system in moving oxygenated blood throughout the body, the disengagement of major posture muscles hinders this work. As a result, fuel production is compromised, as is cell function.

Conceivably, the body could cope with the problem simply by doing less work with less metabolism. After all, our environment is not as rough-and-tumble as it once was. But one system in particular is working as hard as ever—maybe harder: the immune system. The immune system is like a network of fire stations scattered strategically throughout the body. The T-cells and various antibodies are the fire fighters, ready to deploy, when the alarm sounds, to battle invading viruses, toxins, and other conflagrations. An immune system undermined by an inefficient metabolism cannot respond as quickly or effectively. It just doesn't have enough available energy for aggressive fire fighting, as if many of the fire trucks are out of gas and their crews understaffed.

That's why we're seeing the rise of the new "epidemics"—diabetes, asthma, allergies, virulent but heretofore unknown strains of TB, some types of cancer, and the like. This alarming trend coincides with another epidemic—chronic back pain, headaches, bad hips, knee injuries, hurting wrists, and other musculoskeletal disorders. I believe the link between this epidemic and the others is visible all around us. If millions of Americans do not have the strength to stand up straight, to hold their shoulders square and their heads high and level, and to move smoothly without stiffness or pain, how do we expect them to have the strength to fight off disease?

Without adequate musculoskeletal support for the metabolic process, they simply cannot. Around us, the very *embodiment* of health is crumbling.

I'm painting this gloomy picture not to spread pessimism but to inspire faith. We need to regain our faith in the strength of the human body. After all, it got us through two or three million years of BS—Before Suburbia. Rediscovering it can yield a cure for these epidemics.

By recognizing our strength and its source in muscle and bone, we can escape from the modern delusion that health comes only from experts and technology that soon will be crushingly expensive and beyond the reach of all but a few. Down that road lies misery and future epidemics, the horror of which we can't even begin to imagine.

All of us can afford the price of a genuine miracle cure. We were born with potentially strong, aligned bodies. We were therefore born rich.

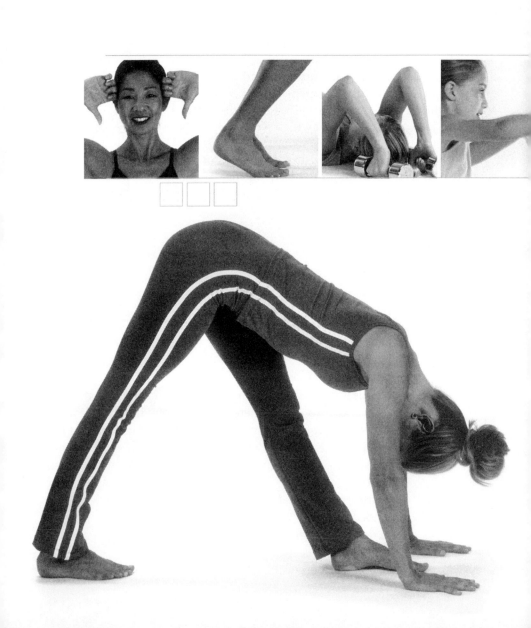

CHAPTER 4

mars and venus,
men and myths

This may come as a shock, if you're easily shocked, but here goes: male superiority is a myth. Men have been legends in their own minds since the first hunter told a tall story around the first campfire. I doubt that women bought it then, and they surely don't buy it now.

Yet I believe some women do tacitly accept elements of the myth. The first whopper that's been swallowed is that men are physically stronger. But how is strength defined, and who defines it?

Clinical kinesthesiologists, who study muscles, have various formulas to measure muscle contraction, length, tension, and force. Still, there's tremendous individual variation. Strength is actually an entirely subjective concept: I'm strong if I can hoist X number of pounds of dead weight; you're weaker than me if you can lift only half of X. But so what? It's meaningless, unless your name is Hercules or Charles Atlas. Rarely if ever has individual well-being depended to a great extent on the capacity to lift heavy objects. (African, Egyptian, and Western Hemisphere slavery are possible exceptions.) The history of manual labor is more often characterized by walking, bending, digging, pounding, pushing, reaching, and grasping. Even those who built the pyramids weren't lifting weight so much as enduring endless toil that kept them on their feet. Friezes and other artifacts recovered by archaeologists show these unfortunate people pushing or pulling on primitive mechanical devices and struggling up incline planes rather than relying solely on unassisted muscular force.

Hence weight lifting is mostly a sideshow stunt, a way to demonstrate manly prowess. It has little military value, and even in athletics, stamina and technical skill have always mattered more than sheer strength. Ironically, as modern male athletes become less skillful because of their musculoskeletal system dysfunctions, they've been turning to weight training as a substitute. It leaves them stiff, clumsy, and accident prone. Meanwhile, when it comes to technique, eye-hand coordination, agility, and grace, female athletes run circles around them.

My own definition of strength is not glamorous; it's nothing P. T. Barnum would have built a three-ring circus around. Here it is: the ability to run one's load-joints—shoulders, hips, knees, and ankles—through a full range of motion over and over again without restrictions, stiffness, or pain.

The next Olympics will not offer gold, silver, and bronze medals for load-joint articulation. But the ability of the load-joints to open and close, within the full parameters of the structure's design, is what championship sports and pain-free living are all about. I can't think of a single legendary athlete who was considered to be the *strongest* man (or woman) for his sport and time. Jim Thorpe, Jesse Owens, Babe Ruth, Margaret Court, Diane Leather, and Walter Patten all possessed sets of skills that rested on musculoskeletal foundations, which in turn rested on load-joints that opened and closed in full range of motion, and did so over and over again without restriction, stiffness, or pain.

I used to define strength as the ability to repeatedly respond to the demands of one's environment without restriction, stiffness, or pain. It's valid enough, but it misled some people into thinking that they were strong, healthy, and functional when in fact their individual environment was undemanding and limited in its range of stimulus. In an undemanding environment, the couch potato is king.

I revised my definition because the body's design requires an environment that offers a full and spontaneous range of demand. In such an environment, you wake up in the morning, and before long you've had to run your major muscle groups and joints through their paces—forward, backward, up, down, and sideways. Such an environment started to disappear at about the same time the wheel was invented. Today in our limited environments, many people routinely and repeatedly respond to only a narrow range of demand or stimulus for hours, days, and years on end. They call it work—typing, ringing a cash register, turning a steering wheel, swinging a paintbrush; or they call it recreation—hitting a golf ball, playing a computer game, watching TV. But only a few joints, and not necessarily the load-joints, are being used.

Accompanying my current definition are several illustrations of two women descending staircases. As you can see in the frontal views, one of them is fully functional—her back is arched, her shoulders are square, and her head is up (Figure 4-1)—while the other has poor posture (Figure 4-2). As the functional woman moves down the stairs (Figure 4-3), she is running her load-joints through the range of motion required. The horizontal and vertical lines of her skeletal grid are parallel as they carry the weight of her body under the force of gravity. Suppose she keeps climbing and descending at a reasonable pace for thirty minutes. The drawing in Figure 4-4 shows what she'll look like after fifteen minutes: no change in posture. Even after a half hour, there's no change.

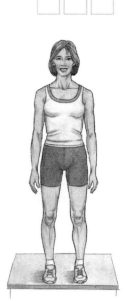

Fig. 4-1

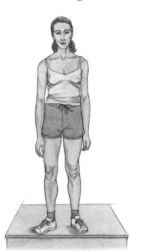

Fig. 4-2

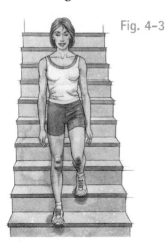

Fig. 4-3

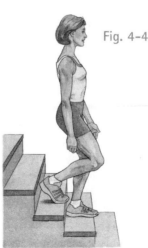

Fig. 4-4

The second woman's dysfunctional posture means that her load-joints are restricted in their movement. Her grid is misaligned, and as she struggles up and down the stairs, she improvises by using whatever joints happen to be the least restricted and whatever muscles are the strongest. Her strength and posture deteriorate with every step (Figure 4–5). After fifteen minutes her posture has worsened (Figure 4–6). She's more stooped and unbalanced, her knees are rotated outward, and her feet are flared. The joints and muscles she started with have been exhausted, and she has recruited others, which explains the change in appearance. It's very unlikely that she will be able to continue on the stairs for the full thirty minutes.

Both women appear to be about the same size, with sim-

Fig. 4–5

Fig. 4–6

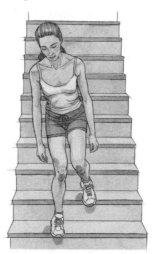 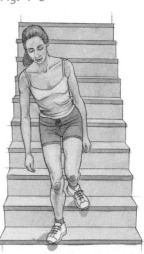

ilar muscle definition or bulk. The first woman could stay on the stairs for a half hour—or more!—if need be, not because she has bigger muscles but because she has better musculoskeletal system functioning. She is, by my definition, stronger. In her stair climbing the right joints are supported by the right pairs of specifically assigned muscles that flex, extend, and stabilize as needed. Her body is functioning as a unit, according to design. She doesn't tire unduly because the movement is the result of the coordinated interaction of powerful muscle groups from head to toe. There's no friction or stress. All her systems are operating at maximum efficiency. This guarantees cardiovascular fitness and stamina.

The other woman doesn't have the same resources. Off balance and overburdened by the force of gravity, she climbs by using a few isolated muscles of her hips, thighs, and lower back. The natural pairing between flexors and extensors has broken down. To compensate for incomplete extension of her legs (which she needs in order to straighten the knee after placing the foot onto the next step), she leans forward and twists her hips, shoulders, and neck. Those muscles aren't designed for that and soon tire and start to hurt. Eventually, since there's no handrail, she'll edge over toward the side wall and use her hand and arm for support. Afraid of toppling forward, she'll begin to ascend and descend sideways so as to shift the work to the adductor and abductor muscles, which run along the outside and inside of her thighs. Those muscles remain powerful because they get a steady workout holding us in an upright seated position, which, second only to the supine position for sleeping, is our most typical modern position.

Perhaps I should have illustrated a functional woman and a dysfunctional man climbing up and down the staircase, rather than two women. The man, who for the sake of argument, does have more muscle definition and bulk, would also be unable to keep up with the—"weaker"— functional woman. He too would end far short of thirty minutes with his heart racing and lungs aching.

The only difference in the women's ability to deal with the stair-climbing test lies not in a subjective measurement of muscle strength, but in their "degree" of musculoskeletal system function. Because of individual differences in lifestyle, work style, and other circumstances, degree of function varies from individual to individual. On a scale of 1 to 10, with the most functional awarded a 10 and the least a 1, we can graphically chart function and dysfunction for an activity by comparing it to the activity's duration (Figure 4–7).

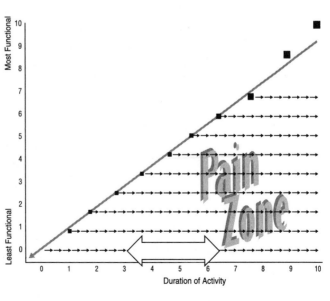

Fig. 4–7

A woman with a functioning level of 10 will complete the stair-climbing marathon without pain. The woman with a 1 will be unable to take the first step or two without stiffness or pain. In between 1 and 10, degree of function determines one's ability to run one's load-joints—shoulders, hips, knees, and ankles—through a full range of motion over and over again without restrictions, stiffness, or pain. For instance, using the chart, a 5 would be able to move without pain for roughly thirty minutes, until her dysfunction caught up with her. A 6 or a 7 could go five or ten minutes longer.

This chart is neither scientific nor based on precise measurements of functions or dysfunction. What I'm trying to do is to get you to see that traditional definitions of strength, fitness, and health are misleading when they fail to account for musculoskeletal system function. Strength without function is a non sequitur. Men and women are equally capable of being either functional or dysfunctional.

Success in sports or the military is a direct result of function. Skill, whether it's dribbling a basketball or flying an Apache helicopter, depends on an individual's ability to run the load-joints—shoulders, hips, knees, and ankles—through a full range of motion over and over again without restrictions, stiffness, or pain. The same goes for business or any other endeavor. Function is not conferred like stock options, partnerships, and corporate directorships. As women continue to make advances, the shattering sound we hear is made by function meeting the glass ceiling. Some will always get to the top by aggressiveness, guile, or luck, but the real deal comes only when full function meets equal opportunity.

Stairs and Chairs

One reason I chose stair climbing to illustrate function versus strength is that it's obviously a specialized activity. The range of motion is limited and repetitive—walk up to the top, turn around, walk down to the bottom, and do it again and again and again. The functional woman was able to engage her load-joints to help do the work without fatigue or pain—it happened automatically. But the second woman wasn't, even though the environment and the task were the same. The difference wasn't in the particular environment where the stair climbing was taking place but in the sum total of

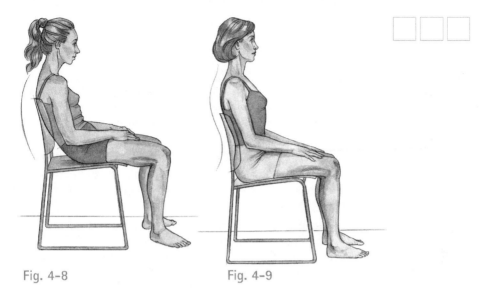

Fig. 4-8   Fig. 4-9

all the specialized environments within which the two women live. These environments are different for each of them. Either by luck (living in the right environment) or by conscientious effort, the functional woman is getting enough overall stimulus to maintain her musculoskeletal system functions and to use them in whatever circumstances she finds herself—climbing stairs, using a computer keyboard, gardening, and so on. The other woman isn't as lucky or as conscientious.

Most modern specialty environments that are created for work, play, and leisure aren't varied enough for people to engage their load-joints and maintain musculoskeletal system functions. Why? Part of the answer is that much of what we do is performed sitting down. This means that half the load-joints—knees and ankles—are usually disengaged. Moreover, the sitting pelvis is more prone to roll under and back, which throws the spine into flexion—that is, it rounds it forward, diminishing the arches of the S-curve. The spine's position pushes the shoulders forward, leaving those load-joints out of alignment with the hips (Figure 4-8). Hence skeletal integrity and function are seriously undermined. Figure 4-9, showing an aligned and functional seated posture, makes for a vivid comparison.

Furthermore, when the misaligned person gets up out of the chair, her muscles, having been deconditioned through lack of use, will no longer be able to hold her body in vertical alignment when she is standing on two feet (Figure 4-10). Because she is more com-

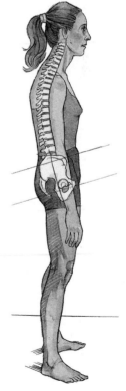

Fig. 4-10

fortable seated, that's the environment she seeks, the one that is created to suit her capabilities. Work is brought to her, and she holds it close to her abdominal area so that she can access it conveniently with a stooped spine and rounded shoulders that are not called on to provide rotation or much arm leverage.

Although I've been using the personal pronouns *she* and *her*, the same goes for *he* and *him*, except he is generally worse off than she is. Here's another myth: that men, because of their rugged, masculine, active lifestyle come to the job better able to handle physical demands than women.

Wrong, for two reasons. Today a disparity between the kinds of work done by men and women is less than it once was. Gender counts for less and less on the job, thanks to changing attitudes, technology, techniques, and material. Secondly, the rugged, active, masculine lifestyle isn't what it once was (and probably never really was to begin with). Most men today are far less active and far more sedentary than their fathers and grandfathers were. Because of tools, transportation, and television, much has changed in only a few generations. In the 1920s, Owen Gittines, my coauthor's grandfather, walked to and from work in Philadelphia. He spent the day as a millwright, using a variety of heavy tools to maintain assembly lines and other systems at the Atwater Kent Radio factory. Today his grandson Roger works at home, sitting down, tapping at a computer keyboard. His load-joints are not participating in the work (unless he makes a deliberate effort to ensure that they engage).

Roger's specialized environment shapes and limits his functions, whereas Owen's was more varied, utilized his load-joints, and induced a wider range of motion. All Owen had to do to remain functional was to respond to the demands of his environment. Still, Owen's world of work and leisure was narrower and offered less variety than did that of his own father and grandfathers, who were Welsh and Pennsylvania coal miners. This trend toward less movement and more homogenous movement has been going on in a major way since the Industrial Revolution began. The effects are so widespread today that it is having profound health consequences.

When it comes to function, women are in slightly better shape because they've had to contend with gender discrimination. Kept mostly on the margins of the workforce for much of the Industrial Revolution, their lifestyle and work style remained more varied than men's and less subject to the restricted patterns of specialized factory and workshop environments. While they were deprived of the physical benefits of some forms of labor that were reserved for men—such as increased muscle mass, upper-body strength, and endurance—they received some positive trade-offs. Running a home, up until the first half of the twentieth century, required walking, bending, lifting, stretching, sweeping, pulling, pushing, and a host of other vigorous movements. The demands placed on a woman were different from moment to moment, day to day. Over the decades "women's work" changed somewhat as labor-saving devices were introduced, but on the whole, women were preserving their functions as men were losing theirs.

But don't gloat. This advantage is fading rapidly.

Motion in a Box

Humankind is not a habitat-immured species—that is, people are not bound to a set range, territory, or terrain, as is a tropical hummingbird or a grizzly bear. We're willing and able to go from point A to point B, no matter where it takes us, as long as we have air to breathe. As a result, we've adapted to many different circumstances, from the steamy equator to the frozen polar regions. This adaptiveness has fostered amazing agility, eye-hand coordination, stamina, and mental acuity. As we roamed far and wide, we became tough and smart. But today even athletes repeat the same limited sequences of moves over and over again. Few ever successfully move from one sport to another—not even Michael Jordan when he tried professional baseball. It's almost as rare for athletes to make a switch within the same sport. When it happens—when Cal Ripken moves from shortstop to third base, for example—it usually means the end of a career is approaching. Where we were once adaptive, habit is making us habitat-immured.

For much of our lives, we are confined to a limited space, be it a chair, an office cubicle, or a computer workstation, which amounts to a box or cell with transparent walls. The box is our habitat, and we take it with us wherever we go. We never use many muscles, structures, and functions because they aren't needed within the box. But once they are disengaged and inaccessible, disused and deconditioned, we are effectively trapped in our box. It takes a special effort to break out. That's why I use the stuffy, archaic word *immured*. It means "imprisoned."

I cautioned you not to gloat about women having superior musculoskeletal system functions, because a one-size-fits-all trend is under way. His box and her box are roughly the same size—and both are shrinking steadily. As women have moved into the workforce, they too have been required to operate in a motion-limited environment that does not fully engage their musculoskeletal system functions. Ironically, some aspects of gender inequality—like the "double work-day"—work in favor of women's health. Many women employed outside the home are expected, once they return home, to carry out the bulk of their family's domestic chores as well: cooking, cleaning, laundry, errands, childrearing, and the like. These chores put them back in a more demanding environment. Thanks to the additional demand, living in these two worlds, however unfair the arrangement may be, enhances women's musculoskeletal system functions.

But modern home life too is becoming less varied and more patterned. Are you busy? Of course. Are you crazed? Probably. Even so, the motion that is required of you tends to be carried on in the invisible box directly in front of you. That's where the car's steering wheel is to be found, the stove, the refrigerator, the TV set, the washer and dryer, and other appliances. It's pretty much the same hectic drill day after day. Consider your own life. What patterns repeat themselves Monday through Friday? What are your weekends like? For all of its seeming diversity, modern America has an amazing social uniformity. Whether they occur in a million-dollar colonial mansion in Bedford, New York, or in a $500-a-month walk-up apartment in Bedford-Stuyvesant, the patterns of day-to-day life are similar—and limited. Few of us are getting anything close to the range of stimulus and demand that our grandparents experienced.

Women's "Special" Health Needs

As we saw in Chapter 1, men's and women's musculoskeletal systems are almost identical. Our physiological similarities too are numerous and fundamental: there's no such thing as a gender-specific kidney, liver, or lung. We part company, of course, with reproduction, but that accounts for only one of twelve internal organ systems. And of the twelve, the reproductive system bears the least direct influence on the second-to-second, hour-to-hour, day-to-day survival of the individual. (The survival of the species is another matter.)

Poetic airs, wild nights, and gentle mother's love notwithstanding, when it comes to individual survival, digestion, circulation, and respiration take precedence. By sheer force of numbers, the essential functions, supporting organs, and tissues that men and women hold in common make us human before we are divided and multiplied by sex. If the essence of womanhood is the womb, that crucible of life, our human essence is blood and brains, bone and muscle, a thick skin, a hard head, and an indomitable will to adapt and endure.

More and more is being written today about the "special" health needs of women. I won't directly dispute that those needs exist, but before we focus on special needs, we need to make sure that the vital necessities that men and women share are recognized and respected. If not, our health will have no foundation, or a shaky one, and even our legitimate special needs will come tumbling down.

Much of what is regarded as falling within the "special needs" and "special treatment" categories deserves to be carefully reexamined. In some cases we may actually be seeing symptoms of musculoskeletal system dysfunction rather than conditions that are unique to women. Musculoskeletal system dysfunctions can take on substantially different characteristics depending on individual lifestyle and circumstances. One person's irritable bowel is another's headache or sleep disorder. Given the lifestyle that is relatively typical for women in the world's more affluent, developed countries, it's possible that a health problem may actually be a social or cultural phenomenon more than a gender-derived condition. That's not to say the problem doesn't hurt or should be ignored. But treatment must be appropriate to the condition, and not be mostly generated by what's politically correct or commercially profitable.

Example: A number of studies show that women who migrate from the underdeveloped world to industrialized countries develop rates of diabetes that are in line with the rates of women in industrialized countries but substantially higher than those of women still living in their original homelands. Based on this information, diabetes among immigrant women may deserve, not so much special treatment based on gender, as a more generic approach that addresses the affluent Westernized lifestyle—more sedentary, with a fatty, high-protein diet. Gender may be a factor, but the same trend appears to affect immigrant men. Before we embark on a search for a treatment that is directed at women's unique physiological characteristics, wouldn't it make sense to try to make changes in diet and exercise first? Such a program, if I had my way, would include restoration of musculoskeletal system functions, which directly impact dietary metabolism and exercise capability. Who knows? We may find that it works for both women and men. After all, they do share the same musculoskeletal system.

It sounds too easy, doesn't it? In a sophisticated, technologically adept society such as ours, complications are what confer legitimacy. And complications are headed our way at warp speed. With the help of burgeoning genetic technology, we are on the cusp of being able to create almost infinite pathological subsets. Microscience and micromedicine can now examine and manipulate the body—which is unquestionably holistic in its functioning—in smaller and smaller fragments. They can even examine and manipulate the "beads" on strands of DNA. But in this complicated process, we are losing sight of the macro aspects of health. If restoration of skeletal alignment through a program of simple and easy exercises will correct joint dysfunction, and thereby lead to an overall improvement in health, tinkering with DNA seems like overkill.

Administering powerful medical treatment for the wrong reasons is a dangerous game. In November of 1999, there was a public uproar over a study that estimated that anywhere from 44,000 to 98,000 deaths a year are caused by medical mistakes in U.S. hospitals. The rate is remarkably low given the huge number of fallible, overworked people involved, the cumbersome health-care structure, and the enormous number of variables that influence medical outcomes. Micromedicine threatens to pelt us with a dust storm of microtreatment options that may or may not be consonant with the closely interconnected overall dynamics of the body. Let's try to remember that microcures, no matter how flashy, must work in a macro context and keep on working over the remainder of the individual's life span. Within each of us there are millions, probably trillions, of microprocesses that are synthesized into macro outcomes. Yet even with all these complications, the solutions to some health problems are relatively simple. Ignore that fact and we may look back fondly on the days when medical mistakes only accounted for *so few* deaths annually. And the tally will probably never record the suffering that's written off as aging, accident, or bad luck when, in fact, it was the result of the wrong weapons being brought to bear on the wrong targets.

Fat as Dead Weight

Men and women do differ physiologically in their body fat: women have more of it. The body of the average woman is 27 percent fat, while the average man's is only 15 percent fat. Since fat is "bad," this statistic seems to imply that men, being leaner, are healthier than women. But if that's so, why is the average life expectancy for women in the United States 79.4 years from birth, as opposed to 73.6 for men?

Given our dread of fat, surely 12 percent more of it would be likely to have profound health consequences. But it doesn't seem to. Fat, in fact, isn't as inherently evil as it's cracked up to be. Soaked in lipids (the genteel term for fat), adipose tissue is an excellent fuel storage medium. One gram of fat holds roughly twice as many calories as a gram of muscle. It's a source of many vitamins, insulation for or-

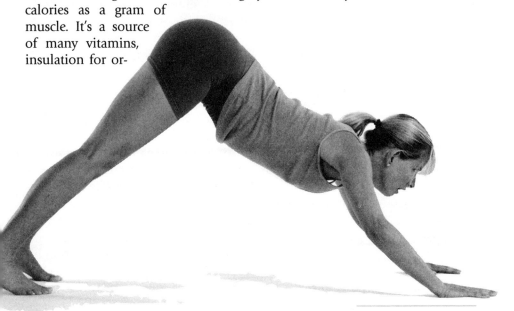

gans, muscle fiber sheathing, and cellular membrane, and it serves as an alternative fuel that allows glucose from carbohydrates to be diverted to sustain the central nervous system, which does not normally utilize fat. Historically, these fat reserves allowed women and men to survive periodic famines, and while that's not much of a threat in modern developed nations, it's nice to know that we have enough fat stockpiled to survive forty days without food next time Earth collides with a giant asteroid. As Natalie Angier notes in *Woman: An Intimate Geography*, a woman can lose 50 percent of her body fat and still recover. But loss of 40 percent of her lean mass, as happened to victims of Nazi concentration camps, means death. Fat provides a bit of a safety margin.

When we take into account bones, organs, water, and the rest of the organic material of the body that is neither fat nor muscle, a woman has approximately a third, or 34 percent of her total body weight, as muscle. Factor in weight difference—160 pounds for the average man and 125 pounds for the average woman—and he has about 8 percent more available muscle tissue, or 42 percent. Based on sheer numbers, he has an extra 13 pounds or so of muscle on average. Theoretically, that gives men a metabolic advantage, since each ounce of muscle can perform work, while fat tissue just sits there.

But distributed equally among the body's roughly 660 skeletal muscles, 13 pounds turns out to be less than a quarter of an ounce of extra lean tissue per muscle. That's not much, is it? And more importantly, some muscles don't work—or work inadequately—because of musculoskeletal system dysfunction. This is where women's legacy of superior musculoskeletal system function makes the difference in life expectancy. Women have less muscle overall, but they use it more efficiently than men. In many cases, pound for pound, the male advantage in muscle tissue is converted into a disadvantage since the muscle adds weight without conferring additional usable strength. Metabolic efficiency, brought about by greater musculoskeletal system function, is one of the major reasons that on average American women live about six years longer than men. Each of the 660 skeletal muscles is an individual organ in its own right. Contracting again and again, the muscles do the heavy lifting of the metabolic process. Muscular contraction lights the fire, keeps it burning, helps distribute the "heat" in the form of oxygen and nutrient-rich blood, and disposes of the waste products. Muscles that are disengaged, because they are bypassed by specialized environments with their restricted patterns of motion, cannot adequately support the metabolic process. The fewer the contractions, the less the breakdown of carbohydrates and protein into cellular fuel; the less fuel, the less work. The result is a less efficient overall metabolism that suppresses the body's immune system, stresses internal organ function, and adversely impacts cell performance.

Musculoskeletal system function is more than just perfect posture and avoiding inconvenient aches and pains. It is the foundation of good health. Women cannot afford to lose this precious legacy—but that's what's happening, particularly among children, teenagers, and women under the age of thirty-five. They are at greatest risk because they've never lived outside of motion-restricted specialized environments and therefore have never developed their important functions to even the most rudimentary stages.

Never—and I mean it. The girls and young women who come to my clinic show a shocking lack of musculoskeletal system function. Their mothers and grandmothers have far more. To jump-start them, we have to take them back to the crawling stage. Imagine—they missed out on a whole chunk of their childhood development! These young women are psychologically ready to become all that they can be, but their bodies won't let it happen. Not because they're female but because they haven't had a chance to develop the *human* musculoskeletal system functions that are their birthright.

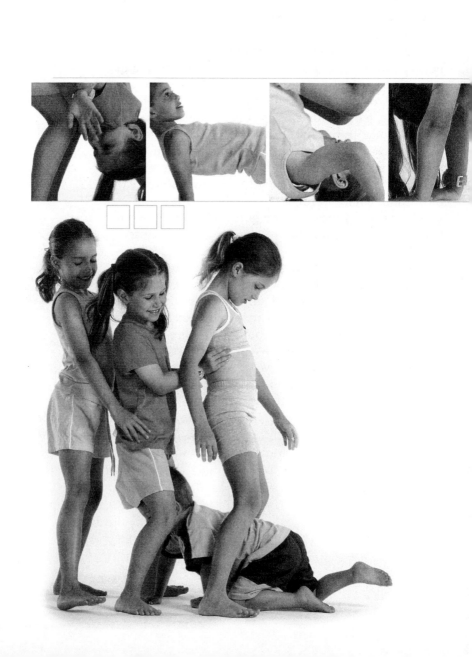

chil∂ren: the magic of motion

I love to watch children play. What a blur! Wiggle, crawl, stretch, run, dance, kick, prance, leap, bounce, roll, pounce, waddle, shimmy, and shake. Go here, go there, and then come back again on tiptoe. Hop like a frog, gallop like a horse, spin like a top.

They never stop. Or so it seems.

The pure joy that children take in moving is truly fascinating. There's nothing grudging or burdensome about it. They seem enchanted, intoxicated, enraptured by motion. There's almost a touch of the supernatural.

Motion is a magic potion, an elixir. Young children crave it and literally can't get too much of it. This truly ancient rite remains unchanged after nearly three million years. It is the equivalent of watching a fledgling eagle take wing, a lion cub tussle with her brothers and sisters, or a gray whale calf frolic at her mother's side. For a moment we are blessed with second sight—and we glimpse the future.

Technically, it's not that romantic. Young children in motion are undergoing a juvenile primate's unmediated response to their environment. Plunked down in the middle of the lawn or living-room floor, a child's reaction—since she doesn't know any better—is to fill this empty space with her presence. She imposes herself on her environment, and in return the environment imposes or imprints itself on her.

Such interactions, although more limited, are experienced by all living creatures. Coming to terms with one's habitat is the very first rule of survival. Where's the food? Water? Shelter? Friends? Enemies? At about two years of age, the little girl on the lawn or the living-room rug is actually well along in this process. But as adults we should start earlier to see how her musculoskeletal system functions develop and how they don't.*

It's the "how they don't" part that worries me. I'm seeing more and more children who do not know the joy of motion. They're not enchanted, not enraptured, not intoxicated. Sober, stiff, and still, they appear old and weighed down by a burden.

I'm going to see if I can change that. My mission in this chapter is to introduce you to the need to adequately *motionalize* your children as well as yourself. If you're not a parent, you'll find practical insights into how you were motionalized as an infant and the many important ways it influences your strength and health as an adult.

Caution: Baby on Board

Humans are at their most vulnerable from birth to about six months of age. In a harsh, unforgiving, hostile world, six months is a very long time—so long, in fact, that it's amazing we ever emerged as the planet's dominant species. Perhaps it was just dumb luck, or smart problem solving.

For most other animals, the early physical-development cycle is generally much faster than ours. There are some exceptions, but not many. Our fellow primates are slow to develop, as are many of the big predators. Still, most other creatures cannot afford the luxury of a long maturation. A newborn bird or rabbit begins to feed and protect itself (hide) within a few weeks. That's certainly not the case with newborn human infants. One reason is that we don't have much time in Mom's womb to get our little acts together. If gestation took much longer than nine months, it would be impossible to fit an al-

*I'll favor the pronouns *she* and *her* and tend to stay with females as examples, but particularly in these chapters dealing with children, most references apply equally to girls and boys.

ready oversize skull, which encases an already oversize brain, through the narrow opening in the female pelvis. Even though it's risky for a mother to be encumbered with such a fragile being and it's certainly dangerous for the child to be so entirely dependent, there's no other choice.

Yet in addition to allowing the head through the birth canal, the "quick" nine-month gestation period has three important benefits. First: since the newborn is not ready to physically engage with her environment in any substantially direct, tactile way, this frail, inept creature is free to use her big brain like a sponge, soaking up perceptions and insights. Letting her mind do the walking enhances her powers of cognition. Second: as the infant's mind and emotions fill out, she simultaneously masters the tactile and physical basics to accompany her rapidly accumulating mental resources. Thus, her mind and body become working partners. And third: since this development occurs outside the womb, Mom is spared a prolonged pregnancy, which is hazardous in and of itself.

In addition, the relatively short gestation period and the infant's resulting vulnerability have an even greater evolutionary advantage. Instead of locking in functions prior to delivery, based on a best guess that some will be more necessary than others, that selection process is left open and subject to change. Thus the postnatal environment—it could be hot, cold, rainy, dry, chaotic, or whatever—shapes the child's mental and physical platform. The result is a uniquely adaptable mind-body combination that is a prime example of the body's wisdom.

There is nothing illogical or irrational about the human body. Nothing. We may not fully understand its logic and its many ramifications, but it's always hard at work. A sequence of problem-solution logic is involved in birthing an infant with a skull that will become too large if it remains in the womb. If we can understand and accept what's going on—accept it as a solution to a problem, not as a lucky accident—then it's possible to see how the logic spins ever outward. That knowledge may let us realize how easy it is to interfere with the body's solutions—its logical processes—either inadvertently or by trying to impose our own solutions, our own version of a process.

Having a Big Head

In the fetal stage, the head can account for as much as 50 percent of body length. At birth, it's down to 25 percent, and by adolescence it accounts for only 12 percent.

As concepts go, this one is important enough to be printed on every package of disposable diapers. Since it isn't, I need to spend some time exploring it fully.

Start with helpless babies. To us, the existence of a vulnerable infant seems illogical, even idiotic (as well as extremely inconvenient for the busy modern parent). The extreme vulnerability of infancy eventually does abate, and children continue to progress toward physical and mental maturity in logical stages that can't be rushed in the interest of quickly achieving the safe and convenient haven of adulthood.

The body's own logic drives a child's development. Fortunately, a newborn's vulnerability helps awaken a ferocious—and there's no better word to express it—maternal instinct. This instinct provides protection as well as almost nonstop tactile stimulation.

Mom cuddles, hugs, tickles, and fusses with her baby. These are expressions of love, but such external stimulation also makes the baby aware of her own body. This awareness is crucial, and in the first six months it steadily builds, providing the equivalent of an electric current that powers the baby's functions. With Mom's help, the baby becomes mindful that she is an actor and not merely an object acted upon (the state the fetus experienced in the womb).

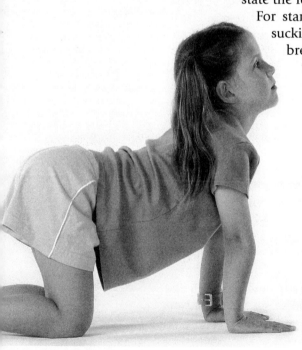

For starters, the child is born with a sucking reflex that is reinforced by breastfeeding, which begins to establish the chain of stimulation-reaction-response that we considered in Chapter 3. Almost right away the baby knows that she is a "player" in the feeding process. And she plays—eats—by moving her muscles.

Where am I going with this? Right where I told you: to the wisdom of the body.

Research has shown that babies who are neglected—who are not picked up when they cry, are not breastfed, are not cuddled, have insufficient aural stimulation, and so

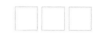

on—experience immediate and long-term health, emotional, and developmental problems. In one classic 1940s-era study at an orphanage, the nurses were not allowed to provide affectionate treatment to the children, and the majority of these children died or became severely retarded.

Short of outright neglect, tactile stimulation is interrupted in other ways. Modern logic has prevailed over the body's wisdom, and we have learned to "manage" our most vulnerable infants. Or to quote from *Dr. Spock's Baby and Child Care* by Benjamin Spock and Steven J. Parker, "Our society has thought up dozens of ingenious ways to put distance between mothers and their babies." This distancing may start with anesthetized childbirth or cesarean section and extend to feeding by way of a commercial formula or such technology as remote crib monitors and special carriers that resemble ejector seats from jet fighters. Spock and Parker note that in many other cultures women keep their babies with them throughout the day; the infants "continue to share their mothers' movement as their mothers go about their regular jobs whatever they may be—food gathering and preparing, tilling, weaving, house care. The babies are breastfed the instant they whimper. They not only hear but feel the vibrations of their mothers' words and songs."

Is your daily pattern of motion compatible with lugging around an infant all day as you work? Probably not—that's why we manage our babies. The starting point is not any lack of maternal instinct but rather the character of our specialized environment, which determines how American mothers move. For a mother to keep the child with her all the time would be not only inconvenient, but physically impossible. The musculoskeletal system functions that are needed to do that *and* to carry out necessary activities have been made inaccessible by our specialized environment.

Here are some examples: a stroller, baby carriage, or car seat substitutes for Mom carrying the child in her arms, on her back, or slung across her chest. These accessories put distance between mother and child, interfering with direct tactile stimulation. If suddenly all strollers, carriages, and car seats disappeared, most mothers in the developed world would be in a quandary. How do they transport the child? Pick her up,

Quality Cuddles

Between the ages of three and nine months, there is a major spurt of development in the frontal cortex of the baby's brain. Researchers have measured an increase in electronic activity there. As a result of the surge, the baby is able to accomplish more coordinated and complex movement. I believe that the extent and power of this electrical activity varies directly with the amount and quality of outside stimulation that the baby receives.

right? But they couldn't. Many women don't have enough upper-body, low-back, or hip function to carry a baby for more than short intervals. In addition, without access to her major functions (which drive her metabolism), Mom is fatigued, overstressed, and irritable.

This problem has nothing to do with bad mothering. Let me repeat: it has nothing to do with bad mothering. Without knowing why, many mothers turn to baby-minding devices because of their own dysfunctions and, in the process, begin the first stages of compromising the baby's future musculoskeletal system functions. A dysfunctional mother almost guarantees a dysfunctional child. I hate to put it that bluntly, but it's true. The child will be less body-aware, less grounded in her tactile senses, and less confident and comfortable with her burgeoning physical prowess. If you're planning to have children or if you already are a mother, I suggest you seriously evaluate your own musculoskeletal functions with an eye to their impact on your child's development. In Chapter 10 you'll find an E-cise menu designed to restore lost functions for women in their childbearing years.

I've found that mothers who have restored their lost functions stop relying on baby-minding devices, not because they're making a statement but simply because they don't need them anymore.

Floor It

Newborn babies come equipped with floppy heads: they don't yet have the spine and neck functions to keep their heads erect. Soon they will, and rather quickly. I'm not going to say how long on average it takes, because the pace varies from child to child. The more an infant is cuddled and held and rocked, the faster the functions will develop, due to the stimulation the child is receiving. But she progresses at her own speed. We must not impose our own management timetable.

I've theorized (half seriously, half in jest) that the floppy head is nature's way of scaring parents so they don't try to put the infant in a vertical position and keep her there, thinking it will encourage her to walk sooner. Babies belong on their backs or bellies, not in a vertical position. The spine isn't yet strong enough to support the head or the rest of the body's weight. From a prone or supine position an infant wiggles and stretches, twists and turns, and—here's the payoff—lifts her head to look around from side to side. These little random movements, all so awkward and cute, serve to stiffen the spine and engage its musculature. Eventually she will have the function and strength to roll over. But none of that can happen if she is kept in a vertical position.

Carriers and other contraptions designed to hold the baby flat on her back or at a slight angle also defeat her need to be on a relatively unrestricted horizontal plane. Strapped into a carrier, she's not going to be able to wiggle and wobble around much. The floor is an ideal place for her to do it, and unlike a crib, Mom can be down there with her. But Mom may not like the floor much, because it requires functions she doesn't have access to. A modern bassinet or crib, like a modern workstation, puts the child into Mom's restricted motion box—about waist high—where she is most comfortable. This leads to restricting the child's movement for safety's sake, so she doesn't accidentally tumble over the edge.

The floor is better for both mother and child, because the more time you spend on the floor, the more you'll grow to like it. I promise. Floor time will help you activate functions that you haven't used for years. Since our specialized environment keeps us either on our two feet or on our butts in a chair for so much of the day, we hardly ever use the joints and supporting musculature that handle the work of getting down on the ground and back up. A functional six-year-old will fall and then bound right back up. But adults, even those in their twenties, and even teenagers, will struggle to get back on their feet. Many people can't get up at all without assistance or without pulling themselves up, hand over hand. Their functions are so inaccessible that even the compensating functions are not available.

By rediscovering the floor and its outdoor equivalent, the lawn, you're breaking out of the box and changing the motion pattern of your specialized environment. You're also less likely to inadvertently impose that pattern on your daughter or son. Once a baby is able to hold her head up, we tend to waste no time in getting her into a vertical position. But here again we are unconsciously managing the baby to allow ourselves to stay in our own motion box. Backpack baby carriers are a case in point. They hold a child vertically and move her through the world at an adult pace. Left to her own

Today Sally is thirty years old. She describes herself as clumsy, uncoordinated, accident prone, and nonathletic. She first came to the Egoscue Method Clinic because she thought she was developing back problems, as she put it, "just like my mom's."

"You may have your mother's eye color or hair," I said, "but it's far less likely that you inherited her bad back." I quickly explained that her musculoskeletal system depends on adequate motion to stay strong, aligned, and fully functional. Sally in response told me that ever since she was a little girl, she preferred reading to running around and playing games.

"Why do you suppose that was?"

"I guess I'm a bookworm by nature," she said with a shrug.

"You enjoy reading?" I asked. "And you don't enjoy sports and games?"

"Basically, yes."

devices, she would remain horizontal, strengthening her spine and other musculoskeletal system functions by gradually turning her twitchiness into more purposeful movement. At about three months, for example, the grasping reflex she exhibited from birth, when an object was put in her hand, gives way to a deliberate reaching and grasping function. Other reflexes are also switching over to voluntary movement as the baby's involuntary and semivoluntary reactions and responses to the stimulation of her environment bring her muscles and musculoskeletal system structures on line.

Part of what's happening has to do with the brain. The cerebral cortex, which handles more complex voluntary motor skills and intellectual processes, is not as developed as the reflex-generating subcortex. The subcortex is the brain structure the fetus relies on in its relatively motionless state in the womb. As the cerebral cortex matures—in direct response to the child's self-generated motion (helped along by Mom's tactile stimulation)—the role of the subcortex recedes. Thus the baby's movement is strengthening not only musculoskeletal system functions but brain functions as well.

I have to repeat that: *the baby's movement is strengthening not only musculoskeletal system functions but brain functions as well.*

In the study of neglected, affection-starved children in the orphanage, which I mentioned on page 65, the death and mental retardation were the result of motion starvation (stimulation-reaction-response starvation) on children's brains and other internal organs.

It's been estimated that 95 percent of a child's brain growth takes place by the age of seven. Is it a meaningless coincidence that this explosion of brain power occurs just at the time when children are little whirling dervishes of movement and energy? I don't think so. Nor is it just hap-

"Okay. Let's turn our attention to working up an E-cise program for your back, and we'll come back to this conversation in a few days."

When we did return to it, Sally had been considering my point. She told me about her mother's child-rearing technique. Naturally she didn't remember it firsthand, but her mother and father had often told the story. "Do you suppose I would have been less of a klutz if I..." The question trailed off. She didn't want to blame her mother, and her mother didn't deserve to be blamed.

"Maybe the reason you didn't enjoy running around and playing games was that you didn't have the physical structure and development to get the most out of those activities," I said. "Are you enjoying the E-cises we gave you?"

Sally shook her head.

penstance that brain power–building trails off at about the time children are entering the first and second grades, where they encounter a socialization process that values sitting still more than moving around.

I can't help myself. I'll repeat it one more time: the baby's movement is strengthening not only musculoskeletal system functions but brain functions as well.

Creeping and Crawling

From about two months on, a baby is usually ready to roll over on her own. At about seven months, give or take, she will be strong and functional enough to sit upright. At first she won't be able to get herself into that position without help, but she'll try, and most parents can't resist lending a hand. It's okay to do so sometimes but not every time; let her also struggle and accomplish it on her own. Don't overdo the sitting either—and never prop her in an upright position. If she needs propping, she's not ready to be upright. A few minutes of sitting on your lap, with her back and head held vertically, are fine. I'm not wild about high chairs because a busy Mom will tend to keep the infant confined to the chair too long, since it puts her in the adult work zone.

Creeping and crawling can start anytime after the first six months. Creeping (dragging along on the belly) generally starts first. It's a wonderful way to activate musculoskeletal system functions. Colorful toys like blocks and rattles scattered around just beyond her reach will encourage creeping. The next phase, crawling on hands and knees, may start a month or two later. Spock and Parker advise that some babies may crawl without creeping first, while others may not creep or crawl at all but just stand up when they are ready. This shouldn't be greeted as a "whatever happens, happens" situation, and it surprises me that these distinguished authors didn't red-flag it. Walking without crawling, I think, occurs only when a child has spent too much time in a vertical position or has been fitted out too early with semihard-soled baby shoes (which I'll discuss in a moment). Close confinement and the sheer boredom that results can also discourage a child from crawling. Once she learns to sit upright on her bottom, if toys are placed close at hand so that she has no need to hunt or explore for them, a baby will be encouraged to anchor herself in one place. Cooping up a child in a

"At first I didn't, but the more I do them, the better I like them."

"Got any theories why?" I asked.

"I'm developing structure and muscles I didn't have before."

"Not exactly. The muscles and structure are already there—you were born with them. Now after thirty years you're finally getting around to beginning to activate them."

"Does that mean I can't be a bookworm anymore?"

"I'm afraid you're incurable on that score. But how about the back pain?"

"Pretty much gone."

"So the E-cises must have altered your genes," I said.

Sally rolled her eyes, and we laughed.

A Floor Show and Function Test

Get down on the floor without using your hands—that's right, no hands. The body is designed to do that. Take your time. Then get back up without pushing off or steadying yourself with your hands and arms.

How did it go?

If it was quick, smooth, and effortless, your knee, thigh, hamstring, and gluteal functions are intact and accessible. The more difficulty you experienced, the more dysfunctional you are. Feel free to turn to Chapter 11 and start those E-cises.

playpen is good management but may adversely effect musculoskeletal system functions.

If you have one of those wind-up swings that suspend an infant carrier or seat like a pendulum and rock it back and forth, consider this: a baby's sense of balance comes from her butt or tummy being on the ground. It's home base. As her functions strengthen and engage, they form around an awareness of what's solid and supportive and what's not. The mechanical swing is completely confusing, since movement is occurring without the baby's voluntary involvement, and she is off the ground without a home base. What's she supposed to make of that? A child's development process should be keyed to her discovering her innate capabilities and putting them to use. What the swing is doing is beyond her power. That sort of confusion only slows the development process by creating uncertainty, at a time when the child is attempting to simultaneously solve thousands of puzzles.

Giving Baby Shoes the Boot

Baby shoes have been a pet peeve of mine now for nearly thirty years. A hard-soled shoe turns a child's foot into a platform that will encourage her to push herself up into a standing position before she is ready. Those soles are so stiff that they act as levers, which gives the child a mechanical advantage not provided by her muscles. Standing usually takes place between seven and twelve months, but you should forget that. If your child is still crawling at thirteen—it's no big deal! She will stand when she's ready.

Upright bipedal motion is so fundamental that we're in a great hurry to get our children up and walking. To that end, much adult and baby playtime centers on holding the baby vertically, bouncing her up and down on her rubbery legs, and playing other games that seem to be conditioning her for that great moment when she can stand on her own. Infants learn by watching and attempting to imitate what they see. Mommy stands up on two feet and walks. The little girl or boy wants to do the same. The bouncing games also signal that the upright behavior is important and valued.

Give a child the assistance of a hard-soled shoe, and she'll put it to work to get upright. The usual route is to pull herself up on a playpen or crib's rails. Or Mom supports her by holding her by the arms, and she sways on her legs. This is all right if the baby is getting plenty of other musculoskeletal system stimulation through creeping, crawling, and a variety of spontaneous and unrestricted motion. But generally I find these days that most babies, as they approach the toddler stage, spend a lot of time doing the same things: sitting in a car seat while Mom does errands, riding in a baby backpack, being pushed in a stroller, amusing herself in a playpen, or being plunked in front of the TV. I suggest that you monitor closely how much *unrestricted* playtime your daughter or son gets. If the ratio of restricted to unrestricted play is on the order of fifty-fifty, you'll need to bump that into the thirty-seventy range or higher. It's not going to be easy—a crawling baby is an exploring baby. But let 'em rip. Unrestricted play is crucial to develop her musculoskeletal system function.

I'm still not finished with my campaign against hard-soled shoes. When a child uses shoes as a platform to pull herself upright, she's really pushing, and her arms don't contribute much. Her leg and hip muscles are doing the work. But those muscles and supporting functions are probably not ready for that work. The human pelvis is designed to let us stand, walk, and run on two feet, but it's got to be ready to do so roughly a year after birth. That means that the baby arrives with a formidable array of musculoskeletal system equipment already in place. To make it down the narrow birth canal without getting hung up, the pelvis allows the baby's legs and feet an extreme amount of latitude to rotate. They'll be able to move almost 360 degrees before reversing and coming back the other way, and all the while the right leg is moving independently of the left. The shoulders and arms, also potential obstructions, have this same malleability. It's the next best thing to creating a rubber baby.

It's better, actually, since rubber never gains strength. The human musculoskeletal system does, and relatively quickly. Once parturition is over, as the child begins to interact with her environment, the hip joints firm up and lose their plasticity. This puts the joints into the proper configuration to eventually support the child's weight on two feet pointed straight ahead (the most favored configuration for locomotion).

But if the shoe gets involved, she tries to stand up

Little Rockers

Babies need to be allowed to rock and roll in the horizontal position. Instead of an elaborate backpack baby carrier, I suggest you use a simple sling that will allow you to carry the baby across your chest. It will keep her in a horizontal position and allow for relatively unrestricted motion. She's also accessible for lots of tickling and touching. You will benefit too. The sling is good for your shoulder and back functions, but if there's pain or stiffness, use the E-cises in Chapter 11.

too early, using the inside muscles of the leg to push herself into an upright position. But the joints aren't ready for the load or to assume the aligned position. The femurs are still rotated outward, and so are the feet. She is extremely unstable. The body doesn't like it, and it will rush to strengthen the inside leg muscles and supporting structures. The more she stands, jiggling and jouncing, the more she conditions her hips, legs, knees, ankles, and feet to lock into this dysfunctional configuration.

Without shoes, parental encouragement, and handy items like playpens that offer support (and boredom), children wouldn't and couldn't get into an upright position until their hip functions were capable of supporting them properly. Dysfunctional hips are a serious musculoskeletal system problem. They lead to poor balance, skeletal misalignment, knee damage, foot and ankle impairment, and lower back pain. Solid, fully functional hips are a foundation for everything else. The more crawling the baby does, the stronger and more functional those hips will be. Shoes can actually discourage crawling by being cumbersome and slippery and denying the child the traction she gets from her bare toes.

Tearing Up the Timetable

There's no optimal age for a child to stand or walk. Neither standing nor walking has anything to do with chronology. The key is stimulation, not age. If the child has been kept out of hard-soled baby shoes, playpens, and other accessories of the vertical world, then any time she stands is the "right" time. And the chances are good that she won't be in a hurry to stand. As an adept quadruped, she has figured out how to get around just fine, thank you. Furthermore, if Mom has been sharing that horizontal world with her, she feels less pressure to go vertical. But if Mom rarely comes down to her level for a visit, it's only natural for her to conclude that standing is more desirable.

Eventually the horizontal world has been fully explored, and the brave new vertical world becomes enticing. That's another reason that I oppose playpens. Strictly confining the child's roaming ability makes her get bored quickly, and she wants out. There isn't nearly enough physical or mental stimulation. To learn, a child must go beyond the known into the unknown, where she can test her perceptions against her collected assimilated experiences, asking, in effect, *Does the world do it my way, or must I do it the world's way?* She can't do that in a playpen.

I know it is easier said than done, but parents have to take pains to create a safe but challenging (as in stimulating) horizontal environment. Then we have to be gutsy enough to allow the child to encounter and explore without our constant intervention. The link between learning and doing is broken when Mom is too quick to assist the toddler by making an experience easier or less frustrating, or to reduce the potential for a bump or tumble. The blander the environment, the more quickly a child will grow bored and restless. Going vertical, ready or not, is a way to jazz things up.

Ironically, using a playpen creates even more pressure to rely on the playpen to keep the child out of trouble. Sadly, it is common to see a toddler hanging on to the bars of a playpen wailing at the top of her lungs, letting the world know how irritated she is at being locked up. Her tantrum is nothing more than a message: *More motion, please!*

The same caterwauling child may also be upset because now that she is standing, she can't figure out how to sit back down again. Mom will gently set her on her bottom, but the child promptly stands up and starts crying all over again. This behavior is another indication that the toddler isn't ready to stand. Braced against the playpen rails, she's pushed herself up, but since there's no way to push herself back *down*, she is stuck. Her muscles and supporting functions are not yet strong enough, and her motor control coordination is not yet sufficient, to do the job of putting her knees, hips, and spine into smooth interactive flexion. Her only option is to squat and drop.

It's cute, if you overlook the fact that the child has learned how to sit down without putting her knees, hips, and spine into smooth interactive flexion. So what? Well, twenty, thirty, sixty years later, she will still be sitting down by squatting and dropping. It's a technique that I would estimate 90 percent of all adults use. They line their butts up over a chair and relax their contracted muscles—the ones along the inside of the thigh that they've been using since they first pushed themselves upright in the playpen—and gravity does the rest. The problem, from a musculoskeletal system standpoint, is that healthy knee and hip functions are lost in the process. When it becomes awkward to get in and out of chairs, adults think they are showing signs of aging. What's really going on is that they haven't grown up and into proper function.

Play's the Thing

Whenever I visit Toys Я Us or any other toy store, I'm struck that almost every game and toy is labeled a "learning tool." There's nothing wrong with learning, but movement—action—precedes learning. The purpose of a game should be to put the child in motion. The obsession with making every game a learning experience often means that movement becomes secondary and is restricted to meet a specific goal. Advanced learning involving higher motor skills—playing a musical instrument, riding a bike, ice-skating, and the like—requires repetition. Excluding random motion in favor of repetitive motion runs the risk of inflicting motion starvation on some musculoskeletal system functions and a surfeit of motion on others.

It's not far-fetched to believe that a child's short attention span is a purposeful mechanism to ensure that she experiences an adequate amount and variety of random motion and movement. A little girl may sit for a few minutes happily scribbling with crayons; then she sees the cat and is off in hot pursuit; the animal escapes but that's okay, there's a sofa to climb on, an imaginary puddle to jump; and where is the cat again? This mélange of activity offers abundant cross-functional stimulation, and by rapidly switching on and off according to the child's shifting interest, it avoids overloading functions that may not yet be ready for sustained use.

Children in motion also experience an interplay between activities that require finer eye-hand coordination and those that call for gross locomotor skills. A toddler may pretend that she is feeding a doll with a spoon and thereby increase her own manual dexterity at dinnertime. A few minutes later she drops the spoon and is hopping up and down on one foot. This "channel surfing" from function to function reflects an instinctive awareness that major posture and locomotor muscles support finer movement. The child switches from more settled, sedentary activities to periods of hypermotion to, in effect, replenish her energy. It's not necessarily that she is bored with feeding the doll, but rather that her functional ability to feed the doll is reaching its limits. The shift to hopping up and down boosts her flagging metabolism by engaging and strengthening major muscle groups, generating glucose production, and facilitating the branching of her neurons.

After a child begins walking, manual dexterity improves markedly. It's my view that until the locomotor functions are up and running, a child will lack the metabolic capacity to support advanced sensorimotor functions. The major posture and locomotor muscles drive the metabolic process hard enough to support the demanding work of neurological development. In many ways the development of locomotor functions continues the process that begins when the baby first started to wiggle, stretch, and arch. Literally with each move, the child is growing stronger and smarter.

Furthermore, achieving manual dexterity depends on having a stable musculoskeletal system platform. Fine motor skills are all about balance. Our body is designed to be symmetrical right to left, front to back, and to maintain balance not only when we walk but also when we use our arms and hands. When we are dysfunctional and asymmetrical, weight and equilibrium are subtly—and not so subtly—redistributed. If a child, for example, is trying to catch a ball with both hands, the left one might arrive just a little slower and less nimbly than the right, and she drops the ball as a result.

Play, therefore, is extremely important, as long as it's

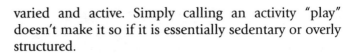

varied and active. Simply calling an activity "play" doesn't make it so if it is essentially sedentary or overly structured.

Babes in E-Land

In the Appendix I'll offer menus of baby and toddler E-cises for moms, caregivers, or concerned aunts. In general, unstructured spontaneous movement is the best way to go. Keep it simple with a variety of small, inexpensive toys, including that old standby the ball that can be tossed and chased after. Avoid formal calisthenics or workouts unless your pediatrician recommends them to treat a specific condition.

But before you turn to the Appendix or even turn this page, I'd like to return to the image I opened with: wiggle, crawl, stretch, run, dance, kick, prance, leap, bounce, roll, pounce, waddle, shimmy, and shake.

Babies and toddlers in motion. These littlest angels bring us surprised delight in remembering something we didn't know we knew: motion makes us strong, makes us smart, makes us happy: "In our proper motion we ascend."*

*John Milton, *Paradise Lost*

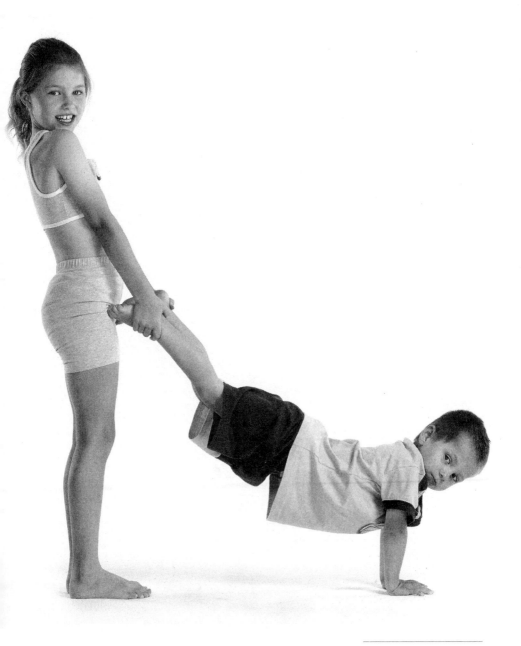

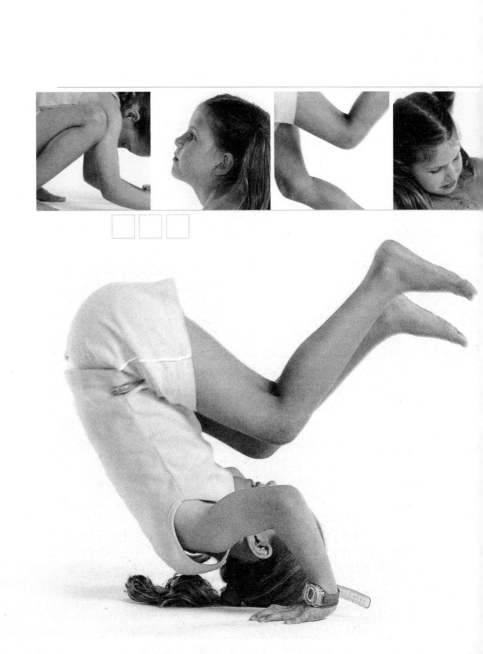

CHAPTER 6

the M&M years (middle and mobile)

Middle childhood (roughly, between the ages of five and twelve) can be a wonderful, rewarding, trying, terrifying, and hazardous place. Let's see what we can do to cut down on the hazards for children and to provide adult women with the insights they need to confront musculoskeletal system dysfunctions that have their roots in this period of their lives.

If all goes well, middle childhood is the time when children become gradually less vulnerable and more independent. Bigger, stronger, and smarter, they can move out of harm's way under their own power, and they have a reasonable (though far from perfect) grasp of what's potentially life threatening and what isn't. Eating, sleeping, dressing, and other bodily functions aren't the hassle they were during infancy and early childhood.

In a primitive setting, probably just enough progress is made in the early stages to lift the burden on Mom and allow her to care for younger siblings or to bear other children. A beneficial distancing between mother and child takes place that works to their mutual advantage. For modern mothers it has rewards too, like allowing them to return to work outside the home or to resume routines and valued activities that have been put on hold. But the child is the bigger winner. Having between the ages of two and five become a master of bipedal motion—we hope!—she can now run, jump, climb stairs, and play all sorts of games on her own or with other kids. She's got the musculoskeletal system equipment in place to vastly expand both her zone of autonomous action and her capabilities.

Even so, countervailing pressure on the child mounts to use *less* of her emerging physical prowess and *more* of her emotional and mental energies—and that's a hazard that concerns me. The intellectual-versus-physical issue—is it better for Johnny and Jeannie to read or run?—has moved back in the child development cycle from adolescence to middle childhood. The battle royal used to be against hell-raising teenagers, when parents incanted: "Settle down," "Grow up," "Act like a lady." Now, although it's not as rhetorical or drenched in rampaging hormones, the quieter conflict starts much earlier. Just when she's getting her "wings," a five- to seven-year-old is expected to mold her actions and activities to a template shaped by adult institutional forces, such as school, after-school care, and other social structures and strictures. If we're not careful, the child will be grounded before she flies, so that she will "be a good girl."

Infancy and early childhood were demanding and difficult on parents, but middle childhood is even harder. Moms with children in middle childhood face at least three major challenges:

1. They need to contrive to keep direct physical engagement and active exploration from being eclipsed by more sedentary behavior patterns that are more in keeping with adolescence or young adulthood.

2. In those children who did not fully develop their musculoskeletal system functions in early childhood and infancy, they need to restore the lost urge to explore.

3. They need to avoid making symptoms of musculoskeletal system dysfunction into a standard for ideal behavior. Passive, incurious, unenergetic children are not first-rate students,

even though they seem easy to teach and assimilate into an orderly adult world.

Bad News About Good Kids

The good news about children is that left on their own, they tend to strike their own balance. This is particularly true if they've managed to fully engage age-appropriate musculoskeletal system functions, which ensures that their mental and physical powers develop in tandem. They go farther afield on two feet, try new things with two arms, two hands, and ten busy little fingers, get into trouble, pull back, ponder mistakes, and try again. Gradually, and rather quickly at that, they'll start fitting the puzzle pieces together. The more they explore, the more they'll be able to make sense out of the experience. The bold body and the bold mind work together.

Do I need to repeat that? It's too important not to: *the bold body and the bold mind work together.*

Step by step and hand over hand, children build mental capacity and competency as they *move.* They go from being unable to understand objects, actions, and causes and effects outside of themselves to comprehending that they must reckon with the external reality of concrete items and information. "Decentering," to use an important term introduced by pioneering Swiss psychologist Jean Piaget, takes place when the child discovers by trial and error that she is part of a larger world and can master the technique of accommodating herself to it. An example of this is learning to pet a cat. If the child is too rough on the animal, it will run off to hide. But if she is gentle, the cat will roll over and purr. The child decenters and accommodates herself to the world of cats.

Accommodation is one of four key learning mechanisms in children that Piaget identified. The other three are perception, assimilation, and cognition, all of which play a huge role in a child's development. A higher form of accommodation, called consolidation, enables the child to structure knowledge to make it accessible, general, and more abstract. She consolidates her experience with one cat, for example, by applying it to all cats, pets, playmates, and maybe even to her new baby brother.

But physical exploration and intellectual consolidation don't always balance out. If the musculoskeletal system isn't fully engaged—if there's been too much playpen, hard-soled baby shoes, insufficient crawling, and not enough tactile stimulation—and if the child, as a result, is less than comfortable exploring the larger external world, then consolidation will take priority. The child will not seek out new experiences. Decentering will be impaired. Instead of going to the world, the child will expect the world to come to her. I believe this is what's happening, as more and more children move into middle childhood with musculoskeletal system dysfunctions.

The child sets up camp, and experience arrives through indirect, mostly adult channels. Still hungry to develop, little Jeannie becomes a "good girl" and little Johnny becomes a "good boy." Consolidators (and consumers) rather than explorers, they sit still and behave themselves. They're appreciated, praised, and rewarded for this "grown-up" behavior. And no wonder—modern life is complicated enough that many of us can do without having a fully mobile, hugely energetic five- or six-year-old smarty-pants running around exploring. The stroller and playpen aren't of use anymore. The "solution" is to resort to learning—adult-orchestrated consolidation—as a child-management device. It can be used to stifle unruly exploration of the kind that's needed to build both body power and mind power.

What I'm saying, to put it bluntly, is: adults hijack the consolidation process. They don't mean to, but that's what happens.

In the 1950s and 1960s, amusement parks had fun houses, where the "carney" would provide visitors with a set of 3-D glasses that distorted everything. When you put them on, the walls shimmied and shook, the floors undulated, and you couldn't tell which end was up. After a while, though, as you got the hang of the crazy perspective and figured out how to compensate with your movements, you'd begin to navigate. Then back outside, it could take several minutes to readjust to reality. At first your legs wouldn't want to work right. You'd stagger around acting goofy. It was a blast.

Think of the 3-D glasses as the adult "take" on the world that's presented to the child. What's offered may be accurate and useful—for adults—but not necessarily for children who were unable to explore the real world *before* they entered the funhouse. The child can adjust, but the adjustment is dicey. It's based on someone else's experience, not theirs, and on other priorities and sets of physical interactions with and reactions to the world. Can full consolidation take place under those circumstances? I don't believe it can.

The reason is that exploration brings on the physiological (including neurological) changes that are necessary to support a decentered mental and emotional structure that can accept second- and third-hand learning. The more the brain is stimulated by new experiences and challenges, the more neural branching and pathway building occurs. But the child who has skipped over exploration is not physically prepared to break out of her me-centered world.

Second- and thirdhand learning needs to come when the child is ready physically, mentally, and emotionally and not on the adult timetable. Middle childhood is hazardous to the degree that it tries to fit kids with adult 3-D glasses. While wearing them, they pick up our version of reality without having the underlying experiences to validate it.

Inadvertently, because they seem so well behaved and "adult," the dysfunctional good girl (or boy) becomes a role model. She makes life so much easier for adults. We persuade ourselves that success later in life is determined by her ability to structure her behavior in socially acceptable ways as a child. That's always been the case. There's never been a society without a mechanism for training—socializing—the young. Our historical contribution to this process has been to strip childhood of many of its last preindustrial, preurban, presuburban characteristics. I see the results in my clinic when the grown-up Jeannies and Johnnies arrive suffering from chronic musculoskeletal system pain, often bringing with them severe emotional problems as well.

Our environment, as I have said, does not encourage movement, and it also doesn't reward movement. Quite the contrary, the less one moves, the more material success accrues. In the era of the double-click billionaire, it's only logical for parents to want their children to avoid wasting time and energy on things that are not obviously productive. Music isn't productive, so cut back on music instruction in the schools. The visual arts aren't productive, so they meet the same fate. Likewise, physical education programs are rolled back right and left. Our bias favors carefully structured, efficient, purposeful repetitive movement. This creates a self-actuating dynamic that selects as leaders and role models those who are the least capable of functional musculoskeletal movement.

Jeannie and Johnny are not at home in the more independent zone of individual action and discovery. That zone is actually a bit frightening and frustrating. For security and self-esteem, they circle the wagons—that is, they circle the adults and adult-sanctioned activities.

They're the "good" kids. What about the "bad" ones? Another response to musculoskeletal system dysfunction at this stage is almost the polar opposite behavior. Unable to smoothly interact with the world in a series of increasingly successful and satisfying experiences, a child becomes cranky, angry, unfocused, and aggressive. She's a little monster. He's a brat. Neither of these patterns of behavior reflects the child's personality or even an illness. They reflect a response to musculoskeletal system dysfunction.

Ode to Disorder

Let's consider the "good girl" some more. Do we really want to change her and then have to put up with more unruly behavior?

That's a tough one, especially since by being "good," the child is making life a lot easier for her parents and other caregivers. But I say yes, because the price of saying no is much too high. I say yes also because the alternative to the "good girl" is not a "bad girl" but rather a better girl. Better in the sense of wellness, better in the sense of being more capable and self-assured.

Middle childhood is a time when disorder should take place, to allow order to appear in adolescence and young adulthood. Order and structure—both physical and emotional—are products of complicated interactions that must be allowed to occur and that cannot be brushed aside or wished away in the interest of child management or "early learning." Children five to eight years old hate structure, as well they should. And adults should love them for it. The "good girl" or "good boy," who seems to be the exception, may in fact be the exception. But chances are, they are dysfunctional children from a musculoskeletal system standpoint. Consolidation has won out over exploration. That doesn't mean that all is lost. Correcting musculoskeletal

Best Behavior

A bolder, action-oriented child is not by definition a problem child as long as we are willing to accommodate her thirst for motion and stimulation with a genuine need to impart social skills and higher learning. These objectives are not mutually exclusive, but modern, technologically dominated societies tend to reconcile them poorly.

"Childishness," as in "full of energy, unpredictability, activity, and spontaneity," is out of place in a world run for machines and by machines.

system dysfunction in middle childhood is relatively easy. And no trade-off is involved between mind and body. In fact, the opposite is true: a functional musculoskeletal system gives the child the power she needs to build intellectual and emotional strength.

Rethinking the Hyperactive Child

The first step that parents should take is to recognize the signs of musculoskeletal system dysfunction in the child. But one thing, I must emphasize, is *not* a symptom of any ailment, disorder, or disease, and that is hyperactivity. I object to this term and the way it's commonly misused and misunderstood. Children from five to twelve years old are supposed to be hyperactive. They are intended to be nearly nonstop motion machines.

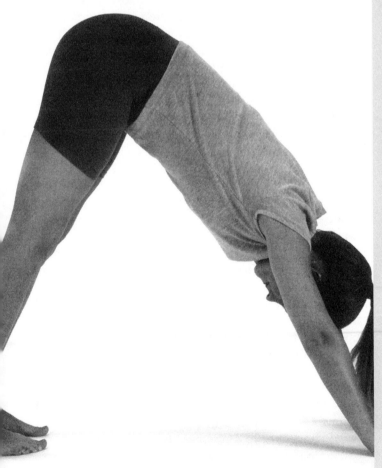

Troi's Story

When Troi was five years old, she spent much of her free time baby-sitting her grandfather. Technically she was the baby and he was the sitter, but it was really the other way around because he was frail and ill. Instead of being outside running and playing, Troi stayed close by so Granddad could watch her from his armchair. Troi learned to play quietly without disturbing him. She was a good, "grown-up" little girl.

Much of Troi's motion-driven physical development took place slowly. Predictably, she went into her teenage years lacking overall strength and structural stability. At age fourteen, while playing tennis, she tore the anterior cruciate ligament (ACL) in her left knee. Her knee joint would pop out without warning. I could tell by looking at the

In the course of a couple generations, we've gone from knowing and accepting that children "can't sit still" and conducting our lives and theirs accordingly, to believing that children who "can't sit still" are sick. As the American lifestyle has grown increasingly restricted in motion, our intolerance for active children has become even more pronounced. Our homes, backyards, play areas, streets, and schools are unwelcoming to active children. In many places the woods, fields, and open lots are gone. Safe bicycling is impossible because of traffic. Even city streets and alleys that once shared commercial activities with jump rope and hopscotch are off-limits.

A friend recently told me that he was driving through a residential neighborhood in the Washington, D.C., suburbs when a boy and a girl about nine or ten years old dashed out of a backyard, madly chasing each other around the house. At first he wondered if something was wrong—why else would they run like that? He pulled over and watched, and then he realized that they were just playing and having a ball moving.

That's how unfamiliar kids in motion have become to us. When we see it, we're startled. Something must be wrong. As a result, the contemporary definition of *hyperactivity* amounts to "any activity that isn't structured." Every neighborhood used to have a grumpy man or woman who wasn't used to kids. They'd complain to your parents or turn the dogs loose. Now we are all grumpy. Children are supposed to sit still and behave themselves. When they don't, we take them to the doctor and drug them.

As many as two million elementary school children in the United States are believed to have attention deficit disorder (ADD) or attention deficit hyperactivity disorder (ADHD), and in the 1990s the number of those receiving Ritalin, amphetamines, and antidepressants almost doubled. Two million is roughly 3 to 5 percent of all elementary school children, but in some parts of the country, the ADD and ADHD rate is anywhere from 8 to 17 percent. No other country has numbers that are remotely comparable to these, and according to news reports, 85 percent of the worldwide production of drugs prescribed for ADD and ADHD is consumed in the United States.

As disturbing is a study released in the winter of

2000 that found that the number of preschoolers ages 2 to 4 taking such drugs doubled and possibly tripled from 1991 to 1995. Bear in mind, none of these drugs, including the powerful antidepressant Prozac, have been approved for children under the age of 6. The study, published in the *Journal of the American Medical Association*, analyzed data from three major health systems located in the Mid-Atlantic, the Midwest, and the Pacific Northwest, and concluded that the figures represent a national trend.

A national trend? 1.5 percent of all children between the ages of 2 and 4 being administered stimulants, antidepressants, or antipsychotic drugs—a group that includes major tranquilizers like Thorazine? In reporting the story, the *Washington Post* quoted Mark A. Stein of the Children's National Medical Center as saying that children are being treated for ADD and ADHD at a younger age than in the past. A few years ago they typically began taking stimulants at age seven or eight. Now doctors often start them on Ritalin at five or six. "As we hurry kids along and put more expectations on them, they're going to display more symptoms of ADD/ADHD and I think there is a tendency to treat them younger," Stein concludes.

Dr. Joseph T. Coyle of the Harvard Medical School criticizes the practice and points out that this age "is a time of extraordinary, unprecedented change in the brain." Indeed it is. By about the age of seven, approximately 90 percent of the adult brain structure has formed. To jump into the middle of a process where hundreds if not thousands of complex, intertwined organic changes are taking place on a daily basis is irresponsibility of the worst sort. As an anatomical functionalist, I have long been alarmed by the use of powerful drugs to treat chronic musculoskeletal system pain. But pain mitigation among adults who are knowledgeable about the side effects and consequences is almost understandable, compared with blindly tampering with a child's brain in the interest of making her behave "properly."

ADD/ADHD are real conditions affecting real people, children and adults alike. There is evidence of a genetic link and indications that nutrition plays a role. But it's difficult to believe that anything close to 3 to 5 percent of the elementary school–age population suffers

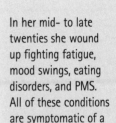

In her mid- to late twenties she wound up fighting fatigue, mood swings, eating disorders, and PMS. All of these conditions are symptomatic of a compromised metabolic process.

But that's now history. Today Troi does a daily routine of E-cises that maintain her strength and musculoskeletal system functions that were restored by a prior series of E-cise menus that I developed for her after we were married in 1990.

She lifts weights, runs, and practices Ashtanga yoga. She has boundless energy and feels great.

from such disorders. ADD/ADHD–like symptoms, yes; ADD/ADHD, no. Hyperactivity, inattention, and impulsiveness are symptoms of childhood. Even so, our preferred definition of childhood has changed radically. We don't want our kids wasting their precious time (and ours) by moving around. Parents who feel frustrated by an unruly child and are genuinely concerned that the youngster is losing ground educationally and socially need to take a hard look at these so-called symptoms and ask questions. Among them:

1. How much energetic free play does the child get each day?
2. If left to choose his activities, does he run, jump, climb, crawl?
3. Does he sleep through the night?
4. Does he get enough sleep?
5. Does his hyperactivity follow sedentary periods?
6. Do his focus and attention span improve after a period of energetic activity?
7. Are you feeding him a diet high in salt, sugar, nitrates, caffeine, dyes, and other chemicals?
8. How many hours of TV does he watch each day?

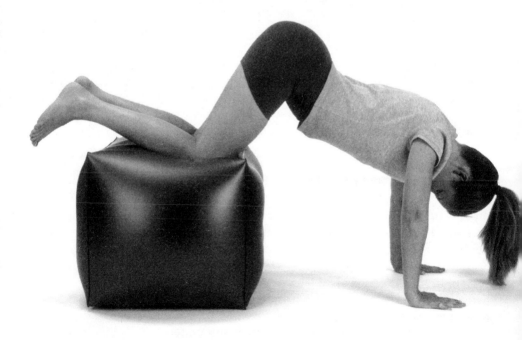

9. How structured are his routine and his environment?

10. As a parent, how much time do you spend with him in energetic, unstructured play and interaction?

This line of inquiry has two purposes. The first is to determine whether the child is just trying to blow off steam and behave like a normal, active, and functional six- to twelve-year-old in a modern motionless world. The second is to find out if the symptoms are caused by musculoskeletal system dysfunction rather than a disorder that requires drug therapy.

I have to admit that there is a downside to functional children. They are a handful, two hands full. The world is their playground. The upside, however, is that they are healthy, strong, and smart. Pam's son Tony is a good example. In early childhood, Tony was an Olympic crawler—his parents gave him plenty of room and encouragement to explore, and they never put him in hard-soled baby shoes or confined him to a playpen. Today Tony is larger, stronger, and more energetic than many of his peers and has more developed motor skills and finer eye-hand coordination.

Even so, when Tony was getting ready for kindergarten his preschool teachers suggested that he might be a little too rambunctious and that his parents might consider drugs to settle him down. In addition, Pam and her husband were told that Tony would not be moving into kindergarten because California, where they reside, has a new law requiring children to learn to read by the end of kindergarten. Few four- to five-year-olds are ready, in terms of their mental development, to be taught to read; that's why reading traditionally isn't taught until first grade. The solution for Tony, and for most other California children his age, is a classic in bureaucratic double-think. Hold them out of kindergarten until they've matured to the level of a first-grader. Then presto! Kids can read by the end of kindergarten!

Meanwhile, Tony, who is ready for kindergarten activities like drawing, being read to, and playing games, is expected to twiddle his thumbs in preschool for another year. He's not the thumb-twiddling kind, and I predict that the pressure on his parents will grow to "do something" about his overly energetic behavior.

What needs to be done is educational reform. We

cannot wave a wand and decree that six-, five-, four-, and three-year-olds from now on will read just because it will make state bureaucrats and politicians look good. While it may seem desirable to accelerate learning, there are physical limitations that cannot be transcended without severe consequences. In many cases—if not most—we simply cannot overcome the lack of brain-structure development. Where it can be surmounted, the unfortunate child is being force-fed instruction at the expense of his physical development, which is more than likely to result in the suggestion that his parents might want to "do something about his behavior." We have two extremes: a functional child may be too active, while the dysfunctional child is too inactive—or depressed, aggressive, or ill. We are designing a catch-22 for our children. If they act like they're healthy, they must be sick and in need of drugs, because to keep healthy children from acting like they're sick, drugs are needed.

The list of questions on pages 88–89 is designed to help parents break out of this nightmarish circular logic. If a child is "hyperactive" because he is functional and normally energetic, he does not need drugs, because the result will be a drugged-out dysfunctional child with another set of symptoms. His learning ability may seem to improve in the short term, but at a price. Musculoskeletal system dysfunction will surely follow because the drugs push the child over the edge into a sedentary behavior pattern that cannot build or maintain proper functions. Next we will have the clumsy child, the accident-prone child, and the moody, angry, or violent child. All are symptoms—not of a disease but of motion starvation.

You may have noticed that during this discussion of ADD/ADHD, I've used the pronoun *he*. That's because boys are said to be more affected by ADD/ADHD. The explanation for this comes in two parts. By the time children hit middle childhood, social patterns of gender differentiation have shaped the behavior of boys and girls in ways that favor boys in terms of building and maintaining musculoskeletal system function. At about six years old, boys can throw a ball better than girls, while girls have superior eye-hand coordination for activities like drawing. But the difference probably has nothing to do with chromosomes. Like it or not, girls still play with dolls and boys play at being G.I. Joe. The toys and games we give our children have subtle and not-so-subtle gender-specific influences. Many of us parent differently based on the child's gender. The disparities may not be as great as they once were, but they exist nonetheless. It's just enough to have a physiological effect.

Boys are diagnosed with ADD/ADHD more often because these functions have kicked in sooner than in most girls and at a time when formal schooling is getting under way. Boys are ready to rumble and run when they are supposed to be reading. Boys' dysfunctional behavior may also be driven by incomplete functions that enable them to "act out" and get into trouble, whereas girls seem more well behaved.

Seem. That brings me to the second part of the explanation: girls have different symptoms. (Boys have them too, but they're hidden behind the larger ADD/ADHD cluster, or ignored.) *She* may be crabby or depressed. The mood swings that start to show up in girls in late middle childhood and early adolescence are the equivalent of ADD/ADHD symptoms in boys. At about twelve years old, many girls begin to lose confidence in themselves, and their schoolwork starts to suffer.

After spending the years from five to twelve concentrating on adult-sanctioned consolidation rather than exploration, a dysfunctional child inevitably begins hurting. It comes out as either emotional or physical pain. As with ADD/ADHD, in an effort to understand what's happening, the problems are defined as diseases and disorders that require drastic remedies, when in fact the child's body is simply crying out for adequate motion and movement.

Free Play

Take another look at the list of questions on pages 88–89. The answer to Question 1 is a key indicator. If the child gets less than ninety minutes a day of energetic *free play*, then there's not much chance that his musculoskeletal system will remain functional. With ninety minutes or more—preferably more, and with the activity broken into morning, afternoon, and evening segments—children, even those who didn't get enough crawling time as infants and toddlers, can develop and maintain full musculoskeletal system function. But free play means free play. Ninety minutes of Little League batting practice or kicking a soccer ball is not free play. It is structured, restricted, and repetitive play. With a little encouragement (and it's amazing how little), young children will gravitate from passive, structured, adult-mandated play that feeds their dysfunctions to free, active play that revs up their functions. A functional child will also tend to choose more physically vigorous play (see Question 2).

As for Questions 3 and 4, if a child is sleeping poorly, I favor the most basic explanation: she's not tired. Without sufficient energetic activity, a child isn't physically ready for bed, no matter what the clock says. When the alarm goes off the next morning, she'll get up stressed and unprepared for the day. Is it surprising that she's unfocused and inattentive at school? Crabby? Depressed?

Let's look at Questions 5 and 6: Does his hyperactivity follow sedentary periods? Do his focus and attention span improve after a period of energetic activity? If the answer is yes, common sense suggests that a disease that gets worse after rest and improves after stress is not following the normal pathological sequence. Most diseases unfold in stages. What's happening here is that hyperactivity ebbs and flows in direct response to the stimulation provided by the environment: low stimulation–high activity, high stimulation–lower activity. Why should it surprise us that a child wants to move after he's been forced to sit still? Likewise, if the child settles down after discharging his excess energy, it's quite a stretch to continue believing that that was just a fluky coincidence.

Question 7—Are you feeding him a diet high in salt, sugar, nitrates, caffeine, dyes, and other chemicals?— was prompted by a conversation my collaborator Roger Gittines had with Karen Harris, a veteran first-grade teacher in Prince William County, Virginia, a suburb of Washington, D.C. She said it's appalling what the children bring to school for lunch. "There's practically no fruit or whole food. My mother used to give me a sandwich and an apple. Today, it's packaged snacks and prepared quick meals loaded with salt, sugar, and nitrates. They're crazed after they eat." How sad it is. We drug these kids with junk food so they are bouncing off the walls, and then we hit them with psychotropics and depressants to bring them back down again.

As for Question 8, about TV watching, I'd like to observe here that in middle childhood the average child watches about four hours of TV a day. Where does that time come from? Sleeping? No. Eating? No. School? No, again. Sitting passively in front of the tube comes at the expense of active play. In one week, it totals up to a loss of twenty-eight hours—more than one full day. Keep figuring. That means more than sixty days a year or about eight and a half weeks of lost playtime—more than an entire summer vacation from school.

Questions 9 and 10—How structured are his routine and his environment? As a parent, how much time do you spend with him in energetic, unstructured play and interaction?—address the core of the issue. Almost every ADD/ADHD–diagnosed child shares the same sedentary environment. What motion exists is restricted and repetitive. You don't need experts to verify this fact. Just take stock of how much free play you personally enjoy with your child. If it's minimal—and it is for most parents—there's not much likelihood that your child is going to get it from other sources.

Fig. 6-1

Between television time, computer time, reading time, and travel time (sitting in a car), the average child winds up with next to no time for the kind of pure, unstructured, spontaneous movement she depends on to build and maintain her musculoskeletal system functions (and brain functions). Television and computers are particularly insidious because they provide an illusion of stimulation—a sense of going someplace and doing something—and can become addicting substitutes for actual motion. This trick of technology robs children of their innate appetite for motion and sets them up for a lifetime of chronic pain, poor health, and unhappiness.

A Symptom Summary

Now that we've ruled out hyperactivity as a disorder, let's take a look at some of the actual symptoms of musculoskeletal dysfunction that may appear in middle childhood.

Start with this set of illustrations. Each child depicted is presenting different physical symptoms of musculoskeletal system dysfunction. All of them are extremely common. In Figure 6–1 the child's feet are toed out. In Figure 6–2 her shoulders are

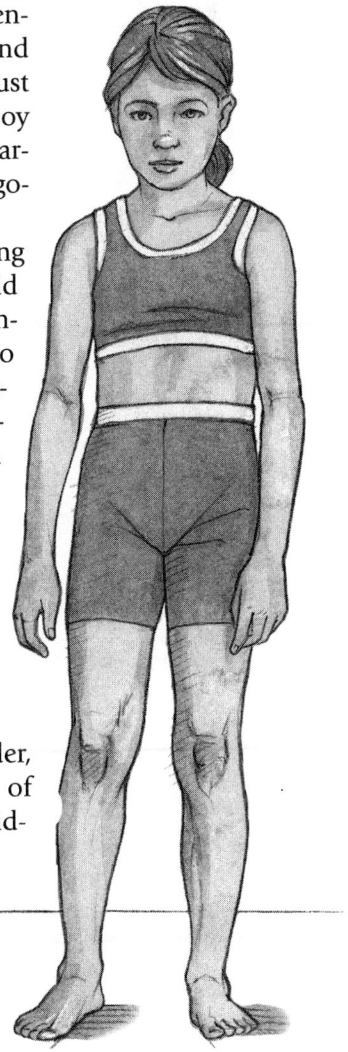

Fig. 6-2

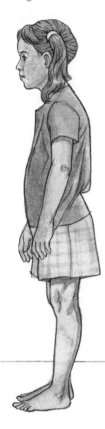

rounded and her head is forward. In Figure 6–3, this girl has lost the S-curve of her spine, and her hips are folded under. And the boy in Figure 6–4 has misaligned shoulders and hips.

Any of these symptoms can be accompanied by one or more of the following symptoms:

▶ **Joint and/or nerve pain.** Chronic musculoskeletal pain is not "normal" in children. Bad backs, knees, wrists, and such should not be regarded as routine occurrences. Likewise, nerve pain tells us that dysfunctions are at work—not heredity, accidents, or just "one of those things." However, mild muscle pain, when it follows strenuous activities, is usually a sign that strengthening is under way, and despite TV ads for over-the-counter painkillers, the best treatment is no treatment. This applies no matter how strenuous the activity level. If Brenda's knees hurt, it's not because she pounds them on the

Fig. 6-3

Fig. 6-4

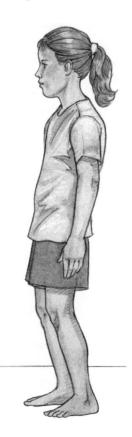

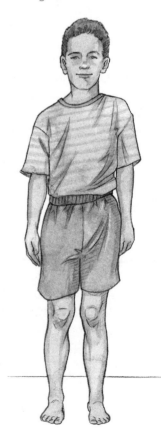

basketball court. That's not the problem. Joint pain and injuries, as well as pulled muscles and persistent muscle and nerve pain, are symptomatic of dysfunction.

▶ **Muscle cramps.** Occasional muscle cramps are usually nothing more than a reflection of the rapid growth process that's under way in middle childhood. Frequent and prolonged muscle cramps indicate musculoskeletal misalignment and the metabolic system's inability to handle the demand that's being put on it.

▶ **Headaches and/or stiff neck.** Both conditions are often associated with the shoulders, neck, and head being rounded forward to the point that the neck muscles are thrown into contraction (a classic computer posture), and thus blood and oxygen flow are restricted.

▶ **Lethargy.** High energy is a natural childhood attribute. Its absence should set off alarm bells.

▶ **A preference for repetitive activities.** In middle childhood kids are activity "shoppers." Their curiosity, creativity, and energy drive them to try a little of this and a little of that. A preference for repetitive activities indicates that adult-style consolidation has taken hold.

▶ **Inattention.** The child's ability to focus her attention should gradually increase through middle childhood. If progress stops or doesn't move past the levels achieved in early childhood, musculoskeletal system dysfunction may be impeding her physical and mental development. There's a direct link between active muscles and an active mind.

▶ **Hyperactivity.** In a varied, motion-rich environment, the stimuli will produce energetic highs broken by calming plateaus. If the child's go-go pace never seems to vary, it may mean he is not capable of reacting to anything but self-generated stimuli.

▶ **Aggressiveness and anger.** Insecurity, fear, frustration, and low self-esteem are by-products of musculoskeletal system dysfunction. Our vehicle for interacting with the world is the musculoskeletal system. If it is faltering, we know it and fear the consequences. There are also metabolic and neurological penalties; children build mental capacity as they move.

▶ **Sleep disorders.** Generally speaking, the human body has a simple reaction to physical fatigue—it sleeps. A disengaged musculoskeletal system does not tire as readily as one that is fully engaged. Too much time spent sleeping, on the other hand, could be a product of extreme stress on a dysfunctional system or the child's fear that she can't handle normal stimulus.

▶ **Poor appetite, digestion, and elimination.** Without the support of an engaged, fully functional musculoskeletal system, the body's metabolic activity declines. Digestion needs a lot of energy production to work effectively.

▶ **Obesity.** A child who does not move much but eats as if he did accumulates excess calories stored as fat. Dysfunctional children also use food to provide the stimulation that a motionless environment does not provide.

▶ **Pronounced and frequent mood swings.** Mood swings may result when the metabolism has been thrown off-kilter. But physical activity produces biochemical compounds in the brain that calm and tranquilize. The less major muscle work a child performs, the fewer biochemical tranquilizers she is producing.

▶ **Accident proneness.** Motor control and eye-hand coordination suffer when the body is misaligned and major functions are disengaged. Balance is also disrupted.

▶ **Allergies and asthma.** The body has systems for neutralizing and filtering out undesirable substances that are inhaled or otherwise ingested. These filters depend on an energy source— metabolism—to stay fired up and operational. But here again musculoskeletal dysfunction draws down metabolic efficiency. Asthma and allergies are different conditions, but they tend to occur in tandem, which leads some researchers to conclude that air pollution, or food-borne or water-borne substances, are to blame. I regard asthma as primarily a symptom of musculoskeletal dysfunction. It's the result of a triple whammy: lung capacity, which is directly tied to the musculoskeletal system, is reduced; lack of oxygen crimps the metabolic rate; and the immune system (part of the body's filtering mechanism) is underpowered and erratic due to the loss of metabolic horsepower, so it forfeits the ability to effectively dispose of unwelcome particles (when allergies trigger asthmatic attacks). In effect, the immune system overreacts by releasing too many chemicals that dilate blood vessels and constrict the bronchial tubes. Absent allergies, an asthmatic attack is brought on by muscle contractions and other physiological responses to oxygen starvation, which becomes acute when an extra stimulus occurs, like excitement, emotional stress, or strenuous activities.

There's one more symptom that doesn't fit on the list. I call it "the straight-ahead kid." Watch good little Jeannie and Johnny. Most of the time they will walk and move in a straight line like adults. Grown-ups have things to do and places to go, so we travel efficiently from point A to point B. Children who are fully functional take on the world like broken field runners—they're all over the place, in reaction to 360 degrees of stimulus. But as they lose function, children settle into a straight-ahead track. Unable to move smoothly to the right and left or to reverse field, they focus on what's in front of them. The straight-ahead kid is growing up and out of her functions.

Reinventing the Imagination

I've outlined quite a problem, so you're probably ready for some specific solutions. In subsequent chapters I'll offer extensive menus of E-cises to remedy musculoskeletal system dysfunction in adults. But like infants and toddlers, children in middle childhood are still too young to be put through a regimen of structured exercises.

They hate them. Even ten- to twelve-year-olds who seem to take to sports drills and workout programs are probably doing it more to please their parents and other adult authority figures than because they enjoy them. If the children are functional, that's okay, as long as they continue to stay functional by getting enough varied, unstructured movement as well. But dysfunctional older children are engaged in a consolidation process at the expense of exploration that can build and maintain overall musculoskeletal system function.

This age group, however, isn't too old for games that are crossed with E-cises. Try some from the menu you'll find in the Appendix.

But in the absence of a motion-rich environment, such hybrid games are only a partial solution. Therefore we must be creative and courageous: turn off the TV and the PC. For older children, going cold turkey won't work. You'll have to wean them by cutting back gradually. Not only are they habituated to TV and the computer, their musculoskeletal system dysfunctions are of longer duration and will be harder to restore.

This creative and courageous act is designed to foster creativity and courage in your children. It will jumpstart exploration again and rectify the consolidation imbalance, because without these two entertainment and learning mainstays, the child will be thrown back on her own imaginative resources. An imaginative mind and an active body work together. The idea is to get the child to play again for the sake of playing—for the sheer joy of moving.

I remember being thunderstruck by a conversation I had with Billy and Eric, two brothers, ages eight and ten, who came to the clinic with their parents. I asked them what they liked to do for fun. They told me all about their great computer games. I asked if they ever played hide-and-seek.

"Hide and what?"

Billy and Eric didn't know what I was talking about. I explained. Billy looked at me like I was nuts. "What's the point?" he asked. I could have been talking to a thirty-year-old. Like a modern adult, this child was outcome-oriented. Eric was more intrigued with the possibilities of hide-and-seek. The beauty of this ancient game is that it has no point or outcome, other than what the children imagine it to be. They can hide from a monster, outsmart an enemy, play a joke on a friend, become invisible, find a missing person, and so on. In the process they're dashing around, clambering under bushes, and climbing trees. And who knows, the hide-and-seek game may one day yield a cure for cancer or another breakthrough in the incredible collaboration between body and mind.

The human imagination is in service to the body. The human body is in service to the imagination.

When you turn the TV and PC off, don't fill the available time with structured activities like music lessons and team sports. Throw the child back on his own resources. He'll grouse and sulk, but after a while he'll take the initiative and fill in the blank spots with his own inventions. What will probably kick things off is reading. To kill time, a child accustomed to inactivity will turn to books. I love books, and I'm not knocking reading. Books are the most *active* sedentary medium ever devised. Words on the page have the magic power to engage the imagination *and* to inspire action. Books have sparked exploration, conquest, invention, travel, love, faith, and all manner of human greatness and folly.

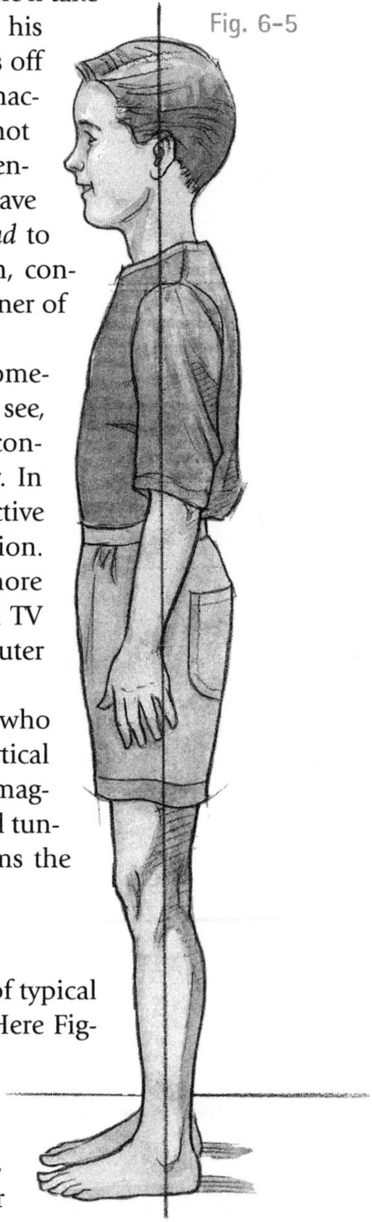

Fired by imagination, a child who draws something, builds something, or goes afield to see, touch, and taste something is exploring *and* consolidating. The mind and body grow together. In due course the TV and PC will lose their addictive power. The child won't need them for stimulation. The world will be providing stimulation of a more satisfying kind. Sure, they'll continue to watch TV from time to time, and they'll use the computer more skillfully than their dysfunctional peers.

More skillfully? You bet. A computer weasel who is functional has better concentration, analytical skills, endurance, eye-hand coordination, and imagination, and she doesn't come down with carpal tunnel syndrome. Being fully functional transforms the computer weasel into a computer athlete.

What You'll See Is What You'll Get

In Figures 6–1 to 6–4, I showed you examples of typical dysfunctional postures in middle childhood. Here Figure 6–5 shows you what to look for as your child moves toward regaining his musculoskeletal legacy. Compare it to the earlier drawings. Note the position of the heads, shoulders, hips, and knees. In addition, as your

Fig. 6-5

child progresses, look for three key indicators to confirm that function is returning and strengthening.

1. Sleep patterns will change for the better. You won't have as much trouble getting her to go to bed or rousting her in the morning. The reason is that the engagement of major muscle groups has caused an uptick in the metabolic rate. She is producing and burning more energy, which means that come bedtime, she's ready to sleep.

2. Spontaneous patterns of learning will emerge. A child who has been relatively oblivious to his surroundings will suddenly start taking an interest. His curiosity and thirst for knowledge will switch on. How dinner is prepared, for example, or how a car works, will suddenly become important issues. Like a three-year-old asking why, why, why, the five- to twelve-year-old is rolling back to an earlier developmental phase to fill in the gaps that were caused by dysfunction.

3. The child will become more physically engaged and active, running up and down stairs, skipping, and jumping around, where she once tended to plod straight ahead. Her moods will level off, without the down periods and the crankiness.

These changes won't happen overnight. But making the effort to reengage a child's musculoskeletal system functions will pay off big-time. Our kids can live in prosperity and good health in the twenty-first century if we have the courage and creativity to help them rediscover the power of a cutting-edge technology that's three million years old.

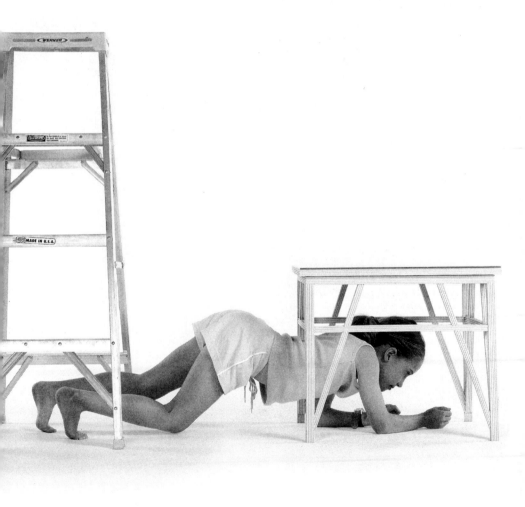

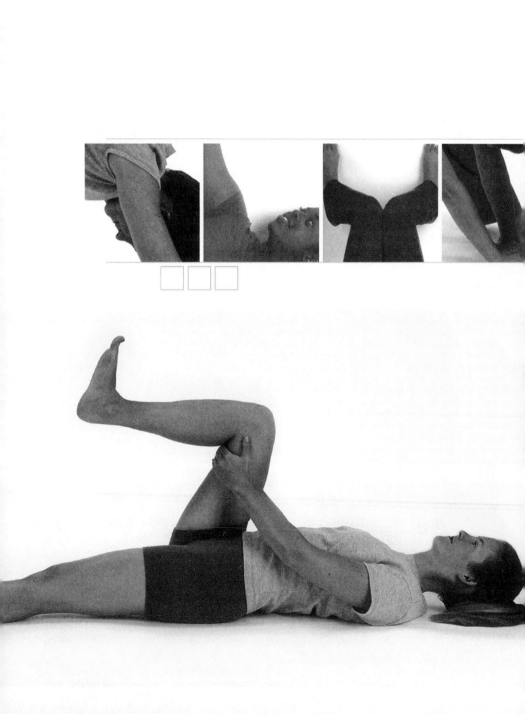

CHAPTER 7

she was just umpteen, *if you know what I mean*

Let's consider the typical teenager, from a musculoskeletal system standpoint. In other words, a teenager who is typically dysfunctional. I rarely see a functional adolescent these days, so that when I do, I often ask them what they're doing differently from their peers.

These functional kids—the ones who have good posture—tend not to be dedicated, hardcore athletes. Some of them are, but most aren't, particularly the boys. They'll play a sport or sports, usually more than one, but they're not consumed by a particular game and its discipline. They have time for a wide variety of other activities.

With functional girls these days, the main difference from boys is that many are athletes, although participation in sports doesn't guarantee function. Title IX, the federal statute that requires equal spending on and access to sports programs in schools for both sexes, has generated unprecedented female athletic involvement, and it has had positive effects on female musculoskeletal function. Participation in sports is now a full-fledged option for girls, whereas it wasn't for their mothers and grandmothers.

Whether these functional teens are athletes or nonathletes, boy or girls, I find that they balance their intellectual pursuits and physical activities, and they're successful in both worlds. By not choosing one at the expense of the other, they've mastered both. They're brimming with energy and self-confidence. I hardly ever detect the sullenness, anger, and alienation that are the signature characteristics of many modern teenagers. Their parents and teachers confirm that these teens control their emotions better and are more independent and well adjusted than their peers. This observation supports my belief that success in life rests on a bedrock of self-confidence achieved through physical accomplishments that set the stage for intellectual development.

Fig. 7-1

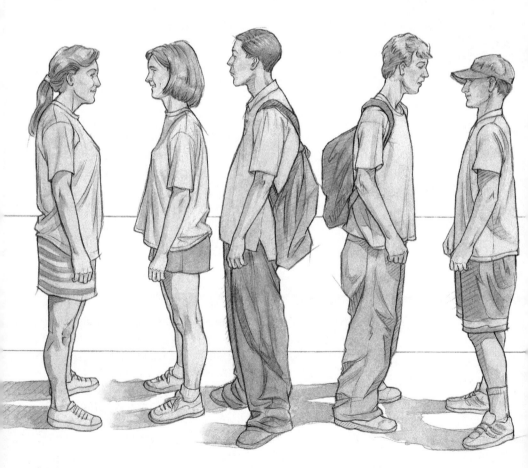

These functional teens aren't freaks. Like their peers, they watch TV, play computer games, and hang out at the mall. Sometimes they have a bad day. The difference is in degree: their TV time tends to last about an hour a day; they can take or leave computer games and Internet chat rooms; and hanging out at the mall is not a daily ritual. Moodiness never lasts very long, since too much other stuff attracts their curiosity and interest.

It sounds too good to be true, I know. But when it comes to teenagers, many "typical" patterns of behavior—alienation, anger, lack of purpose, and the like—are often actually symptoms generated by musculoskeletal system dysfunction.

Picture Imperfect

Let's look at the evidence. The teens in Figure 7–1 are drawn from snapshots that I've taken at San Diego–area high schools in recent years. As far as I'm concerned, this display confirms comedian Flip Wilson's great line: "What you see is what you get."

What we're seeing and getting here are learning disorders, eating disorders, antisocial attitudes, depression, lack of self-esteem, drug and alcohol abuse, rebelliousness, and premature sexual activity. We are also seeing children who are in pain. When I examine head position alone, I can understand why a million school days a year are lost because of headaches. Our teens' musculoskeletal system structures are so misaligned and weak that many of them can't hold their heads up enough to maintain adequate blood and oxygen flow.

They look unhappy—and they are.

They look uncomfortable—and they are.

They look fearful—and they are.

They look ill—and they are.

Here's why. The primary posture of dysfunction among teenagers is that of flexion. Their hips, backs, shoulders, necks, and heads are rolled forward and down. Notice that with their arms at their sides, the backs of their hands face forward. In a functional person, both thumbs will face forward as the palms face the thighs. Today's teenagers' bodies have been shaped and molded by school chairs, family-room sofas, and car seats. Their tools, toys, and control devices are arrayed waist-high. All they do is bend at the hips and reach out—again and again. They are the *embodiment* of their environment.

More than twelve years of restricted, repetitive movement takes a toll physically, mentally, and emotionally. And now, the teenager must contend with rapid growth, burgeoning responsibilities, higher expectations, the quest for an independent identity, and a flood tide of hormones. It makes for tough going, very tough.

Fig. 7-2

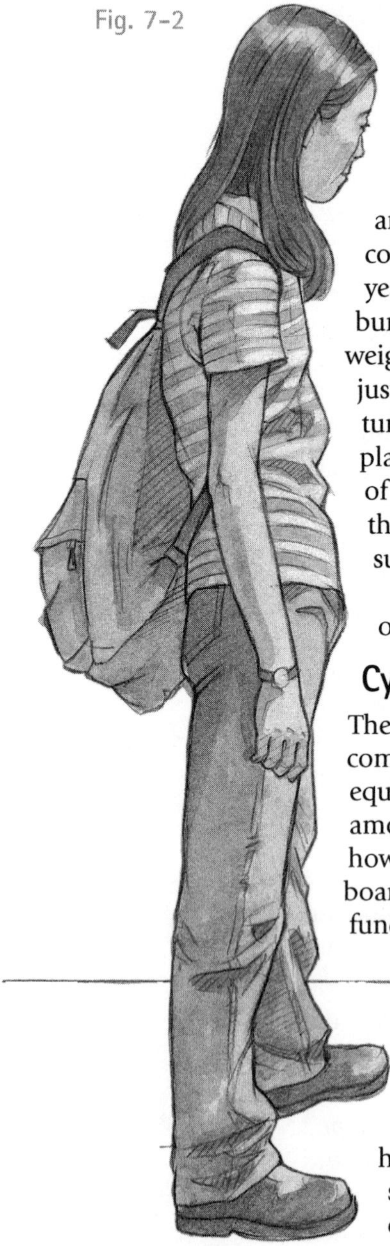

Let's consider the least of their worries first: books and backpacks. When I read newspaper and magazine articles about the terrible burden that young children and teenagers must endure as they trudge to and from school under the weight of backpacks bulging with books and laptop computers, I chuckle. Under normal conditions the human spine at twelve or thirteen years old has the structural integrity to bear the burden of several pounds of dead weight (and live weight) without undue stress or damage. But as I just mentioned, flexion is the typical teenage posture. Now that the chair-hugging C-curve has replaced the classic spinal S-curve, the body's center of gravity descends through the lower portion of the thoracic back, bypassing the hips, which are supposed to be carrying the weight.

Figure 7-2 gives you an idea of what's going on. The backpack isn't the problem; the back is.

Cyberpain

The same posture is also brought to the personal computer, which has become standard academic equipment, not a luxury but a necessity, particularly among middle-class and affluent students. Here's how the posture looks seated at a computer keyboard (Figure 7-3). This time the spine's dysfunctional C-curve isn't being weighed down by "heavy" books; instead, heavy hands, wrists, and arms are the culprits.

Heavy? Very.

When the back and its grid of supporting load-bearing joints are out of alignment and stressed by friction and limitation, then hands, wrists, and arms are burdens. In this position the tendons of the wrist and forearm drag, the elbows and shoulders lose their

Fig. 7-3

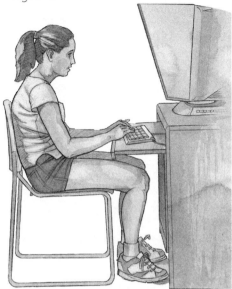

Fig. 7-4

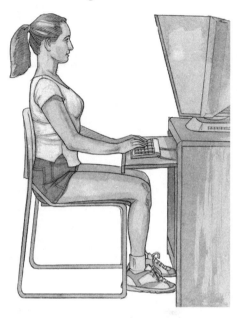

smoothly working kinetic linkage, and the peripheral muscles take over most of the work. And it's a lot of work—it takes tens of thousands of individual muscular contractions to type a term paper or chat on the Internet. But these movements don't seem like work, so the fatigue and the pain get blamed on the PC's design.

As long as these dysfunctional postures persist, no amount of ergonomic tinkering—not a foot mouse, not voice recognition, not robotics, back braces, wrist supports, or eye-movement-detection devices—will cure the typical teenager of her typical pain symptoms. Furthermore, as the PC supplants the three-ring binder and the pencil box in every schoolroom in the land, they'll occur earlier and earlier. The real cure—the only cure—is to restore the body's structural integrity (Figure 7-4).

Kids instinctively know when something is wrong with their bodies. I believe that's the reason baggy, loose-fitting clothing has stayed in fashion for so long. Kids are hiding and camouflaging their otherwise-visible dysfunctions.

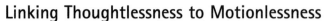

Linking Thoughtlessness to Motionlessness

Parents often tell me that their teenage boy or girl is "fifteen going on twenty-five." While that may be the case in terms of the pressure to grow up quickly, I think they've got the timeline wrong. Many teenagers are fifteen going on five or six. Their brain and body structures remain incompletely developed well past the chronological point when certain motor skills, behavioral norms, and cognitive abilities were once expected to emerge.

Having been deprived of adequate motion in middle childhood, the teenager loses out on the physical and mental growth opportunities that come in response to the stimulation that motion provides. In its initial form, an action (or reaction) is a thought: *I act, therefore I am.* The ball rolls into a busy street, and little Jeannie chases after it. It doesn't matter that the act is dangerous and downright stupid. Thinking about acting comes later in the development cycle (as does thinking *instead* of acting).

Eventually, given enough direct, hands-on experience, thought spins off from action and becomes a separate entity. In effect, thanks to the burgeoning brain's ability to store memories and access them, thought emerges as a substitute for action. Jeannie can anticipate the consequences before she acts. This leads to pattern recognition, organized internalized action, and a budding system of abstract thinking.

This extremely complex process is not fully understood, but structural changes in the brain most likely precede the separation of thought from action and make their coexistence possible. These changes, however, don't occur as a matter of course. Something must happen to make them happen.

And what might that be? I believe it's our old friend motion. My take is that roughly half of all teenagers—those who account for the most extreme forms of antisocial and self-destructive behavior, such as excessive risk taking, drug and alcohol abuse, depression, suicide, violence, classroom disruption, and sexual promiscuity—do not possess age-appropriate concrete operational thinking ability, another concept formulated by child psychologist Jean Piaget. They haven't moved from "action is thought" to "thought is action" because musculoskeletal system dysfunction has impeded their ability to take a wide variety of actions in response to a wide variety of stimulation. Their memory bank is not up and running.

As a result, these kids arrive at adolescence looking like teens but thinking—and controlling their emotions—like much younger children. They are extremely narcissistic, easily frustrated, prone to anger and impulsiveness, easily bored, and isolated. They do what any five- or six-year-old would do: they act without thinking about the consequences.

Now, all teenagers—good, bad, and in between—test the limits, cross the line, and get into trouble. Exploration and consolidation (more Piaget) are still under way. But I'm convinced that the most successful teens are those who have had the full benefit of motion-driven physiological and neurological development.

The Unhappy Camper

Musculoskeletal system dysfunction makes adolescence, difficult under the best of circumstances, even more painful and disruptive. That was the situation for sixteen-year-old Steve, whose father enrolled him in the Egoscue Method Clinic's annual summer athletic day camp eight or nine years ago.

"His mother and I are desperate," Steve's dad told me over the phone. "We can't do anything with him. He's totally uncooperative, uncommunicative, and unruly. He's running with the wrong crowd, and we think he may be dabbling in drugs." Day camp was just getting under way, and the man begged me to take Steve, who was a high school sophomore.

"Sounds like we'll have to chain him to a goal post," I said. The dad promised that he would personally deliver the boy each day and make it clear that going AWOL was not an option.

Steve arrived the next day. Our athletic camp is world-famous for mixing top professional and amateur athletes with promising high school and college players. Young and old, men and women, they come from all sports backgrounds. The common denominator is a desire to improve their performance or to augment mainstream medical therapy for an injury with an intensive twenty-eight-day application of the Egoscue Method. Steve had no interest in athletics, and when they arrived, his dad had to literally pull him out of the car. He wouldn't look at me; he kept his head down and his shoulders slumped. The body language was unmistakable: "I hate you and I hate myself."

The first day Steve stayed aloof. He refused to interact with the other campers and staff, some of whom a more sports-savvy teen would have recognized from the pages of *Sports Illustrated*. He was unable to decenter and join the group.

But we insisted that Steve participate in all the physical activities: miles of running, obstacle-course workouts, special sets of E-cises to enhance balance and agility, and our own brand of strength training. There's a lot of camaraderie, cutting up, and competition. I advised the other campers about Steve's attitude and urged them to encourage and mentor him. Little by little he started to come around. The more physical challenges he faced and surmounted, the more socially engaged he became. As he discovered that his body was getting stronger and more capable of keeping up with the others, Steve became more confident and outgoing. As the musculoskeletal system dysfunctions peeled away, his body stopped being a liability and became an asset.

Steve wound up coming to camp for three summers in a row. He became one of our stars. By his senior year in high school, he was playing varsity football, and he continued to excel both as a scholar and as an athlete in college. Steve and his father are convinced that the only thing that pulled him back from self-destruction was that opportunity to jump-start his musculoskeletal functions. Could it have been a coincidence? Perhaps Steve was just ready to grow up, but I doubt it. The body (like all living things) is subject to coincidence and random occurrences; accidents do happen, but the prevailing operative mechanism is cause and effect. Something caused Steve to snap out of his teenage isolation and anger. His home life, friends, and other influences remained the same; what changed for four hours a day over the course of twenty-eight days was that the boy went from being nearly motionless to being motionfull. We know the effect—Steve got his act together. I think we know the cause too.

The story is heartening because it suggests other teenagers could have the same experience—and they don't have to enroll in the Egoscue Clinic camp. While Steve missed important brain-and-body-building opportunities in early and middle childhood, he was able to go back and recover the lost ground in a relatively short period of time. During that first summer, he spent roughly 112 hours in motion working to engage his musculoskeletal system functions. A teenager who conscientiously does the E-cises in the Appendix for a half hour or so each day for four months, then graduates to the menus in Chapter 9 for another four months, can make similar progress. (If they're conscientious, they'll rack up 168 hours over the course of a year.) There's no reason that they can't keep using those teen E-cises as the core of their fitness program for decades to come.

The Accidental Teenager

By early adolescence, teenagers are big and getting bigger by leaps and bounds. But because they didn't do much leaping and bounding in middle childhood, their physical age has not kept up with their chronological age. Stranded somewhere in the zone of middle childhood, they are adding inches and pounds to a musculoskeletal structure that is weak and unstable. It's simply not ready for prime teenage time. While no reliable figures have been collected as yet, there appears to be a dramatic rise in the number of orthopedic injuries for teenagers, athletes and nonathletes alike. Adolescents have always been considered clumsy, coltish, and gangling. Now they must also contend with poor balance, lack of resilience, stiffness, and a shortage of stamina and energy. As a result, accidents happen.

The incidence of scoliosis, commonly referred to as curvature of the spine, also seems to be on the rise. In some kids, during their adolescent growth spurt, the spine outruns the capacity of the back's supporting musculature to keep it straight. Because a dysfunctional musculoskeletal system loses its bilateral symmetry, stronger muscles on the right or the left will pull the spine in that direction. Drastic treatments are often prescribed for scoliosis—among them braces and implanted metal rods—but the most effective approach is to rebalance the spine's musculature equally on both sides.

Girls develop this muscular imbalance more than boys do, for two reasons. First, boys still are traditionally encouraged to take part in activities that build and maintain upper-body strength. Little things make a big difference, like helping carry grocery bags from the car, swinging a baseball bat, or climbing trees. Hence their spinal muscles are stronger and more capable of keeping the vertebral column straight. Second, at the onset of puberty girls undergo a pronounced shift in activities more often than boys do. The so-called tomboy will suddenly lose interest in the rough-and-tumble games she played with her brothers and become more of a "lady." The transformation can go the other way too: the girl whose idea of a workout was wheeling her dolls around in the carriage can develop a passion for competitive sports.

Whichever way it breaks, the change in stimulation takes the body by surprise at the same time a major growth spurt is under way. The newly minted soccer or basketball player will suddenly be taking part in daily kicking or shooting drills, thereby increasing the demand on selected muscles. Strengthened by the activity—repetitive and specialized as it is—the muscles begin to overpower those that aren't involved in the stimulus. It makes for a one-sided tug-of-war in which the spine is caught in the middle.

What's going on is similar for the teenage girl who stops being a tomboy. Her new lifestyle—think *stimulus*—won't maintain the muscles and functions that she's been using to run and climb trees. The iron rule of muscles is "Use 'em or lose 'em." Unused, as they lose strength, these muscles also give up the ability to keep the spine straight, as other sets of muscles—the ones that *are* being stimulated—take over.

I recommend the E-cise menus that begin on page 401 of the Appendix as a way to rebalance the teenage musculoskeletal system, for girls and boys alike. You'll notice in the instructions that when an E-cise is done on one side of the body, it is always repeated on the other. The idea is to spread the work evenly. Otherwise some muscles and other musculoskeletal system components will be overworked and others underworked.

Go Girl(s)

Title IX, as I mentioned, has had a huge impact on girls' participation in sports. But it's also had a downside.

When I went to high school in the bad old pre–Title IX days, my school had varsity programs in track, basketball, football, baseball, and wrestling. We didn't have a single women's program. Not one.

One afternoon my track team was practicing behind the school building, and seventeen-year-old Helen Burton was heading home by taking a shortcut across the field. The guys gave her a lot of lip, teenage stuff, like "Get a move on, girl, or you're going to be roadkill" and "Run baby, run," exactly what you expect from jocks and jerks. Helen wasn't intimidated. She was a farm girl who worked alongside her dad and her brothers. She made some disparaging comments about the team's athletic prowess. So our star runner promptly challenged her to a race. "Name it," Helen retorted. "The hundred-yard dash," he shot back.

Helen accepted without a flicker of hesitation. Our star—let's call him Joe, because I can't recall his real name—was fast. He had been a state finalist the year before. The guys made much merriment at Helen's expense. Unfazed by it all, she kicked off her school shoes, rolled her skirt above her knees, and crouched down on the blocks.

You know how this ends: Helen waxed the guy. She blasted past him, and he never got close. And he never lived it down. Beaten by a girl! His excuse was that she jumped the gun and he slipped. Right!

Our coach heard about the incident—how could he help it?—and tried to get permission to sign Helen to the team. But the Utah state athletic authorities flatly refused. I didn't realize it at the time, but it was my first lesson in how gender-blind human anatomy is when it comes to functional movement. Helen was totally functional, thanks to her upbringing on the farm. Even without training she could run just as fast as—faster than—any boy on that team.

What about Joe's advantage in lean muscle mass?

What about it?

What about Joe's superior size?

What about it?

What about Joe's testosterone?

What about it?

Helen's only disadvantage was a society that wouldn't let her compete. Title IX changed that. In the early 1970s the federal government ordered schools to provide equal access to sports programs, triggering a slow-motion revolution. Slow, because it took almost thirty years for the full effects to be felt. The regulation ended the era of lavish stadiums for men's football and weedy back lots for women's field hockey.

But in the years since Title IX, fewer and fewer Helens are around who are capable of kicking off their shoes and whomping the high school smart aleck. Teenage girls may have athletic talent, but what's missing is function. Today Helen might run and win, but her career would be a short one because her knees or ankles would soon start hurting.

The success of women's basketball and soccer has brought more girls and young women to organized athletics than ever before. The prestigious Olympic spotlight on gymnastics, track and field, and figure skating has generated a lot of interest too. With our own eyes, stopwatches, and scoreboards, we're finally seeing that women are as talented and capable as men, and better in many ways. I'd much rather watch women's basketball, since men can't come close to their grace, agility, and heads-up playing.

Even so, I'm afraid that success may ruin women's sports. Many of the girls and young women who are flocking to sports come with limited musculoskeletal system function. As they train and play, they use up this shallow functional reserve. Remember how it works: a misaligned musculoskeletal system is structurally weak, unstable, restricted, and under stress. Putting more demand on it doesn't change that situation for the better; it only gets worse unless function is restored.

Musculoskeletal system dysfunction is an accident waiting to happen, and as it happens to more and more girls and young women, the level of interest and participation in women's sports may begin to wane. When it comes to athletic injuries, an odd form of gender bias comes into play. A guy gets hurt, and there are many rationalizations. One of the favorites is that the injured player's opponents are tougher and stronger and harder hitting than ever before. *No wonder he smashed an elbow or blew a knee!* But the woman who's hurt on the court or playing field is immediately tagged as a victim of her own female frailty.

During basketball season I must read a news story every week about how vulnerable women's knees are to damage. But the structure of the male knee and the female knee is identical. The supporting component of the joint that's most commonly damaged is the ACL, the anterior cruciate ligament. Women tear them and so do men—for the exact same reason, which has nothing to do with gender. Weak, misaligned hips mean that when the athlete pushes off to jump or land, the knee rotates laterally rather than flexing and extending. The ACL, which forms an X behind the knee, is violently torqued and twisted from side to side.

While it's true that more women basketball players tear their ACLs than men, they are no more frail than men; nor do wider female pelvises cause the injury. The difference is that men, due to lifestyle, bring more functional hips to the game. Furthermore, male and female training regimens are different in emphasis. Women's coaches are aware that their players are structurally weak, and they work on muscle building. The effect is to strengthen the muscles that carry out the damaging rotation of the knees and hold the hips in misalignment.

Stress fractures are another symptom of skeletal misalignment. A few years ago the service academies—West Point, Annapolis, and the Air Force Academy—noticed that a disproportionate number of women were experiencing stress fractures in sports and physical training programs. The brass immediately concluded that the programs were too rigorous. They eased the requirements and made estrogen therapy available to the women.

Estrogen therapy for nineteen-year-olds! Those young women don't need extra hormones to strengthen their bones. They need an aligned musculoskeletal structure. You cannot pound on a misaligned skeleton without doing damage. They need a systematic, rigorous strength-training program that will build both muscles and bones on top of a solid foundation.

Instead what happens is that an effort is made to fix female "abnormalities." If we're not careful, this mindset will sink women's sports just as they are beginning to develop real buoyancy. How many parents will encourage their daughters to play basketball if they are convinced that women have weak knees or need estrogen to avoid bone fractures? Not many. An additional danger is that teenage girls will lose the buzz they get from being physically active and will stop playing because of dysfunctional, in-pain bodies. They'll drop out and return to relatively sedentary activities.

Crowd Control

In our society most teenagers do the bulk of their social interaction with other teenagers. This isn't the case everywhere—in some places teenagers apprentice or join the workforce, where they are surrounded by adults who directly supervise them. Where this pattern prevails, there tends not to be much disruptive, antisocial teenage behavior.

One reason is that they're exposed to positive adult role modeling. These cultures tend to be less developed than ours and require more hard labor and physical activity day in and day out. Therefore the adult role model for a teenager is probably going to be more functional from a musculoskeletal system standpoint. By mimicking adult behavior to win acceptance and to fit in, the teenager's functions are engaged and strengthened. The kid stuff drops away. He has no need to blow off steam by causing trouble. Her competence and accomplishments give her a satisfying identity, confidence, and pleasure.

American teenagers, by contrast, are at a double disadvantage. They are by and large cut off from adult role models, and those they do have contact with tend to be musculoskeletally dysfunctional because of their lifestyle and work style. On top of that, their adolescent peers are also dysfunctional. So teens wind up forming groups that share similar dysfunctional characteristics. They run in packs whose members look and act alike, because otherwise they would be "different" and out of place.

In such a peer context, a functional teenager is going to be different. She won't fit in and will be pulled out of her group's orbit—that's the downside. But the upside is that full function brings her confidence and competence. She will gravitate to other groups made up of kids with stronger and more engaged musculoskeletal system functions, for the same reason she was formerly pulled toward dysfunctional peers: they act and look more like she does.

At the same time, the functional teenager will be more independent and capable of resisting peer pressure. The group will lose some of its power. She'll have a better idea about who she is and what she wants, and she'll be ready to go get it on her own. As far as I'm concerned, that's the definition of a genuine "teen queen." And since peer groups serve as transitional vehicles to sexual relationships, her elevation to Queen of Hearts may bring on a reign that features more rose petals than tears.

Early Puberty and the Hormone High

When the Queen of Hearts in *Alice in Wonderland* bellowed "Off with her head!" she could have been making a wry observation about puberty. Teenage boys and girls do seem to lose their heads. But what else is new? Adolescents have always gone through turbulent times as their adult sexuality takes its mature form. Well, what's new is that puberty is occurring earlier than ever and is having profoundly disturbing effects on the mental and physical health of teenagers. In the mid–nineteenth century, puberty probably began at around sixteen and a half. On average, the onset of puberty in girls now begins at the age of ten or twelve. For boys, it happens about a year to eighteen months later.

Strictly speaking, puberty starts to occur when the pituitary gland secretes certain hormones—among them estrogen and progesterone in females, testosterone and adrenal androgens in males—in sufficient quantities to activate their reproductive systems and cause other physiological changes. This doesn't happen by accident: subject to the closest scrutiny by the body's internal monitoring systems, the individual is deemed smart and strong enough to survive on her own and to bear and successfully nurture offspring. The right organs, brain structure, muscles, bones, and neurons are in place. The requisite physical and mental maturation is the cause, and puberty is the effect.

There's no scientific consensus on why puberty is arriving prematurely. Perhaps synthetic hormones are leaking into the food and water supply from agricultural uses. Insecticides may be culprits, as well as contamination from plastic wrap to cover children's sandwiches and leftover food. Drip by drip such hormone pollution could be enough to prime a child's endocrine pump.

I don't discount those possibilities, but my hypothesis is that the body is reacting defensively to a pair of troubling and potentially dangerous anomalies. The first is the fact that children in the industrialized world are taller and heavier than ever. To the body's inner monitoring mechanism, they seem older. Second, they are generally sedentary, so the body-weight-to-muscle ratio is badly skewed. They have a low proportion of lean tissue—muscle—and brain-stem development and other neurological mileposts are lacking. By launching puberty early, the body is making a last-ditch effort to boost the muscle production that an adolescent will need to make his or her way in the world.

Lack of muscles and lackluster metabolism are at the heart of the second anomaly. Pronounced musculoskeletal system dysfunction results in metabolic dysfunction because a low energy demand yields low energy output. Sensing that the child is approaching the final period of her development—one that brings with it significantly higher levels of demand—the body triggers a hormone surge as a way to bring the deficient metabolism up to speed and take the place of the absent musculature.

A case can be made that today's teenagers are on a historically unprecedented hormone high that is the consequence of modern motion starvation. The body is manufacturing batch after batch of powerful chemicals as an alternative fuel to run systems that were designed to be sustained by the energy by-products of motion.

Young female athletes who undertake strenuous training regimens, like marathoners and gymnasts, often experience delayed puberty. Having limited functional capacity to begin with (like most modern athletes, they have overspecialized to the detriment of full function), extremely low body fat, and draconian diets, these young women have drawn down their metabolic resources to dangerous levels. The body forgoes activating the reproductive system, which would overtax its ability to meet both the heavy athletic demands and the basic requirements of keeping the heart beating, the lungs pumping, and the other systems operating. The least essential system is put on hold: reproduction.

Teenage boys are also affected by the sedentary

lifestyle, but their symptoms are different. The vast majority of juvenile criminal offenders—at last count more than a million of them were in long-term institutional care—are boys with histories of troublemaking that start as early as third grade. Many fit a common profile: they have low verbal and intelligence quotients and poor grades and are impulsive and emotionally cold; half have relatives who are in prison or have been in prison. I suspect that nurturing and stimulation have been minimal, and that metabolically they are running on empty. Their hormones—principally testosterone and adrenaline—are kicking in big-time to keep them going. Male hormones are supposed to be building muscles and testicles. But since the boys aren't moving much, their muscles don't get the benefit of the hormone high; and testicular growth is being held in abeyance in order to divert whatever testosterone is being produced to fuel the body's metabolically deficient physiognomy and brain. Caught without proper neurological development and the social skills that come with it, these boys are aggressive and violent.

The Period and the Dollar Sign

Menarche, the onset of menstrual bleeding, usually follows the first definitive physical signs of puberty in girls, such as the development of breasts and pubic hair, by about two and a half years. Twelve and a half or thirteen used to be the norm; now it is occurring sooner. Obesity, a symptom of inactivity and dysfunction, may be a factor. Athletic and physically active girls tend to menstruate later, but nowhere near the extreme delay experienced by gymnasts and marathoners. It may have something to do with fat. The more fat the body has stored away, the greater the energy reserves for pregnancy. In *Woman: An Intimate Geography*, Natalie Angier notes that girls pubesce when they weigh roughly 100 pounds, which means that if a quarter of the total is fat, that constitutes 87,000 calories. Angier calculates the energy demands of pregnancy to be 80,000 calories. Therefore the baby is ready to have her own baby.

If that's true, then what's still missing in a dysfunctional teenage girl who has accumulated the requisite fat is the active muscle work to burn it. Here a hormone comes into play—adrenaline—as an ignition source. The adrenal hormones heat up the ovaries, which in turn finish the job of sexualization by pouring out their own hormonal cocktails. As a result, girls in menarche experience an almost immediate hangover in the form of PMS, menstrual cramps, heavy bleeding, and bloating.

In a 1997 study reported in the *Archives of Pediatrics and Adolescent Medicine,* 93 percent of the girls who participated said they experienced discomfort during menstruation. Only 40 percent of all women are believed to be affected by some form of premenstrual syndrome.

PMS and menstrual discomfort are different conditions. PMS is a group of physical and mental symptoms that appear from seven to fourteen days before menstruation and subside about twenty-four hours after menstruation begins. But it has become a catchall term to describe menstrual problems in general and as such has become a hot-button issue. I'm raising it because the hormone-metabolism-function link is at its most vivid during the teenage years and should be seen in the context of musculoskeletal system dysfunction.

Menstruation is not an abnormality, a disorder, or an illness. But to the detriment of women, it is being cast as such by those with an interest in cashing in on women's "special needs." Seventy percent of the teenagers in that 1997 study used over-the-counter medicine to manage their menstrual discomfort. Do the math, and multiply tens of millions of teenage girls who reach puberty each year times twelve or more dosages a year, and multiply that by thirty to forty years until menopause. PMS is a bonanza for the drug industry.

I'm fascinated by the numbers. If 70 percent of the teenage girls in the study used over-the-counter medication, what about the other 30 percent, including the 8 percent who reported no menstrual discomfort? Are they all just lucky? Blessed with good genes? A high pain threshold? Not so coincidentally, the number is about what I'd roughly estimate the truly functional portion of teenage girls to be. Similarly, consider the 40 percent of the general population of women believed to be affected by some form of PMS. What about the other 60 percent? The process of ovulation is the same from woman to woman. Can a major internal system possibly be so quirky that it works well for six out of ten women and goes haywire for the rest? It's possible, but other explanations are more probable.

I'm not suggesting that menstruation has no side effects or that it cannot cause inconvenience and, in some cases, real suffering. My point is that the symptoms of PMS tend to shadow the symptoms of musculoskeletal system dysfunction. Once a month a system that's already pushing the limits of its capacity to handle day-to-day demand is—thanks to the extra demands of ovulation—toppling over the edge into discomfort, pain, or other miseries. Take away the stress caused by the musculoskeletal system dysfunction, and PMS may lessen or disappear altogether.

The Dark Side of Adolescence

Here's a frightening list of problems that constitute the dark side of adolescence today:

- Teen pregnancy
- Drug and alcohol abuse
- Eating disorders
- Violence
- Sleeping disorders
- Depression
- Suicide

Teenage pregnancy and sexual activity may be the result of a permissive society that affords adolescents too many opportunities to use their genitals rather than their heads. Or it may be another indication that children are reaching puberty without the mental and emotional resources necessary to explore their sexuality—exploration that *every* generation has done—and to avoid scarring their lives in the process. Sex is not a new invention. Our mothers and fathers, grandfathers and grandmothers managed to partake of it, and many of them either had the discipline to control and manage their earliest sexual gropings well enough to stay out of trouble, or abstained long enough to finish high school or college, or were lucky enough to get away with it.

Today dysfunction is making discipline, abstinence, and luck awfully hard for most teenagers. As functions decline and take with them self-confidence and self-respect, the need for intimacy, identity, and validation grows exponentially. Sex feels good when the body doesn't. When a kid senses he or she is trapped by physical limitations, sex offers escape. When the world is unsafe and frightening, sex is a safe haven. For someone who cannot focus long enough to see projects through to completion, sex is an accomplishment. Sex is a way for a child to grow up.

In 1997 Dr. Robert Blum, director of the division of general pediatrics and adolescent health at the University of Minnesota, published research that found that 17 percent of seventh and eighth graders had had sexual intercourse. We have no earlier figures for young teenagers to use for a then-and-now comparison, but the trend for high school students is definitely toward having sexual intercourse at a younger age. In the early 1970s, less than 5 percent of the fifteen-year-old girls and 20 percent of the fifteen-year-old boys had engaged in sexual intercourse. In 1997, the last year for which data is available, the figures were 38 percent of the girls and 45 percent of the boys.

In an article exploring this issue in *The New York Times*, a thirteen-year-old boy was quoted as saying, "Sex is pleasurable. Why not now?" His father or grandfather might have asked the same question, but at that age they were probably too busy enjoying the other pleasures of youth that were accessible to fully functional people.

The effort to wrest pleasure from a body that doesn't supply it is also a root cause of teenage substance abuse. Drugs and alcohol are ways to manage a system that has lost its ability to coherently deal with stimulation. Without an efficient and finely tuned metabolic process, the child takes matters into his own hands to create a buzz or to mellow out.

Eating disorders spring from the same source. From junk food bingeing to anorexia and bulimia, teenagers are desperately trying to reignite a metabolic process that in many cases is perilously close to flatlining. Salt, sugar, caffeine, and nicotine are cheap, crude, and powerful stimulants. If they don't work, other options are gorging or starving. Bulimia and anorexia have psychological components related to lack of self-esteem, but in both conditions the victim's behavior aims unconsciously at a metabolic target. The bulimic is overdosing her body with food, hoping to jump-start it and feel a rush; then when the rush doesn't materialize or fades quickly, she purges. The anorexic approaches the verge of starvation—and sometimes goes beyond it—in order to surf on the adrenaline that the crisis-wracked body produces to prevent the metabolism from switching off altogether.

A Wake-up Call

If your teenager has trouble sleeping, she's probably not about to become anorexic. But sleep disorders are serious, relatively common, and symptomatic of musculoskeletal system dysfunction (for adults as well as adolescents). In recent years teachers and school administrators have noticed that many adolescents have trouble waking up in the morning, come to school late and/or in a fog, and fall asleep during class.

This has given rise to the theory that teenagers have different body clocks and biorhythms from adults. What they really have are young bodies that are not being physically stimulated enough during the day to tire them out by nightfall. They stay up late seeking stimulation wherever they can find it, and they fall into bed finally to sleep shallowly and fitfully.

Some educators suggest that school should start later in the day, to accommodate the teenage body clock. But I believe kids would show up at noon just as foggy and groggy as they do today at eight A.M. The time change will merely shift the search for stimulation deeper into the wee hours of the morning, and what little sleep teenagers get will continue to be shallow and fitful.

Another important factor in sleep disorders is a stressed-out metabolism. As metabolism drops off toward basal levels and rings warning bells in the endocrine system, periodic spikes of adrenaline keep the teenager awake or only on the surface of sleep. If metabolism falls low enough and shuts down, the teenager will die. The adrenaline spikes jab the metabolism in order to keep it operating.

Deep sleep evolved as a bodily necessity when our primitive ancestors forged a strong social bond within a family or tribe that allowed individuals in an otherwise hostile environment to feel secure enough to temporarily relinquish consciousness. In deep sleep our skeletal muscles are so disengaged that we dare not rest perching on the edge of a cliff or on a tree limb. Instead of crawling into a burrow, we historically found safe haven in the midst of a trusted group.

But many adolescents are alienated from their family group and are experiencing feelings of self-doubt and insecurity. Their sleep is the broken, restless sleep of the vigilant and the isolated. Here again musculoskeletal dysfunction is at work, reinforcing and compounding the sleeping disorder that stems from understimulation.

The Chemical Equation

Mood changes provoked by hormonal shifts and imbalances have always been associated with adolescence. But as we've seen, today's teenagers are subjected to a torrent of hormones that far exceeds that which affected previous generations. Their metabolism fueled with hormones rather than muscles and motion, teenagers are swamped with waves of multipurpose biochemical depressants and stimulants.

Hormones have frequently been described as chemical messengers, traveling through the bloodstream, but the messages they carry involve more than reproduction and sexuality. They involve growth, cellular nutrition, blood composition, fluid balance, skin color, digestion, heartbeat, and *many* other activities. Neurochemicals perform similar roles via the central nervous system.

Think of neurochemicals and hormones as off- and on-switches. Those that act as depressants are off-switches. Those that act as stimulants are on-switches.* As functions lose their ability to respond to stimuli, the off-switches are flicked simply because the body learns that it can't rely on those disengaged functions. The predominant messages are those sent by the off-switches: *Don't try, it won't work; better hide because you can't run.* Essential musculoskeletal and internal system functions are shut down, and the hormones and neurochemicals lock them down.

---

*To be accurate, hormones and their close relatives, neurochemicals, are largely stimulants even though the stimulation may have the effect of depressing or suppressing an activity. A stimulus is an agent that produces an altered state or activity.

Ironically, the body's constant drive for balance between stimulation and depression accentuates depression by trying to flip the on-switches even though the functions do not respond. So to counteract pointless stimulation, the off-switches activate all the more. After all, depression is a protective mechanism. It is next of kin to doubt, alarm, and fear. Our hunter-gatherer ancestors became sadder but wiser from the chemical frisson they felt when the saber-toothed tiger growled at dawn and the off-switch flicked to keep them hunkered down in the cave.

Sunshine and Shadows

Suicide is the fifth leading cause of death for those five to fourteen years old. From ages fifteen to twenty-four it is the third leading cause of death, ranking behind car accidents and homicides. Girls attempt suicide more than boys by a ratio of four to one. Boys successfully commit suicide four times more frequently. Overall about five thousand teenagers kill themselves each year.

Stress, isolation, identity problems, family conflicts, physiological changes, and depression are all implicated. Researchers have found low levels of serotonin, a neurochemical, in the brains of suicide victims. Since serotonin appears to function to a large extent as an antidepressant and mood elevator, something may be blocking its distribution to the brain. That something, as far as I'm concerned, could well be muscular disengagement.

When serotonin was first discovered, it was thought to be involved in just a handful of activities, among them the contraction of smooth-muscle tissue and the dilation of major blood vessels. Based on current research, however, serotonin may have more assignments than any other neurochemical. Still, it's the muscular-contraction angle that interests me. Could it be that as major muscle groups fall into disuse, the serotonin output related to smooth-muscle contraction is being proportionally reduced? If so, given the body's tiny volume of naturally occurring serotonin, it may be enough to blunt the chemical's antidepressant message to the brain.

Sunlight is believed to be central to the synthesis of serotonin. An acutely dysfunctional, sedentary teenager tends to spend his or her time indoors, where the stimulus is most predictable and manageable. Could this fact be responsible for the lack of serotonin? The suicide of five thousand teens a year is painful to contemplate, but is our modern, walled-off, roofed-over, and motionless lifestyle edging all of us closer to depleting our serotonin and condemning millions to drive on empty, and to travel ever deeper into darkness and despair?

These questions deserve to be thoroughly researched for the sake of our children.

Robert Frost once wrote, "I go to school to youth, to learn the future." But exactly what do we learn at this school? The young teach us that the past is very much alive. It is under siege but enduring.

The world has changed, but we are essentially the same. Our musculoskeletal legacy endures. It's there in both crying babies and restless teens. But in this changed world—a place that doesn't oblige us with enough wind, waves, and rainbows to ride to far shores where we are tested and tempered—we must learn new ways to access and engage our vast wealth of muscle and bone. And learn we will.

If you have doubts and need convincing, just find a toddler, and watch her take her first steps. If she can do that, she can do just about anything.

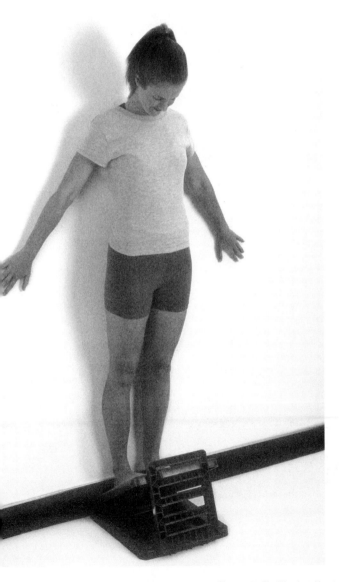

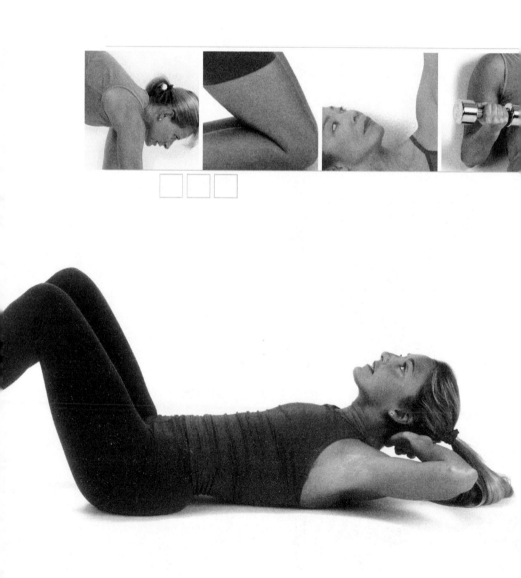

tools

CHAPTER 8

on easy-cise street

□□□

In this short chapter, I want to explain how you can get the most out of the Egoscue Method's principal tool: the E-cises. I'm assuming that you might turn to the chapters that pertain to your own age group. I hope you don't—you'll miss a lot of valuable background material. But if you do, here are the ground rules and fine points for Easy-cise Street.

First, each subsequent chapter includes an E-cise menu. Notice I said a "menu." By that I mean to convey an important concept: the individual E-cises are not intended to stand alone. They are carefully arranged in a sequence to achieve maximum results. Nothing bad will happen if you pick and choose at random, but the full benefits will be diluted.

Here's why. Because the body is a closely interrelated unit, its muscles and joints work in close cooperation and coordination. When these partnerships are fully functional, you have no pain, no problems. But when they're dysfunctional, these supporting alliances break down and/or get a little screwy. To replace primary movers that have become disengaged, for instance, a misaligned joint will borrow peripheral muscles. These misalliances can get very tangled and difficult to straighten out. That's why the menu sequencing is important: layer by layer, each E-cise further sorts out the snarl and restores function. In short, please do the E-cises in the order presented.

The E-cises in this book are largely preventative and holistic. If you have chronic musculoskeletal pain that's affecting a knee, a hip, or a shoulder, please consult my book *Pain Free*, which serves as a body-part-by-body-part, head-to-toe guide to nonsurgical, nondrug pain-abatement techniques. That book also offers E-cise menus, and once those have relieved your pain for at least six weeks, you can switch back here and begin a preventative program.

If you are following a menu and a specific E-cise causes pain—as opposed to the tightness or ache that can come from a workout—drop it from the menu, and go on to the next E-cise. In a day or two, try the offending E-cise again; chances are, you'll be able to do it without pain because of a structural adjustment brought about by the rest of the menu. If not, skip it again. But keep trying to sneak it back into the program. If the pain persists—listen to your body. It's telling you not to do that E-cise!

▶ Do the E-cises in your stocking feet unless the floor is slippery or there is a traction issue.

▶ Any E-cise performed on one side of the body is always performed on the other. This is a hard and fast rule, even if you think that your right leg, for example, is weak and the left is strong. Functional balance is extremely important. By working only one side, you're going to overpower the other. A strong left leg and a weak right leg are probably equally dysfunctional and will benefit equally from the E-cise. In the remote possibility that the left leg is stronger, the E-cise will bring the right one up to strength without overstimulating the left. Eventually they will equalize and function together.

▶ Do the same number of repetitions called for in the instructions on both sides.

▶ Perform the E-cises slowly and smoothly.

▶ Keep your back arched, your shoulders square, and your head up (unless the instructions say otherwise).

- Relax your stomach muscles, and breathe from your diaphragm.

- If you aren't strong or stable enough to complete an E-cise, do as much as you can. Try to go a bit longer each day until you can finish.

- After each E-cise walk around a little, breathe, and relax.

- Have a partner watch you (particularly at first) to make sure you're following the instructions.

- Do the menu every day. If you miss one day, the sky won't fall. But miss two or more, and you'll lose whatever gains you've made.

- If you're doing a multiphase menu and lose more than a week, drop back to the preceding phase and start over. Stay with that menu for at least a week before upgrading back to the phase you were originally in.

- Pay attention to how you feel both while doing the E-cises and after you're finished. "I feel lousy" changing to "I feel better" is significant news. If you don't self-monitor, your gains may go unnoticed, and you'll cheat yourself of the motivation to continue.

- Turn off the TV or remove the headphones while you perform the E-cises. Listen to your body. It's sending you important messages.

- If your menu calls for a time-consuming Supine Groin E-cise, I'm sorry about the time involved, but don't skip it.

- Most E-cises don't require equipment, but in some cases you may have to improvise with a common household item, like a rolled-up towel. I'm not trying to generate business, but some items are available on my Web site, www.egoscue.com.

- If you'd like to combine E-cises with other activities, do the whole menu first to engage and stabilize your structure, and then go play.

- Finally, do the E-cises for the rest of your life. Yup—it's a life sentence. You will never be cured from the need for adequate design motion.

Motion begets motion. A sure sign that the E-cises are working is that more motion is creeping back into your life. As dysfunctions recede, it's more enjoyable to walk, take the stairs instead of the elevator, go dancing, and the like.

To establish a benchmark to measure your progress, set up a motion "date" at least twice a week. For example, spend twenty minutes walking every Tuesday and Saturday. After a month of these dates and simultaneously doing the E-cises each day, take stock. Do you always keep your dates, or do other things get in the way? Rather than just two motion dates, are there extras? Or are you spending more time than the original twenty minutes?

As the E-cises kick in and reengage your musculoskeletal system functions, as I said, you won't be able to resist the temptation to move more and more. It's an addiction. But if you answered "no" to my benchmark questions, you're not addicted. It may be because you've been sporadic about doing the E-cises. Your body needs its daily requirement of motion. Not every *other* day, not a couple of times a week, not when you think of it— *every day*. Another possible explanation is that you've been window-shopping through the various E-cise menus. Resist the temptation. The menu sequence is carefully arranged to address layers of dysfunction. The only time to edit a menu is when an E-cise causes you pain. Then drop it and move to the next one.

Here are some other benchmarks to establish as you begin an E-cise program:

▶ Rate your energy level on a scale of one to ten.

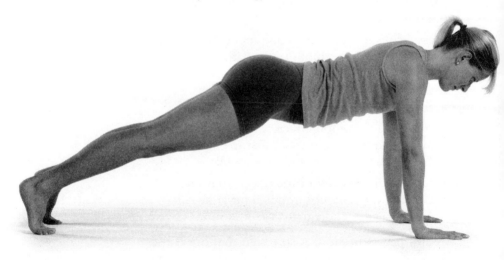

- Rate your stress level on a scale of one to ten.
- Are your moods steady, or do they swing widely?
- How much water do you drink?
- Do you need to push with your hands and arms to rise from a chair?
- Do your feet point outward or straight ahead when you stand or walk?
- Can you balance on one foot with your eyes closed? For how long?
- Do you sleep soundly at night?
- Do your feet hurt?
- Is there joint pain or stiffness?

Write down the answers and tuck them away for future reference. Each item on the list is a measure of function and dysfunction. In six months or so, the list will help remind you where you came from. Most of us have gotten so used to our dysfunctions that we don't notice them to begin with, and ironically we don't notice when they go away either.

In the clinic a client will sometimes tell me that her E-cise program isn't working.

"Does your knee still hurt?" I'll ask.

"It feels weak."

"But it no longer hurts the way it did for the last year?"

"Well—yeah, I guess so."

"So the E-cises aren't working, but your knee has stopped hurting. What do you suppose is going on?"

"I don't . . . know."

What's going on is stimulation and the gradual restoration of function. We expect our muscles and joints to work smoothly, and when they do, the memory of pain quickly vanishes. That's as it should be. To me, this form of amnesia confirms that the body's resilience and healing power are so well established that it sees no need to store these musculoskeletal system pain memories. What's stored—or should be—are memories of function: how good it feels to run, jump, twist, and turn. The fading of those memories is a sure sign of prolonged dysfunction. Even worse is when the pleasurable motion memories aren't implanted in the first place. I'm afraid that many of today's children, teenagers, and young adults are caught in that predicament because their experience of motion and its pleasure is so limited. They don't expect to be without pain or some level of discomfort.

Nonetheless, the body copes. If the absence of pain doesn't register, something else may. Not only does pain recede as function returns, but less obvious symptoms change too. Improved sleep, declining stress levels, better mood management, and higher energy mean that dysfunction is releasing its hold. Enhanced balance is another key indicator, as are feet that begin to point straight ahead. Increased water intake suggests that the body is putting more demand on its resources. And getting in and out of chairs without a struggle is a positive sign.

All in all, it's best to use more than one benchmark and not rely solely on the presence or absence of pain. You might use a marking pen to highlight my next sentence: *the abatement of pain alone should make you very wary.* Treating pain is actually easy—simply immobilizing an injured joint or muscle usually alleviates it. But the cause of the pain still remains. Likewise, drugs and surgery bypass dysfunction and forcibly switch off the pain symptoms. The continued presence of nonpain symptoms, like those we've been discussing, is evidence that musculoskeletal system dysfunction remains extant.

If you don't have one already, a video camera is a good investment. Put on a T-shirt and shorts, and have a friend tape you walking, climbing stairs, sitting in a chair, and standing up. Ask the camera person to tape you in profile from head to foot and straight on. Also, keep the camera rolling while you do your E-cise program. (It will help you spot mistakes or inadvertent shortcuts.)

In the clinic we use videotapes sent in from around the world to diagnose musculoskeletal system dysfunction and to create individualized E-cise programs. I don't expect you to be able to make a diagnosis based on your tape, but you can use it as a basis of comparison by taping another after several weeks of doing E-cises and looking at them both. You should be able to see a noticeable difference in the ease of movement and the erectness of your posture.

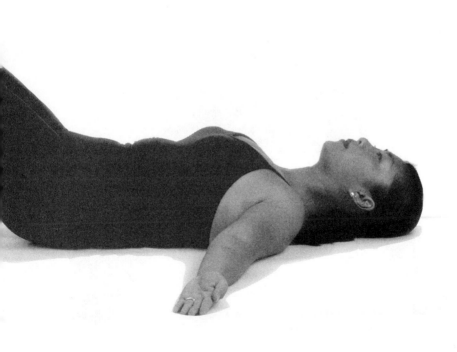

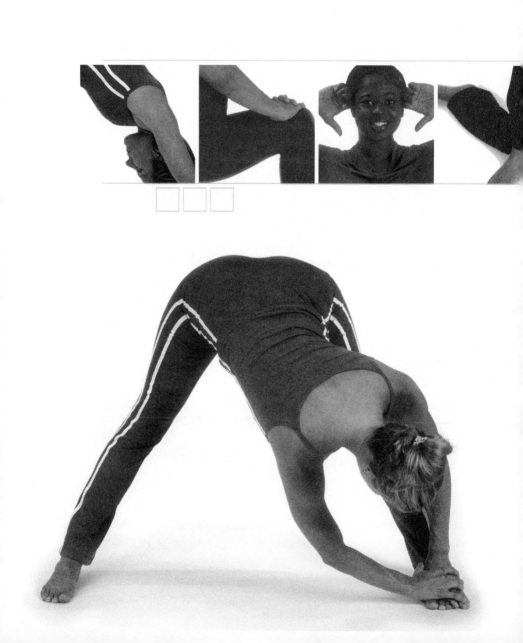

young adulthood

CHAPTER 9

compound growth

How tall are you, and how much do you expect to grow in the next year or two? Most young adults—those roughly between the ages of twenty and thirty-five—would be able to tell me their height to the nearest fraction of an inch without having to check their driver's license or any other record. They'd also say, "I stopped growing when I was seventeen [or whenever]; I'm as tall as I'm going to get."

They would be both right and wrong. Right, in that the long bones of the human skeleton do stop lengthening in late adolescence, as the volume of pituitary growth hormone trails off. But it's wrong to regard that fact as evidence that we are "all grown up." Growth continues—if we let it—for a lifetime.

If we let it is a big *if.* Other than height and weight, there's no handy and physically obvious definition of growth, so it's easy to forget that it takes place constantly throughout the body. Millions of cells are produced each second in the marrow of our bones, in the brain, and in other organs and tissues to maintain and strengthen our vital functions. But by the time many of us reach our twenties, we have become skilled in ways to interfere with this growth. Not only does the adolescent bequeath her young

Cells grow by division, but not all of them are capable of dividing. Some split into two identical parts continuously and have life spans of just a few hours; others never divide after birth. Between those extremes is a vast degree of variation, depending on a cell's specific role and other circumstances. As a general rule, the cells of tissue that is subjected to intense stimulation, like the intestines, divide the most frequently. My view is that there are far fewer nondividing cells than is commonly believed. Their replication mechanisms may be switched off or suppressed by hostile environmental factors like dehydration, toxins, viruses, or other destructive agents.

adult self a physiological platform that may prove inadequate, but her habits, attitudes, and lifestyle may form the basis for continuing patterns of destructive behavior.

Don't get me wrong—the teenage werewolf you used to be did not permanently wreck your health. But the transition from adolescence to young adulthood is extremely significant because it marks the point at which the individual becomes responsible for her own health. Thanks to the very characteristic that we're discussing—growth—it's possible to overcome years of adverse health effects by making mature decisions to change our ways now.

These mature decisions roughly group under four headings. The first, obviously, is motion. Without adequate motion all the body's systems are compromised, if for no other reason than the musculoskeletal system's role as an oxygen pump. Motion starvation leads to oxygen starvation throughout the body.

The second heading is food. I'm not a nutritionist and this is not a diet book, but I need to call your attention to a few issues. Scientists long ago concluded that human height is influenced by nutrition in childhood. Within limits set by the genes, the more abundant and healthier the food a child eats, the taller the individual will be.

For most of the nineteenth and twentieth centuries, the average height of Americans crept upward to about 5 feet 8 inches, but since the early 1970s it has remained unchanged. The halt coincides with the trend toward increased childhood obesity, the decline in the nutritional quality of the American diet, and the falling off of activity levels. Ours is a salty, sugary, starchy, snacky, sit-down, and drive-by culture. As a result, kids are getting wider rather than taller—and so are young adults.

Research verifies that exercise increases the output of the body's pituitary growth hormone. Sixty percent of the American public does not get regular exercise, but they eat as if they did. Not only does this role of food consumption add inches to the national waistline, it subtracts from their overall skeletal growth and makes American men and women shorter than they would otherwise be—and slower-growing in general. When it comes to childhood and adult obesity, I think physical activity plays as large a part or larger than sheer caloric intake. When we do not exercise, not only do we not burn off excess calories, we cannot produce the growth hormone needed to build a skeletal framework large enough and strong enough to carry our extra weight. In due course, this lifestyle also has an impact on continued tissue growth.

Historically, access to an abundant high-quality food supply made for an industrious, active populace. The more people moved around—hunting, gathering, farming, herding—the better they ate. Growth and strength followed. Movement brings a nutritional reward, and nonmovement brings a penalty. Today the penalty is obesity, associated diseases like diabetes and heart disease, chronic pain, and a host of other conditions. The leveling off of the steady increase in average height—which continues to increase elsewhere in the world—is another disturbing symptom of musculoskeletal system dysfunction that is triggered by lack of motion and aggravated by poor nutrition.

Consider the 10 percent average height difference between men and women. Since nutrition has such a strong influence on height and since American women seem to enjoy the same access to the food supply, why the disparity? Genes and male hormones could be factors, but more likely the slight edge in activity levels among boys in their middle childhood and teenage years may tip the scales and trigger just enough extra growth hormone to make a difference. I'm also inclined to think that nutritional inequality helped give men a head start that they still hold. From a social standpoint, male dominance has meant that men claim a larger share of the available resources, including food. With the same logic that dictates that the rich get richer, similarly the tall get taller and the strong get stronger.

Today in the developed world, aside from pockets of poverty, the nutritional gender gap is probably more a matter of cultural convention than stark "my fork is bigger than your fork" dinner-table inequality. In late middle childhood and early adolescence, girls become more conscious of their appearance and begin managing how they are perceived by their peers and the opposite sex. For various reasons smaller—as measured by weight—is regarded as more desirable. To keep their weight down, many teenage girls and young adult women routinely diet. Studies have concluded that in the vast majority of teenage girls and young women, this obsession with weight leads to eating disorders. In many cases they declare war on their bodies, attempting to override by sheer force of will such gender-specific biological facts as the lopsided ratio of fat to lean tissue in women as opposed to men. They chase after "ideal weights." And they take no prisoners at mealtime—food is the enemy. But there are no victors in a war like that, only losers.

In early and middle childhood boys and girls grow and put on weight at about the same pace. In the first months and years of adolescence, girls spurt ahead, and they tower over boys the same age. But the boys soon catch up and grow for three to five years longer. One reason is that their testosterone kicks in and builds muscle, which in turn creates denser, heavier, faster-growing bones. But as most parents can confirm with a slew of grocery store receipts, boys' growth spurt is accompanied by a huge surge in appetite. This growth spurt coincides with a growth slowdown on the part of girls, giving us good reason to believe that nutrition is one reason skeletal growth comes to a stop in girls earlier than in boys.

Women have more control over their physical development than they are led to believe by the "big man/little woman" myth. Unfortunately, many often use this control to impede their own continued growth. Physical activity levels and proper nutrition are important throughout all stages of a woman's life. If you shortchange yourself at thirteen, you will feel the consequences at thirty and beyond. Research indicates, for example, that teenage girls, on average, have a daily calcium intake of 60 percent less than the USDA recommended daily requirement. That deficit occurs right in the middle of the last skeletal growth surge. To me, it helps explain why most girls do not grow as tall as boys. Meanwhile their compromised bone density sets the stage for bone loss later in life.

I was in a Starbucks recently that's in the same neighborhood as an exclusive girls' prep school. The place was swarming with teenagers ordering cups of coffee in midafternoon. But caffeine hammers the adrenal glands and has been linked to bone loss.

Farther along up the same block, another group of girls were slurping down soft drinks in a snack bar. But the artificial sweetener in sodas can block intake of the potassium and magnesium needed for bone building. (Many sodas also contain caffeine.) That's two strikes.

Strike three comes in the common low-fat diets that are high in sugar. These diets have been found to decrease "good" HDL cholesterol in children by as much as 20 percent.

These habits (and their consequences) will carry over into adulthood, and they are habits women can live without, considering that osteoporosis cripples millions and that heart disease is the number-one killer of women each year.

Soda Pop: Liquid Candy

As we have seen, an understimulated, metabolically inefficient body will seek artificial stimulation. That's what's happening with all the caffeine, the soft drinks, and the sugary low-fat diets: teenage girls and women are trying to jolt their systems to increase energy, concentration, and strength while at the same time staying slim by avoiding bulky whole food and "bloating" water consumption.

I'll come back to the myth that equates water with bloating. First, let's look at some hard figures on soft drinks, which in modern America have become food substitutes. In 1997, according to the beverage industry, the equivalent of 576 standard twelve-ounce cans of soft drinks were consumed by every man, woman, and child in the United States. That's 14 billion gallons. Since 1942, when the AMA issued a warning, in the "interest of public health," that "it is desirable to especially have restrictions on such use of sugar as represented by consumption of sweetened carbonated beverages . . . which are of low nutritional value," consumption is up ninefold from just 60 cans per capita a year. Got that? Sixty is closing in on 600 in less than six decades.

Women in their twenties are ahead of this curve. They drink an average of two cans a day, or 730 a year. The rate has doubled since the late 1970s, and it's probably even higher since many people, when they participate in surveys, tend to underestimate their intake of junk food. Also, the trend appears to be heading upward because the serving size of soft drinks (once six ounces) has grown: the twelve-ounce unit is now being replaced by "supersize" proportions that run twenty ounces and larger.

Big gulps of soda beget smaller gulps of other beverages. As teenagers dramatically increased their soft drink intake, they cut their consumption of milk by more than 40 percent. In 1996, among twelve- to nineteen-year-olds, only 36 percent of the boys and 14 percent of the girls consumed 100 percent of the recommended amounts of calcium and vitamin A. Think back to your teenage years. Was this you? Maybe it still is.

For all adults, soft drinks are the fifth largest source of calories. As far as weight control is concerned, empty calories are still calories. They have scant nutritional value, and they are stored as fat. Worse, they take the place of essential vitamins and minerals that come from legitimate nutritional sources. And the mischief-making doesn't stop there. The brain, to function evenly, needs a reasonably steady supply of glucose. Too much glucose triggers insulin production, which induces the cells to absorb and store the excess. Too little means that another substance called glucagon goes to work releasing glucose from storage. Chugging regular nondiet soft drinks produces rushes of insulin followed by counter rushes of glucagon. This cycle greatly strains the control mechanism and may eventually cause it to function erratically or break down entirely.

Slaying the Vampire of "Ideal Weight"

I'd love to pound a stake through the heart of the "ideal

weight" vampire. This monster will not die, even though there is no such thing as an ideal weight. The human body is designed to fluctuate in weight according to how much fuel it consumes and how much work it performs. A fixed ideal weight would constitute an evolutionary disaster. It assumes a fixed, unfluctuating environment—no way!—and a fixed, unfluctuating response to it. Sounds like Planet of the Robots to me.

So what's your ideal weight?

You responded almost instinctively, didn't you? Most people have a number in their heads, and that's okay as long as everyone understands what's going on. That number probably comes from one of three sources. Perhaps it's associated with a happy time in your life—"I was in college, having a great time, making lots of new friends, traveling in the summer." Or perhaps the number stems from popular culture, as conveyed by films, magazines, and the fashion industry. The third possible source would be the height and weight tables ginned up by the insurance industry. Whichever one it is, women end up chasing a mirage.

Associating your ideal weight with past moments of happiness and satisfaction sets you up for frustration and failure. Even if your struggle to achieve that weight is successful, it will not turn back the clock and yield commensurate happiness. Times have changed, and so have you. Hence there won't be any reward for the effort. Furthermore, that past weight reflected the fuel that you were taking in at that time and the work you were putting out. Like it or not, this is an iron rule of weight dynamics and management: the fuel intake–energy expenditure equation must be in balance. Otherwise a drastic curtailment of what you eat, without a simultaneous reduction of your work expenditure, will be at best a half measure and at worst a health risk.

In the same way, a media-inspired ideal weight is also out of reach. What's right for Hollywood actress Charlize Theron may be fine for her (although I doubt it), but it's not for you. Finally, the height and weight tables are a total dead end—literally. They were originally based on measurements taken from cadavers. Some ideal weight!

H2O Is Good4U

You may think water is bloating, but that's a bad rap. The way to avoid water retention is to drink more of

Drying Out

Water accounts for 55 percent of the average woman's body weight. But the amount varies dramatically with age, from a high of 75 percent in infants to 45 percent in the elderly. But I regard this difference as function-related, not strictly age-related. The more functional an individual—of whatever age—the higher the ratio of water to body weight. Why? See the next sidebar, about water's role in chemical reactions.

Waterworks

What is man? What is woman? A veritable fireworks display of chemical reactions. Trillions of them blast away nonstop. Water is the medium in which these chemical reactions occur. Inside each of us is a river of fire. As the volume of water fluctuates, the nature and frequency of the chemical reactions change too. Likewise, water quality, not just quantity, is likely to be important. Another point about water and function: a functional musculoskeletal system has more active skeletal muscle, which holds more water than most other tissue.

it, not less. The body has no real reserve or storage capacity for water. But if there is a shortage, it will try to improvise by rationing and holding as much as possible.

When your kidneys process waste and toxins, they depend on water to dissolve, dilute, and transport the material out of the body. If you're dehydrated, that cleansing function is impeded, perhaps drastically so.

Water may be the best-kept diet secret of them all. It helps metabolize fat (burn it off), and because it is calorie-free but high in mineral content (hard water, anyway), it is an appetite suppressant, an anticancer agent, and a heart health builder.

Water tones the skin and muscles and gives hair more body and sheen. Joints are more limber and have better cushioning. Imagine what would happen to your spine if all the water leaked out of the vertebral disks. It can never drain off entirely, but a dehydrated body robs water from these spongy cushions and the rest of the musculoskeletal system, which only worsens misalignment.

There isn't a single bodily process that doesn't depend on water. The lymph system uses it to sluice out the glandular holding tanks and transport waste; the digestion needs it to break down food; and the circulatory system relies on it to get oxygen to the brain.

You bet "a river runs through it"—from head to foot. But for most people it's at drought levels. I rarely see a new client in my clinic who appears to be fully hydrated. Most people are dehydrated. Paradoxically, the body tells us when we're starving, but not when we're in danger of dying of thirst. Being "thirsty"—having a parched sensation or a dry mouth—tends to fade the thirstier one becomes. Thirst has plenty of other symptoms, but most of us don't recognize them until it's nearly too late. Want to see one? Late in the afternoon, look around your school or office, and examine your colleagues' eyes. That glazed-over, dilated look is not boredom or genuine fatigue but dehydration. It's aggravated by chugging soft drinks and coffee all day, and being confined to a dry, climate-controlled environment. If we exclude dedicated athletes from the mix, I'd guess upward of 90 percent of the population isn't drinking nearly enough water.

How much water is enough? It depends on your size

and your activity level. But no matter what, eight to ten glasses a day is the minimum. Each of us must replenish about two and a half quarts each day. If you think that means a few more trips to the bathroom, you're right, but only after you first raise your water intake to its proper levels. Within a few weeks your body will adjust. You'll urinate less frequently, but the volume will be larger each time.

Slumber Party

Lack of sleep is not only a stand-alone malady: it's also a symptom of lack of motion, poor nutrition, and dehydration. A body that lacks motion has a valid reason for not sleeping (it isn't physically tired), and one that is severely stressed by poor diet and dehydration also ends up suffering from sleep deprivation. Often this stress will so stimulate the body's systems that they will go into a hypercrisis mode. It's like trying to nap through a five-alarm fire. As sleep deprivation grows acute, the internal systems lose their ability to function properly, which aggravates the crisis to the point that the body regards a sound sleep as a precursor to death.

The young adult party animal and workaholic needs to ask herself whether existing on four hours of sleep a night is proof that she is superwoman, or a symptom of illness. Since research indicates that humans are hardwired to sleep from eight to ten hours out of each twenty-four-hour cycle, I suggest she take stock of her motion, nutrition, and water intake. Believe it or not, some people are surprised to hear that colas and other caffeinated or sugary drinks are not ideal bedtime libations; likewise a pint of ice cream and gooey desserts act as stimulants, not relaxants. If you can't sleep, maybe you are not getting enough physical exercise during the day. Mental and emotional exercise are different. Your musculature needs a workout; otherwise the body doesn't release endorphins and other neurochemicals that set the stage for a good night's sleep.

Self-Service

After the age of twenty, everyone is in charge of their own health. It's one buck we can't pass to others.

Under twenty is another thing. A dysfunctional child is reacting to the stimulus of her parents' environment and the environment created by society. So is a teenager.

Time Out, Not Time Off

One theory about the role of sleep is that it allows the body an eight- or ten-hour period to focus its resources on doing energy-intensive jobs like digestion, metabolism, cellular housecleaning, and the like. Without the need to expend energy to walk, talk, and otherwise directly interact with the world, the body is able to efficiently rejuvenate itself.

But at twenty, we're old enough to know that help starts with self-help. It's hugely inconvenient, but we can't buy musculoskeletal system function, and we can no longer expect it to just happen on its own. Musculoskeletal system function is now strictly do-it-yourself. It's the work of a lifetime and a lifetime of work.

Here as in every chapter hereafter, I'll write a motion prescription that will enhance musculoskeletal function. From this vantage point—motion and full musculoskeletal system function—we can also deal with conditions that don't seem related, like diet, dehydration, sleep disorders, and many, many others.

You'll notice that there's no Egoscue Method diet program; nor are there Egoscue Method hydration and sleep programs. I'm often asked for advice on those topics and others, but apart from general commonsense guidance, my response is always this: restore and maintain your musculoskeletal system function *first,* and these other things may take care of themselves. At the very least, a strong and fully functional musculoskeletal system will provide a platform to support other therapeutic approaches, without which even the highest of high-tech remedies will surely fail. You need to make mature decisions.

Construction Zone

The two E-cise menus in this chapter are designed to build, restore, and maintain musculoskeletal system function. You'll need to spend from twenty to thirty minutes a day on them. The investment of time will pay huge dividends. You'll feel better, look better, and have more energy, and your work and play time will be more rewarding. There isn't a profession, sport, or recreational activity that isn't enhanced by full function.

As a rule, you should do the E-cises in the order I've presented them. Don't edit the menu to eliminate those that you dislike or feel are wrong for you. The one exception is if an E-cise causes pain (see Chapter 8). Your muscles and joints will let you know when they are working harder than they are accustomed to. When that happens, what you're feeling is growth and accumulating strength. But outright pain that increases in severity as you utilize the muscle or joint means you should stop. Skip to the next E-cise. Come back and try it again the next day. Often as you begin a new menu, your musculoskeletal system is shifting around and will eventually accommodate itself to all the E-cises. If not, check with your doctor. Pain warns that there is a problem.

The body is designed to be symmetrical on both sides. If an E-cise calls for repetitions on one side, it will always be matched with the same number of repetitions on the other. Give both sides equal treatment.

Do the Young Adults Restoration Menu daily for two to three months and then switch to the Young Adults Maintenance Menu. If the second menu is too difficult generally or some individual E-cises are beyond your ability, return to the first menu until you can make a smooth transition. Why the two different menus? Each has a different job. The *restoration* E-cises will restore alignment and reengage your proper muscles. The *maintenance* E-cises will strengthen your musculature, build stability, and provide full range of motion.

[Young Adults Restoration Menu]

▶ FOOT CIRCLES and POINT/FLEXES (Figure 9-1 a, b, and c)

PURPOSE This E-cise reminds your knees, ankles, and feet how to interact according to their designs.

Lie on your back with your left leg extended flat on the floor and your right leg bent toward your chest. For the Foot Circles, clasp your hands behind your bent right knee to hold it in position while you circle your foot clockwise (a). This motion emanates from the ankle, not from the knee. Keep your knee still, and try to make full circles with your foot. (You may tend to make half circles; it will help to slow down and concentrate.) Meanwhile, keep the left foot pointed straight up toward the ceiling, with the left thigh muscles tight. Do forty repetitions, then reverse and circle in a counter-clockwise direction (b). Do forty repetitions. For Point/Flexes, keep your legs in the same position while you flex your right toes back toward the shin. Then reverse direction and point the toes (c). Do forty repetitions. Switch legs and repeat.

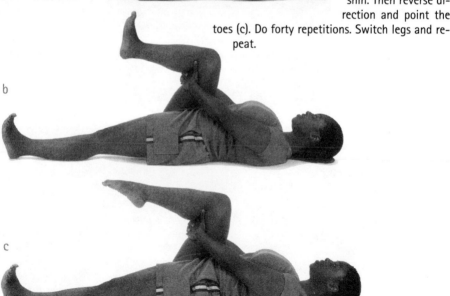

a

b

c

▸ CATS and DOGS
(Figure 9–2 a and b)

PURPOSE This E-cise works the hips, spine, shoulders, and neck in coordinated flexion and extension.

Get down on the floor on your hands and knees. Make a table by aligning your knees with your hips and your wrists with your shoulders. Your lower legs should be parallel with each other and with your hips. Your weight should be distributed evenly. For the Cat, smoothly round your back upward and let your head curl under, to create a curve that runs from your buttocks to your neck—like a cat with an arched back (a). For the Dog, smoothly sway your back down while bringing your head up (b). Make these two moves flow continuously back and forth. Exhale as you move into the Cat position; inhale during the Dog. Do one set of ten repetitions.

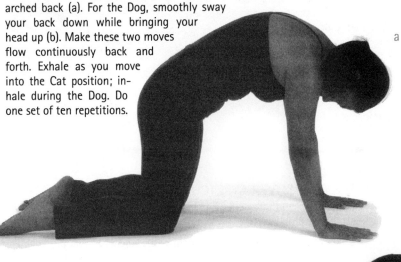

a

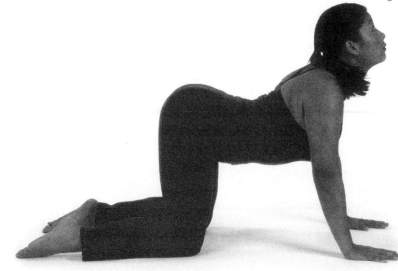

b

▸ HIP LIFT
(Figure 9–3)

PURPOSE This E-cise repositions and levels your hips.

Lie on your back with both knees bent and your feet flat on the floor. Cross your left ankle over your right knee, and press your left knee away from your body. While maintaining this position, lift your right foot up off the floor, bringing both your legs toward your chest. Make sure your hips stay square and on the floor, that your left knee is still pressing out, that your right knee is in line with your right shoulder, and that your hips are still on the floor. Hold this position for one minute. Reverse your legs, and repeat on the other side.

▸ HIP CROSSOVER STRETCH—PALMS UP
(Figure 9–4)

PURPOSE This E-cise counteracts hip rotation on both sides.

Lie on your back with both knees bent and your feet flat on the floor. Place your arms out to each side at shoulder level. Cross your right ankle over your left knee, and rotate the ankle/knee junction in that same direction to the floor. Turn your head so that you are looking in the opposite direction, and relax your shoulders. Press your right knee away from your body with the right hip musculature. Hold this position for one minute. Repeat the E-cise on the opposite side.

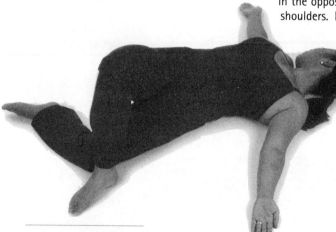

▶ ABDUCTION-ADDUCTION
(Figure 9–5 a and b)

PURPOSE This E-cise engages the muscles on the inside and outside of the thighs, which often interfere with muscle function on the front and rear of the thighs.

Lie on your back with your knees bent at ninety degrees and your feet on the wall. Set your feet parallel to each other on the wall, three or four inches wider than your hips, with your toes pointing up toward the ceiling. Now bring your knees together slowly (a), then move them apart so your feet roll laterally (b). As your feet roll, the bottoms of your feet will leave the wall while the outside edges remain on it. Keep your upper body relaxed. Do three sets of ten repetitions each.

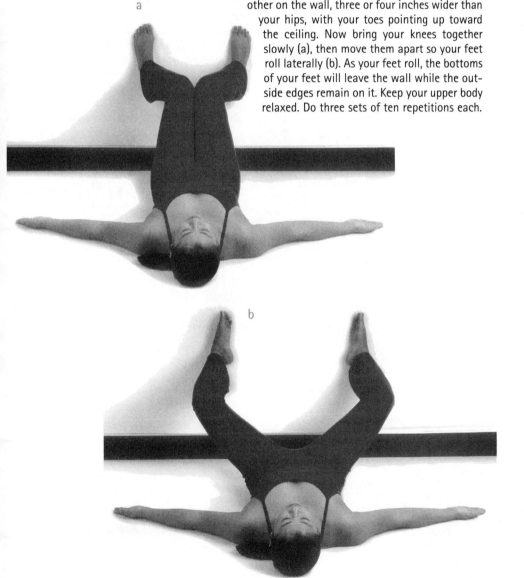

a

b

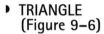

▶ TRIANGLE
(Figure 9–6)

PURPOSE This E-cise puts all the load-joints onto the same vertical plane, where they belong.

Stand with your heels against a wall and your feet parallel, pointed straight ahead. Turn your left foot outward, and take a big step sideways so that your left foot is parallel to the wall, about three inches away from it. Raise both arms at your sides to shoulder level and extend them; keep them against the wall with your palms out. Rotate your hips so both buttock muscles are against the wall. Turn your head to the right, so that you are looking in the direction of the right foot (the one that didn't move). Slide your right hip to the right (keeping it on the wall), while sliding your arms and shoulders up and over in the opposite direction. Look up at your raised right palm, keeping your shoulders and head against the wall, and tucking your left arm and hand behind the left knee. Your arms and shoulders should form a straight line that extends upward from the back of your left hip. Tighten your thighs, and hold this position for one minute. Reverse, and repeat on the other side.

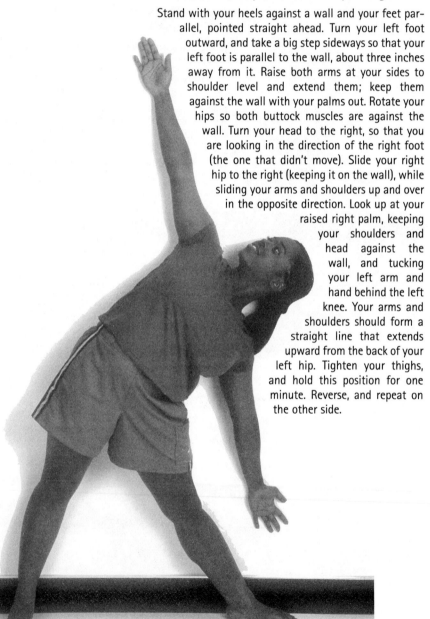

▶ CATS and DOGS
(Figure 9–7 a and b)

Follow instructions that appear earlier in this menu.

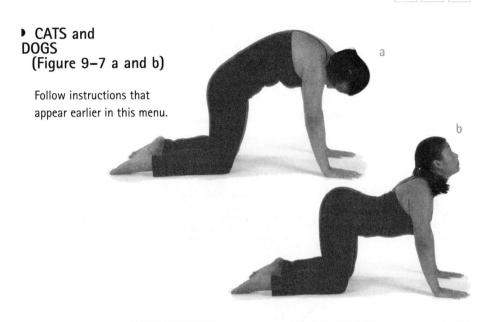

a

b

▶ KNEELING GROIN STRETCH
(Figure 9–8)

PURPOSE This E-cise works to rebalance your hips and shoulders.

From a kneeling position, place your left foot out in front of the right with the knee bent. Place your interlaced hands on the top of your forward bent knee. Lunge forward, but don't let your left knee go beyond the ankle. Keep an arch in your back and your head up and back. Your left foot must point straight forward, and the toes and top of the right foot need to be on the floor pointing straight back. You should feel this E-cise in the groin. Hold this position for one minute. Repeat on the other side.

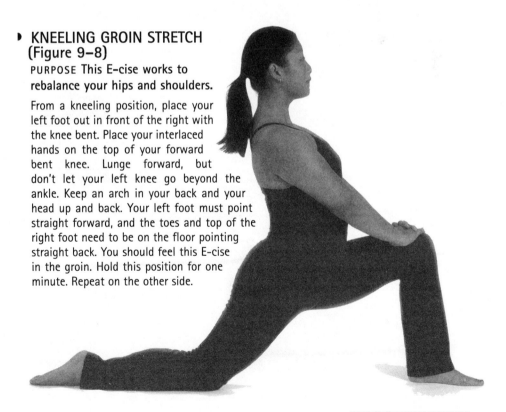

▸ CATS and DOGS
(Figure 9–9 a and b)

Again, follow the instructions that appear earlier in the menu.

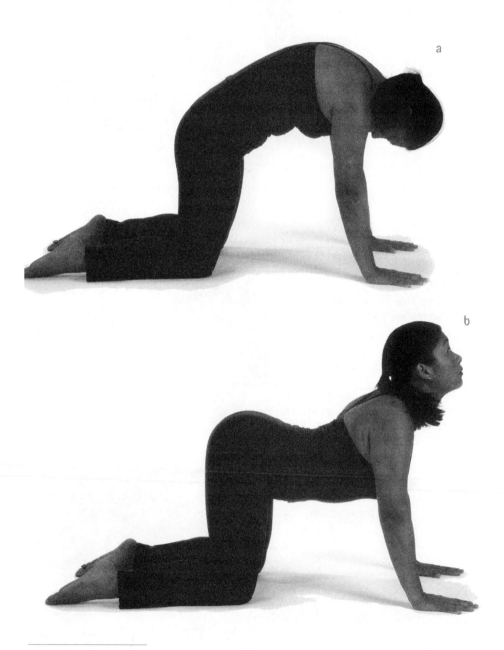

a

b

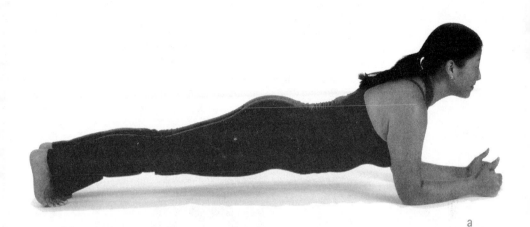

a

- **CORE ABDOMINALS** (front and back only)
  (Figure 9–10 a and b)
  PURPOSE This E-cise gives your deepest layer of
  abdominal muscles a workout.

Position 1: Lie on your stomach propped on your elbows; your
chest is off the floor, and your head is up. Look straight ahead.
Loosely curl your fingers inward on the palms, and extend your
thumbs straight up. Pull your toes under, and bridge your body
off the floor. Your weight is resting on your toes and elbows
(a). Press down and outward on your forearms without moving
your elbows. Roll your hands outward at the wrists, and let
your shoulder blades collapse together. Hold for thirty seconds.

Position 4 (Positions 2 and 3 are not used in this version): Lie
on your back with your legs straight, your heels down and together. Prop your elbows under your shoulders, flex your toes,
and lift your pelvis off the floor (b). Hold for thirty seconds.

b

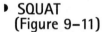

▶ SQUAT
(Figure 9-11)

PURPOSE This E-cise forces the shoulders and hips to remain in alignment while the back goes into extension.

Stand facing a doorjamb, a column, or anything else that you can safely grab on to and that is about chest height, with your feet about six inches apart. Holding the column, keep your elbows straight and tilt your pelvis forward to create an exaggerated arch in your back. Hold this hip position as you bend your knees. When your knees, thighs, and hips are in line and parallel to the floor, stop. Hold this position for one minute.

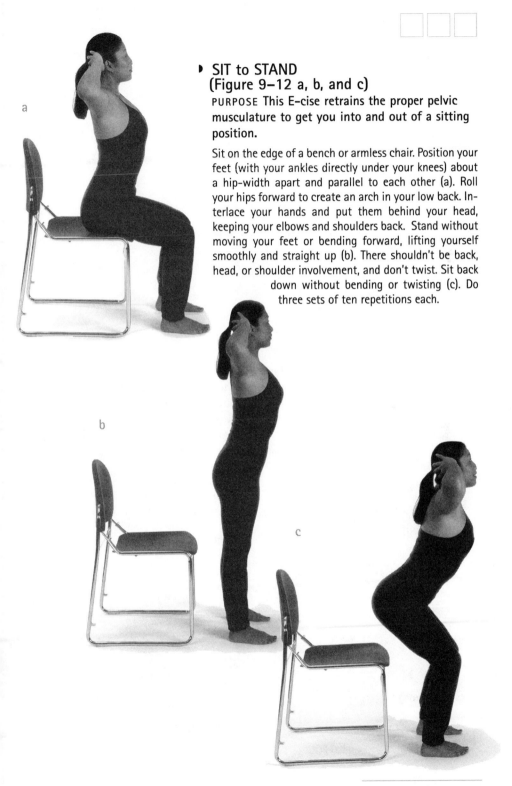

▶ SIT to STAND
(Figure 9–12 a, b, and c)

PURPOSE This E-cise retrains the proper pelvic musculature to get you into and out of a sitting position.

Sit on the edge of a bench or armless chair. Position your feet (with your ankles directly under your knees) about a hip-width apart and parallel to each other (a). Roll your hips forward to create an arch in your low back. Interlace your hands and put them behind your head, keeping your elbows and shoulders back. Stand without moving your feet or bending forward, lifting yourself smoothly and straight up (b). There shouldn't be back, head, or shoulder involvement, and don't twist. Sit back down without bending or twisting (c). Do three sets of ten repetitions each.

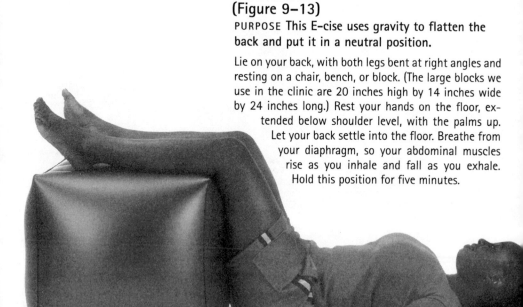

▶ STATIC BACK
(Figure 9–13)

PURPOSE This E-cise uses gravity to flatten the back and put it in a neutral position.

Lie on your back, with both legs bent at right angles and resting on a chair, bench, or block. (The large blocks we use in the clinic are 20 inches high by 14 inches wide by 24 inches long.) Rest your hands on the floor, extended below shoulder level, with the palms up. Let your back settle into the floor. Breathe from your diaphragm, so your abdominal muscles rise as you inhale and fall as you exhale. Hold this position for five minutes.

▸ SUPINE GROIN PROGRESSIVE
(Figure 9–14 a and b)

PURPOSE This E-cise unlocks tight hip flexor muscles.

You'll need to improvise two pieces of apparatus to duplicate the large foam blocks and steps we use in the clinic. I recommend an armless chair or bench and a stepladder. Lie on your back with your right leg resting on the chair or bench, bent at a ninety-degree angle. Extend the left leg straight, placing the heel on the fifteen-inch rung of the ladder. Your foot should be pointed straight at the ceiling; prop it against a book or another heavy object to keep it from flopping to the side. Make sure your feet, knees, hips, and shoulders are in alignment. Hold this position until your low back settles down into the floor (a), which will take ten to fifteen minutes. Then move your foot to the next step down, about ten inches, and hold it there until the back settles (b). Repeat on the five-inch level, and finally do it one last time on the floor. Always, always, repeat the entire cycle on the other side. This E-cise may take as long as an hour, but it's worth it. The more frequently you do this E-cise, the less time it will take for the hip flexors to let go. Eventually, a few minutes at each level will be enough.

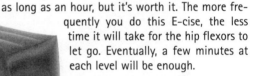

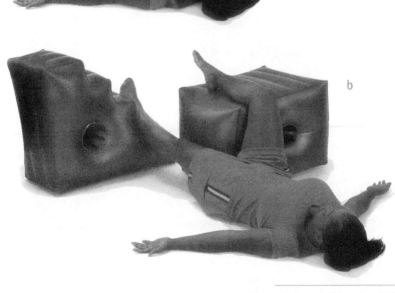

a

b

▸ PELVIC TILTS
(Figure 9–15 a and b)

PURPOSE This E-cise breaks your hips out of their flexion fixation and shows them how to move again from flexion to neutral to extension and back again.

Lie on your back with your knees bent and your feet flat on the floor hip-width apart. Keep your upper back relaxed and your arms out to your sides just below shoulder level, palms up. Make sure your hips, feet, and knees are aligned. Roll your hips backward toward your feet to flatten your back to the floor (a). Then roll your hips away to make an arch in your lower back (b). Remember to breathe in concert with the hip movement—inhale up, exhale down. Do one set of ten repetitions.

a

b

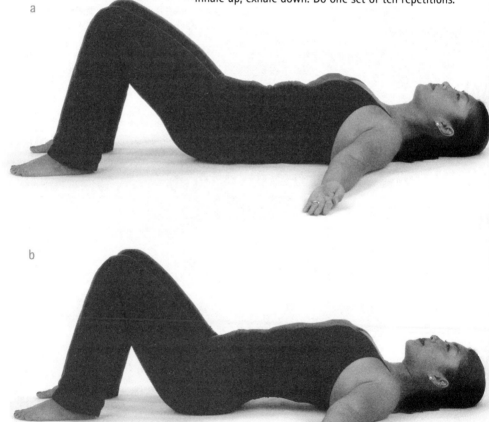

> **STANDING ARM CIRCLES
> (Figure 9–16 a and b)**
> PURPOSE This E-cise
> strengthens the muscles of
> the upper back that are
> involved with the shoulders'
> ball and socket function.

Stand facing a mirror with your feet parallel, about a hip-width apart, your arms at your sides. Curl your fingertips into the pads of each palm (the fleshy area at the base of the fingers), and point your thumbs straight out. This hand position, called the "golfer's grip," is imperative to the success of this E-cise. Squeeze your shoulder blades together, and bring your arms out to your sides at shoulder level, elbows straight. With your palms facing down, thumbs pointing forward, circle up and forward for forty repetitions (a). Now with your palms facing up, circle up and back for forty repetitions (b). Remember to keep your wrists and elbows straight and your shoulder blades squeezed together—the circles must come from the shoulders.

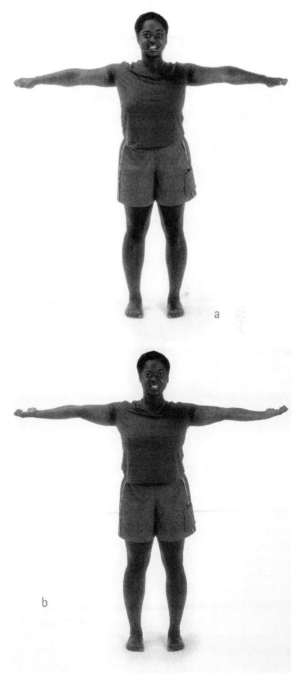

a

b

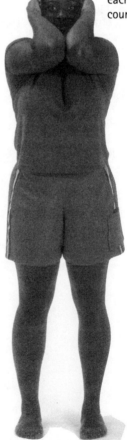

a

▸ STANDING ELBOW CURLS
(Figure 9–17 a and b)

PURPOSE This E-cise reminds the shoulder's "hinge" what full flexion and extension feel like.

Stand with your heels, buttocks, upper back, and head against a wall. Your feet, pointed straight ahead, are about a hip-width apart. Raise your hands in the "golfer's grip" (see Standing Arm Circles), placing your knuckles along your temples, thumbs extended down your cheeks (a). Bring your elbows together to meet in front (b). Make sure your elbows meet in the middle of your body (and are not skewed to the left or right, which would mean that one shoulder is flexing more than the other). Then pull your elbows back even with your shoulders to touch the wall. Your head should remain still, and your knuckles should not lift off your temples. Do one set of twenty-five repetitions; each time your elbows touch counts as one curl.

b

‣ FOOT CIRCLES and POINT/FLEXES
(Figure 9–18 a, b, and c)

PURPOSE This E-cise reminds your knees, ankles, and feet how to interact according to their designs.

Lie on your back with your left leg extended flat on the floor and your right leg bent toward your chest. For the Foot Circles, clasp your hands behind your bent knee to hold it in position while you circle your right foot clockwise (a). The Foot Circles emanate from the ankle, not from the knee. Keep your knee still, and try to make full circles. (You may tend to make half circles; it will help to slow down and concentrate.) Meanwhile, keep the left foot pointed straight up toward the ceiling, with the left thigh muscles tight. Do forty repetitions. Then reverse direction and circle your right foot counterclockwise. Repeat forty times. For the Point/Flexes, keep your legs in the same position. On the bent right leg, bring your toes back toward the shin to flex (b), then reverse the direction to point your toes (c). Switch legs and do forty repetitions of both Foot Circles and Point/Flexes with the left foot.

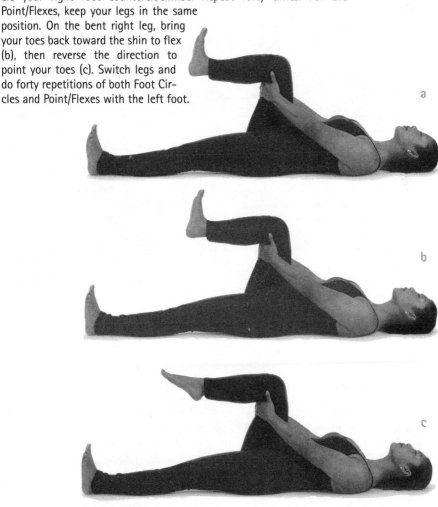

a

b

c

▸ FLOOR BLOCK
(Figure 9–19 a, b, and c)

PURPOSE This E-cise makes use of the shoulder's ball and socket functions, which tend to be neglected.

Lie on your stomach, facedown, your arms over your head. Elevate your arms by four to six inches by placing books or a small foam block under your hands, which you hold in the "golfer's grip" with thumbs pointing toward each other. Lock your elbows, then rotate your arms at the shoulder so your thumbs point at the ceiling. Hold this first position for one minute (a). Move both arms (and blocks) out to forty-five degrees and repeat (b). Finally, move both arms to ninety degrees, and repeat (c). Your hips should be relaxed so your feet are big-toe-to-big-toe, with the heels dropped out to the sides. Hold each position one minute and repeat three times.

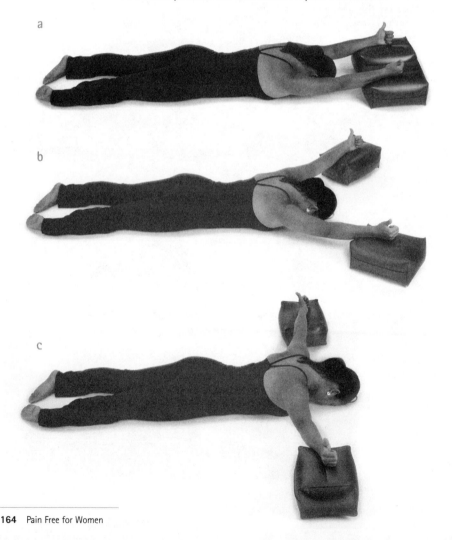

a

b

c

► SITTING FLOOR TWIST
(Figure 9–20 a and b)

PURPOSE This E-cise teaches the spine that it can rotate while the hips remain in place.

Sit on the floor with your legs extended straight in front. Bend your left leg, and cross it over the right, placing it flat on the floor just outside of and slightly below the right knee. Place your right elbow outside the left knee. Roll your hips forward to create an arch in the low back. (Hold this arch throughout.) Now twist your upper body to the left, using your back muscles to rotate your spine. Turn your head to the left as you twist. Support yourself with your left hand on the floor off to the side and behind. Hold this position for one minute and breathe. Your straight leg should be tight, with the toes flexed toward your knee (a). Repeat on the other side (b).

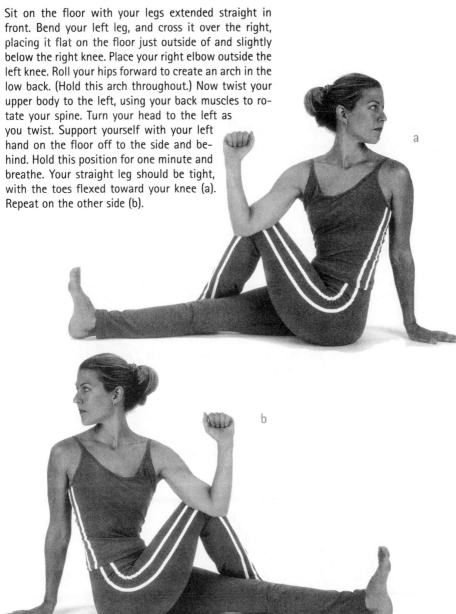

a

b

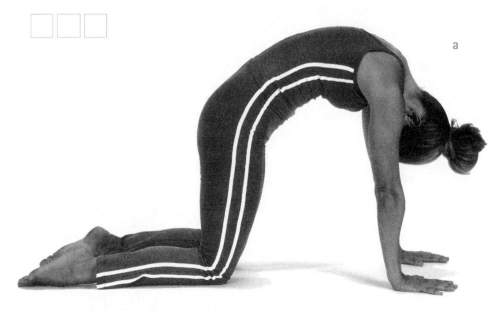

a

CATS and DOGS
(Figure 9–21 a and b)

PURPOSE This E-cise works the hips, spine, shoulders, and neck in coordinated flexion/extension.

Get down on the floor on your hands and knees. Make sure your knees are aligned with your hips, and your wrists with your shoulders. Your lower legs should be parallel with each other and with the hips. Make sure your weight is distributed evenly. For the Cat, smoothly round your back upward as your head curls under to create a curve that runs from the buttocks to the neck—this is the cat's arched back (a). For the Dog, smoothly sway the back down while bringing the head up (b). Make these two moves flow continuously back and forth. Do one set of ten repetitions.

b

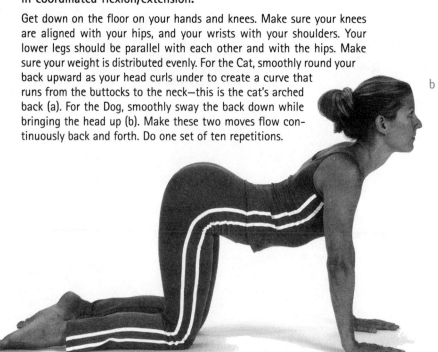

▸ CORE ABDOMINALS
(Figure 9–22 a, b, c, and d)
PURPOSE This four-position E-cise gives your deepest layer of abdominal muscles a workout.

Position 1: Lie on your stomach propped on your elbows; your chest is off the floor, and your head is up. Look straight ahead. Loosely curl your fingers inward on the palms, and extend your thumbs straight up. Pull your toes under, and bridge your body off the floor. Your weight is resting on your toes and elbows (a). Press down and outward on your forearms without moving your elbows. Roll your hands outward at the wrists, and let your shoulder blades collapse together. Hold for thirty seconds.

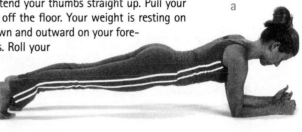

Positions 2 and 3: Lie on your left side propped up on your elbow, feet together, and legs straight. Keep your shoulders, hips, knees, and ankles in a straight line (b). Hold for thirty seconds. Switch sides, and hold for another thirty seconds (c).

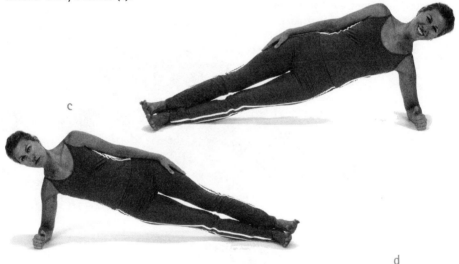

Position 4: Lie on your back with your legs straight, your heels down and together. Prop your elbows under your shoulders, flex your toes, and lift your pelvis off the floor (d). Hold for thirty seconds.

▸ QLO STRETCH
(Figure 9–23 a and b)
PURPOSE This E-cise promotes the lateral stability of the torso.

Sit on the floor with your legs straddled. Make sure you are sitting straight up over your hips and that there's no rolling backward. Flex your feet, so that your knees are pointing straight up. Bend your left elbow, and place it along the inside of your left leg near the knee with the palm facing up. Slide your hand under the left calf. Extend your right arm over your right ear, bending sideways over your left leg and twisting your upper torso slightly. Try to touch your toes with your right arm. Hold for one minute and breathe, making sure your knees and toes are pointing to the ceiling and your thighs are tight (a). Reverse and repeat on the opposite side (b).

a

b

▶ PELVIC TILTS
(Figure 9–24 a and b)

PURPOSE This E-cise breaks the hips out of their flexion fixation and shows them how to move again from flexion to neutral to extension and back again.

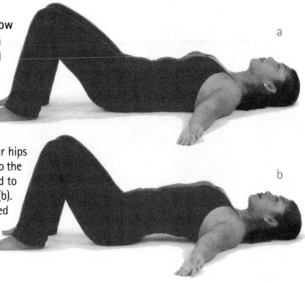

a

Lie on your back with your knees bent and feet on the floor hip-width apart. Make sure your hips, feet, and knees are aligned. Roll your hips backward to flatten your back to the floor (a). Then roll them forward to put an arch in your lower back (b). Keep your upper back relaxed and your arms out to your sides just below shoulder level, palms up. Do one set of ten repetitions.

b

▶ ACTIVE BRIDGES
(with a pillow)
(Figure 9–25 a and b)

PURPOSE This E-cise strengthens the primary hip flexors and lumbar erector muscles.

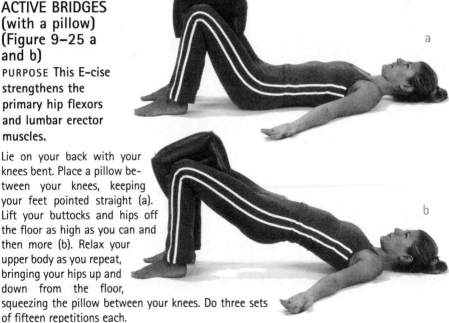

a

Lie on your back with your knees bent. Place a pillow between your knees, keeping your feet pointed straight (a). Lift your buttocks and hips off the floor as high as you can and then more (b). Relax your upper body as you repeat, bringing your hips up and down from the floor, squeezing the pillow between your knees. Do three sets of fifteen repetitions each.

b

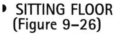

‣ SITTING FLOOR
(Figure 9–26)

PURPOSE This E-cise reconnects and aligns foot, knee, hip, and shoulder functions.

Sit against a wall with your legs straight in front of you. Your buttocks and upper back should be against the wall the entire time. Squeeze your shoulder blades together; do not lift the shoulders—squeeze them back and down. Tighten your thighs, and flex your feet so your toes are pointing back toward you. The keys are to keep your shoulder blades pulled together, your thighs contracted, and your feet flexed. Hold for three minutes.

‣ ABDUCTION-ADDUCTION
(Figure 9–27 a and b)

PURPOSE This E-cise engages the muscles on the inside and outside of your thighs, which often start interfering with the function of the muscles on the front and rear of your thighs.

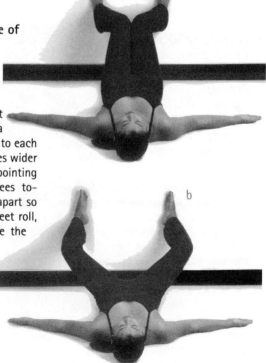

Lie on your back with your knees bent at ninety degrees and your feet on a wall. Keep your feet flat, set parallel to each other on the wall, three or four inches wider than your hips, with your toes pointing toward the ceiling. Bring your knees together slowly (a), then move them apart so your feet roll laterally (b). As your feet roll, the bottoms of your feet will leave the wall where the outside edges remain on it. Keep your upper body relaxed. Do three sets of ten repetitions each.

◗ SPREAD FOOT FORWARD BEND
(Figure 9–28 a, b, c, and d)

PURPOSE This E-cise puts your hips into a neutral position and allows your prime movers to do their jobs without secondary muscles getting in the way.

Stand with your legs spread about as far as they will go without your feet flaring out. Go to the limit on this one. Bending forward at the hips will help get you into the stretch.

Position 1: Bend forward at the hips, and with both hands touch the floor in front of you (a). If this is too difficult, use a small block or book for elevation. Tighten your thighs, and relax your torso toward the floor. Hold this position for one minute.

Position 2: Without straightening up, slide your hands in front of your left foot, keeping both thighs tight and the torso relaxed (b). Hold one minute.

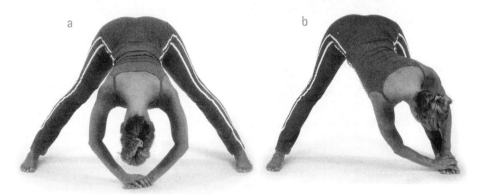

Position 3: Move your hands back to the starting center position briefly, then slide them in front of the right foot, keeping the thighs tight and torso relaxed (c). Hold one minute.

Position 4: Slide your hands back to the center starting position, keeping the thighs tight and torso relaxed (d). Hold for one minute.

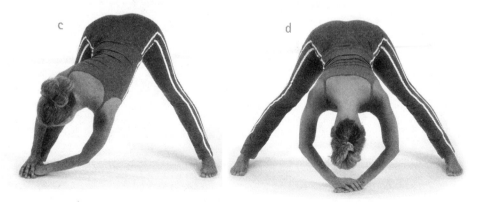

▶ RUNNER'S STRETCH
(Figure 9-29 a and b)

PURPOSE This E-cise reminds the body that when the pelvis extends on one side, it flexes on the other (and vice versa).

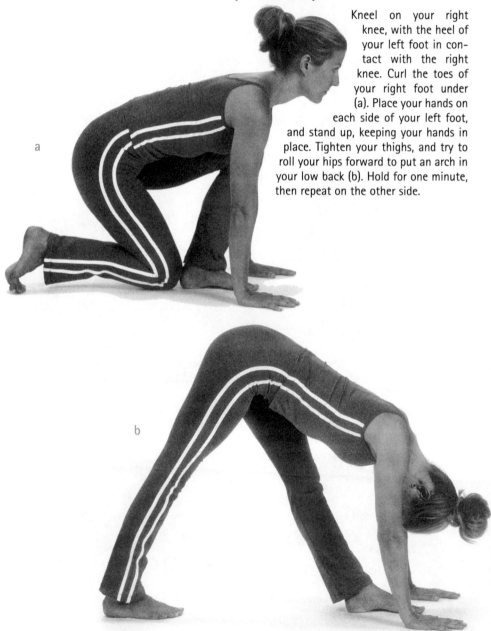

Kneel on your right knee, with the heel of your left foot in contact with the right knee. Curl the toes of your right foot under (a). Place your hands on each side of your left foot, and stand up, keeping your hands in place. Tighten your thighs, and try to roll your hips forward to put an arch in your low back (b). Hold for one minute, then repeat on the other side.

▸ DOWNWARD DOG
(Figure 9–30 a and b)
PURPOSE This E-cise reestablishes linkage from the
wrist to the feet.

Assume the Cats and Dogs position (a). Curl your toes under,
and push with your legs to raise your torso until you are off
your knees and your weight is resting on your hands and feet.
Keep pushing until your hips are higher than your shoulders
and have formed a tight, stable triangle with the floor (b). Your
knees should be straight, your calves and thighs tight. Don't let
your feet flare outward; keep them pointing straight ahead in
line with your hands, which need to stay in place—no creeping
forward! Your back should be flat, not bowed, as your hips push
up and back into the heels. Breathe. If you cannot bring your
heels flat onto the floor, get them as close as possible. Don't
force them. It may take several sessions before they go all
the way down. Hold this position for one minute.

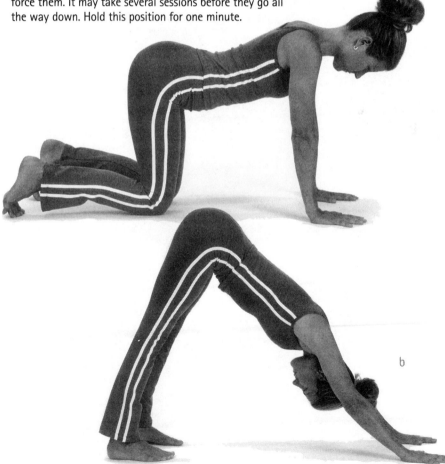

a

b

▶ SUPINE GROIN PROGRESSIVE (Figure 9–31 a and b)

PURPOSE This E-cise unlocks tight hip flexor muscles.

You'll need to improvise two pieces of apparatus to duplicate the large foam blocks and steps we use in the clinic. I recommend an armless chair or bench and a stepladder. Lie on your back with your right leg bent at ninety degrees and resting on the chair or bench. Extend the left leg straight out, placing the heel on the fifteen-inch rung of the ladder. Prop the foot against a book or some other similar object to keep it from flopping to the outside. It should be pointed straight at the ceiling. Make sure the feet, knees, hips, and shoulders are in alignment. Hold this position until your low back settles down into the floor (a). It will take ten or fifteen minutes. Now move your left foot to the next step down, about ten inches. Hold it there until the back settles (b). Repeat on the five-inch level, and finally one last time on the floor. *Always, always, repeat the whole cycle on the other side.* It may take as long as an hour, but it's worth it. The more frequently you do this E-cise, the less time it will take for the hip flexors to let go.

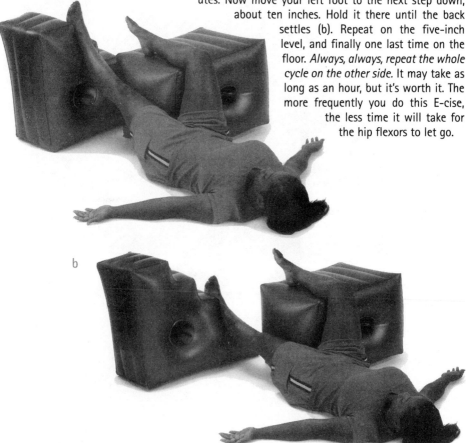

a

b

▶ PELVIC TILTS
(Figure 9–32 a and b)
Follow instructions that appear earlier in this menu.

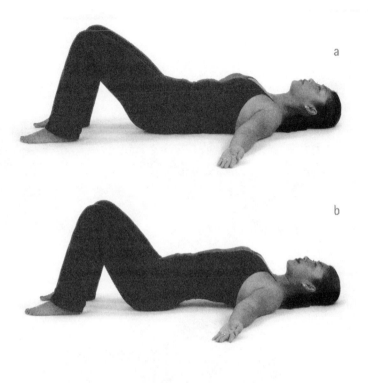

a

b

A few final points about procedure. You should do these E-cises every day. After the first three months, if you miss a day here or there, it's no big deal. More than that, however, and you'll notice that the menu will take longer and be more physically demanding. A long layoff may mean you're giving in to your dysfunctions.

As a father of three daughters, I know it's not always possible to build an ideal future for our youth; things turn out differently from what we'd planned. But by regaining musculoskeletal system function, young adults can build themselves for the future.

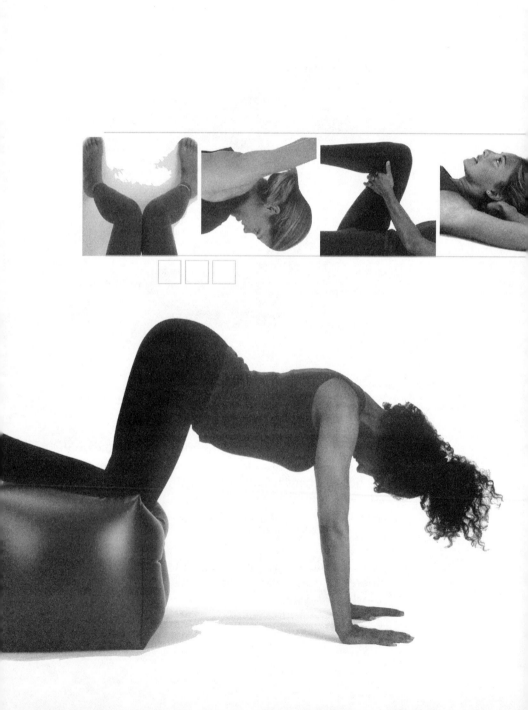

CHAPTER 10

birth right

Hang on. I'm about to challenge conventional wisdom—big-time—with my belief that the musculoskeletal system plays a fundamental role in conception, pregnancy, and parturition. Increasingly, thanks to an ever more motionless environment, young women today arrive at the threshold of motherhood in desperate need of the muscular and skeletal strength and structure that allow them to step through the gateway to a new life and mission without facing unnecessary risk, complications, pain, and the very real possibility of having their dreams shattered. I believe musculoskeletal system dysfunction is a factor in infertility, miscarriages, difficult pregnancies and deliveries, premature birth, birth defects, and postpartum problems. As alarming as these statements sound, this chapter will tell you not only what the risks are and why they exist but what you can do to eliminate them.

In the Loop

The human body is crammed full of extremely sensitive built-in transmitters and receptors (the exact number is unknown) that are constantly monitoring every internal sys-

A Suggestion

Perhaps you're not planning on motherhood and are just passing through on the way to a chapter that seems more relevant to your circumstances. If that's the case, you might hang around long enough to learn about the body's intricate communications network (in "In the Loop" and "Twists and Turns"). This health asset is possessed by all women. Also, my unorthodox take on the mechanics of conception, pregnancy, and parturition may provide insights that you'll want to pass along to family members, friends, and colleagues who are headed for motherhood.

tem and process, from skin rashes on the surface to the deepest inner workings of the organs. The data stream flows from head to foot, much like the river of water that is constantly washing through us (and that plays a key part in moving data along as well). The body is so closely interconnected and interrelated that it depends on this elaborate information network for precise coordination on both the macro and micro levels.

Keep this in mind when you notice in the mirror that one shoulder is higher than the other or that your upper torso rotates slightly to the right or left. It takes a practiced eye to see these symptoms of musculoskeletal system dysfunction, but the body knows all about them (Figure 10–1). Your body, as you gaze into the mirror, is making countless adjustments, from muscle tone to metabolism, from red blood cell formation to lymphatic flow. Close your eyes, and you will probably notice subtle shifts and movements in your knees or hips, as proprioceptors (the specialized receptors of the musculoskeletal system) register the information that your ocular senses are switched off. If we could tune in to this communication loop, we'd be deafened by the racket and the roar. The soundtrack would blow the speakers off the bookshelf.

While every part of the body may not be aware in real time of what every other part of the body is doing, it's safe to say that they operate on a need-to-know basis. In a healthy body, no piece of vital information fails to get through to receptors that have a primary interest in what's happening elsewhere. A simple example is a runny nose caused by cold or wet feet. The temperature change is signaling the mucous membrane of the sinuses to dilate and flush the nasal passages to expel viruses and foreign particles.

This process is stimulus and response in action. No stimulus goes

Fig. 10–1

unnoticed or unresponded to. That sentence may not be grammatically correct, but it conveys a fact. Another fact is that the musculoskeletal system is as plugged in to the information network as any other system and perhaps more so. Only three internal systems provide platforms for total sensory networks. Like the circulatory system, with its canal work of veins and arteries, and the central nervous system, with its neural branches and tendrils, the musculoskeletal system crosses all borders and enters every region of the body. Proprioceptors scan every skeletal muscle, tendon, and joint. As pervasive as it is, when the musculoskeletal system responds to a stimulus, it has an impact throughout the body. Stub your toe, for instance, and your eyes may instantly tear up. News travels fast and is shared between separate "circuits" of sensors. When the news is dysfunction—such as "This muscle is not capable of performing the task you are about to assign it"—the rest of the body responds to the stimulus through this information-sharing process. Hundreds of minute and gross adjustments are made, such as in blood pressure, hormonal flow, respiration, and the like.

Thus the musculoskeletal system and the rest of the body's systems know when an athlete is not ready to run a marathon or balance her way across a ford at Rock Creek in Washington (like Yolanda in Chapter 3). But it knows when a woman is not ready to conceive and give birth. It doesn't check blood chemistry or assess uterine function. That's the job of enteroceptors, which watch the inner workings of the organs. Rather, it knows when the muscles, joints, and bones aren't up to the job. It's that information (stimulus) that gets passed on to the rest of the body for processing and response.

Twists and Turns

Moms and expectant moms are athletes, perhaps the ultimate ones. After millions of years of experience, the female human body knows how demanding a "sport" childbirth really is. The top priority of all living organisms is survival, and the human body is no exception. We do not give up without a fight. An ingenious arrangement of overlapping layers of redundant systems allows the body to improvise its way around and through potentially life-threatening situations. If one route is blocked, it chooses another. This arrangement accounts for much of humankind's ability to endure and flourish.

Consider the body's primary digestive system. If something like a famine interferes with it substantially, another system takes over to break down and metabolize fat that has been stored away for emergency fuel. Breathing is another example. The lungs are designed to fill with air when the muscles of the diaphragm contract and then relax to create a vacuum as the lungs expand in the direction of the abdominal cavity. But if that doesn't happen (and for many people with skeletal misalignment it doesn't, because the hips get in the way), the body switches to raising and lowering the shoulders to pump the chest cavity like an old-fashioned bellows to allow air to flow in and out of the lungs.

Like Odysseus, the Greek warrior and wanderer, the human body is a thing of "many ways," of "twists and turns." But this adaptability has its limits, and when those limits are reached, the body puts on the brakes to prevent destruction. Many cases of female infertility are exactly that—cases of slamming the brakes.

Out of every hundred cases of infertility, thirty to forty involve sperm inadequacy or gonadal deficiencies in the male partner. The rest are the result of ovulatory or hormonal problems, chemical imbalances in the vaginal or cervical environment, disorders of the fallopian tubes, or unknown causes. Are these conditions merely bad luck and confirmation that the body is fragile, or are they a response to stimulus that's coming from other sources? In short, is infertility a disease or a symptom?

I really don't know the answer for sure. But I do know that, in the general population, most women who are treated for infertility also have major musculoskeletal system dysfunction. It's entirely possible, even likely, that their bodies are reading the data stream and being told that, with major muscle groups weak and disengaged, deficient bone density, poor balance, minimal metabolic activity, pandemonium in the endocrine system, and other negatives, the fertilization of an egg and its implantation in the uterine wall would jeopardize the life of the mother and/or the embryo. Hence, the body stops the conception process before it can go too far.

Does it happen to every woman with musculoskeletal system dysfunction? No. But the right combination of dysfunction, severity, duration, general lifestyle, and other factors could push a woman over the edge into this *protective* infertility. Yes, there are other words to attach to infertility, like *heartbreaking* and *frustrating*. But let me explain what I mean by *protective*.

Pregnancy is not a nine-month disease; nevertheless it is a major event that requires enormous effort and entails no small amount of physical trauma. The body is programmed to know the implications and the requirements for success. It only makes sense (and everything about the body makes sense) that a fail-safe mechanism would kick in to defend a woman from the clear and present danger of conception in order to allow her time and opportunity to recover from the musculoskeletal system disorder so she can successfully bear children later. This recovery option is an essential part of the protective mechanism. It's predicated on evolutionary precedent. Time and time again musculoskeletal system function has been restored as women interacted with their changing environment; for example, the famine ended, or some other communal or personal crisis abated. The danger passed.

The problem today is that our environment is static. What we're doing today is pretty much like what we'll be doing tomorrow or the next day. So the musculoskeletal system disorder and the dangers remain. It's not a woman's *fault*, or a doctor's *fault*. Fault is not the issue. But as infertility specialists and their desperate patients attempt to work around these symptoms of disorder, they are in effect searching for a way to disconnect the protective mechanism without correcting the underlying problem that triggered it in the first place. They are switching off the blaring smoke detector, but the fire is still burning. The body is reading the transmission from the musculoskeletal system's proprioceptors loud and clear. There may be other medical reasons for a woman's infertility, and just as I would expect an infertility specialist to remedy them tirelessly, I would like to see a woman's musculoskeletal system being used in behalf of conception, not against it. The body is a unit, and its functional *unity* is paramount. By shrugging off the manifestations of ill health—which is exactly what the symptoms of musculoskeletal system dysfunction amount to—we are losing the opportunity to explore *all* the possibilities for solving the problem and restoring fertility.

Modern medicine is capable of miracles, but we don't need miracles to restore musculoskeletal system function. A little knowledge, a little effort, and a little diligence will do nicely. We shouldn't be trying to force the body to ignore the stimulus it's receiving from the muscles, joints, and bones. We can change the stimulus—and the response—by getting the body moving again according to its basic design. (See the E-cise menus in this chapter.) That may or may not be the entire answer to infertility, but the musculoskeletal system's message, at least, will change from "No way!" to "Good to go!"

Keeping Count

What about male infertility? I was afraid you'd ask. Not because the answer will be inconsistent but rather because it involves veering toward the darker, gloomy side of the street. The average male sperm count appears to be dramatically declining in various parts of the world, including the United States and Western Europe. One controversial study in the early 1990s, which analyzed the data from sixty-two separate sperm-count projects, spotted a 50 percent decline in the previous fifty years in the industrialized world. The decline did not appear across the board, though; some areas showed no change at all. Skeptics question the study's methodology and scoff at dire predictions that, if the trends continue, American men will become totally sterile by the year 2020.

I wouldn't want to bet one way or the other, but whatever its precise magnitude, a decline in sperm count and semen quality does appear to be taking place, and it is a cause for concern. The production of human sperm is an energy-intensive process. A healthy man can produce 500 million sperm with each ejaculate. Like every bodily process that requires energy production and utilization—and they all do—the manufacture of sperm requires a robust metabolism.

Men whose major muscle groups are disengaged do not have an efficient metabolism, and that has an impact on their sperm production. In keeping with the body's demand/response nature, if there's no demand to build major muscles, then there will be limited production of testosterone, the muscle-building hormone that, like sperm, is a product of the male testes. Testosterone is also involved in spermatogenesis. But if it is in short supply because there is no muscle demand, there's that much less of it to contribute to sperm creation.

Protection at a Price

This figure is a shocker: it's estimated that from 40 to upward of 50 percent of all pregnancies (all fertilized eggs) end in miscarriage, or what's also known as spontaneous abortion. Most of these miscarriages usually occur before the woman knows she is pregnant. Among known pregnancies, the miscarriage rate is approximately in the range of 10 to 15 percent.

The almost routine occurrence of what should be a relatively rare event is alarming. Historically, miscarriages were treated as unusual and serious health mishaps. And they are. Having failed to block conception, miscarriage is the body's last-ditch effort to protect the life of the mother and possibly to deny life support to a defective embryo or fetus. While far more drastic, this too is a protective mechanism.

When the body spontaneously aborts, it is not malfunctioning. It's doing its job, albeit a sad, painful, and potentially dangerous one. But the fact that it is being called on to do it for roughly half of all pregnancies indicates that something is wrong. The human body is not wasteful. It is designed to efficiently use scarce resources. Casually throwing away reproductive resources doesn't make sense.

Many women who suffer repeated miscarriages fear that they have anatomical problems, but the majority, when examined by a physician, are told they do not. Their cervix and uterus are normal. But actually those women probably *do* have an anatomical problem: their pelvises are out of proper design position to conceive and bear children without difficulty. Although women with various degrees of musculoskeletal system dysfunction do deliver healthy babies, the difficulties created by this dysfunction may contribute to the high rate of miscarriage, as well as to birth defects and childhood disorders like autism.

To illustrate how important a factor this is, I'm going to provide a full page of drawings, but first I want to offer an analogy that may seem a trifle strange, but helps explain what's going on with the pelvis.

Consider, by analogy, the sinus cavities. When the spine's S-curve is lost to misalignment and the head tips forward and down, the sinuses cannot drain properly. Gradually, as the dysfunction becomes more and more pronounced, it changes the pH of the membrane (the measure of its acidity or alkalinity), altering the viscosity and flow. With less acidity, the sinuses are on the way to becoming a sweet, swampy breeding ground for minor irritations and major infections. The environment in the sinus cavity may become more or less toxic—all because of musculoskeletal dysfunction.

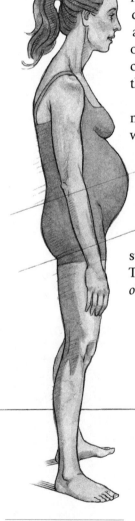

Fig. 10-2

Similarly, skeletal misalignment and muscular weakness often tip the pelvic cavity or bowl back, up, and under (see Figure 10-2). This position can change the abdominal, uterine, and vaginal flows as well as the pH of the membranes. Like the sinus cavity, they can become hostile environments, and possibly they may taint the embryo's amniotic cavity, or "swimming pool."

To say that there is a conclusive direct link between miscarriage or birth defects and tainted amniotic fluid would be going way too far. But the issue is certainly worth putting on the table for your consideration, particularly since prior to or during a pregnancy, such pelvis disparities can be remedied with E-cises.

Another reproductive structure that's possibly put in harm's way by skeletal misalignment is the placenta, the lifeline from the mother to the embryo-fetus that supplies respiration, nutrition, excretion, and hormones. The danger is summed up in *Human Anatomy and Physiology*, a popular text for medical students:

> Previously it was thought that the placenta constituted an impervious barrier, preventing all deleterious substances in the mother from reaching the developing individual. Scientists are now of the opinion that most, if not all, chemicals and drugs ingested by the mother, hormones, and even certain viruses may cross the placenta. . . . Typically, these potentially harmful agents must achieve a harmful concentration before they result in damage to the embryo or fetus. It is no longer a question of whether or not an agent will cross the placenta, but rather whether or not it reaches the tissue of the unborn in a harmful concentration.

Embryo-fetal development is therefore taking place with a permeable placenta that's immersed in possibly toxic buildups in the pelvic cavity. More often than not, human fetuses survive their nine-month marinade in amniotic fluid, and seemingly healthy babies are born; tragically the endings, and beginnings, are not always happy, and cherished babies are lost or delivered with serious birth defects.

Rock-a-Baby

The place where human babies come from is best described as the "pelvic cradle." But the incubator of life is no placid petri dish; it is right in the center of the action. Not only does the pelvis protect the fetus with its bony armored plating, it ensures that the fetus receives 360 degrees of stimulation, agitation, and fortification. It's nine full months of shake, rattle, and roll.

There are much quieter places to locate a nursery, but none of them would offer the combination of amenities provided by the pelvis. It serves a dual purpose as the place of insemination and gestation. Located near the base of the spine, it has no shortage of neural babysitters to monitor every nanosecond of development. It offers space to grow and move, warmth, ready access to fuel supplies, plumbing to remove waste and refresh vital fluids and hormones, a convenient nearby exit when the time comes, and in the meantime beaucoup action—lots and lots of action. As Mom walks, bends, twists, and turns, the zygote-blastocyst-embryo and then (after eight weeks of development) the fetus is bumped, jostled, sloshed, shaken, and otherwise goaded into human form. Sherwin B. Nuland in *The Wisdom of the Body* remarks on the wondrous process of combining three primitive layers of cells into all the right bits and pieces.

> For this to happen, various cell groupings . . . will migrate, twist, turn, glide, fold, bend, lengthen, branch, fuse, split, thicken, thin, dilate, constrict, hollow out, form pockets, pinch off, adhere, separate—it's all like some Busby Berkeley movie sequence, but on a much grander scale. Hundreds of millions of dancers appear and they all participate, forming themselves into the shapes of various tissues and organs.

This dance wouldn't occur so perfectly without the action-oriented pelvic environment powered by major muscle groups. They rock the cradle back and forth, from side to side, and up and down. As the abdominal muscles contract and relax, they act like fingers kneading dough.

Musculoskeletal system dysfunction, however, can turn the cradle into a dead zone. As the pelvic structure goes into a state of dysfunctional flexion, it tips back, under, and down. The hip components, which are designed to move forward and back together or individually, actually jam in the forward position, and that reduces the volume of the pelvic bowl, dampens and stifles the motion-rich environment, and constricts fetal movement. Try this experiment: Walk around with your feet pointed straight, your shoulders back, and your back arched. Put your hands on your lower abdominal area as you walk.

What do you feel? Your abdominal muscles are hard at work. There's a lot of activity under way. Now turn your feet out, let your head and back slump, and walk around some more. All the muscle work shifts away from the pelvic cradle, to the periphery of the hips and thighs. Much like the mischief that the changed head position causes in the sinus cavity, the fresh fluids in the uterine environment stagnate and alter in chemical character. The fetus, thanks to musculoskeletal system dysfunction, is now both understimulated and overexposed to toxins and other hazards. It helps explain why 200,000 babies a year—7 percent of all live births—are born with defects.

Too Little, Too Late

The number of premature births is rising for the same reason.* As in a miscarriage, the body's sensory system picks up on the changing pelvic climate and reacts to it by attempting to expel the fetus before it reaches full term. Depending on how toxic the environment is or the possible extent of the damage, the timing of the expulsion varies and can be delayed long enough to increase the child's chances of survival outside the womb despite his or her lack of development. It would be

*The overall rate for premature births in the United States rose by 0.3 percent from 1989 to 1996, according to the Centers for Disease Control and Prevention. The 8 percent increase for white women was offset by a 10 percent decrease among black women, and smaller declines for Asians and Hispanics. Even so, black babies were still more than twice as likely to be born premature as white ones.

comforting to think that the body is rescuing the fetus, but the motive is actually a rescue mission on behalf of the mother.

The body is powerless, however, to reverse the ultimate structural impediment to birth that's created by musculoskeletal system dysfunction. Tipped back, under, and up (Figure 10–3), the pelvis is in the wrong position for the baby to smoothly drop into the birth canal and slide through the pelvic opening to the outside world.

Fig. 10–3

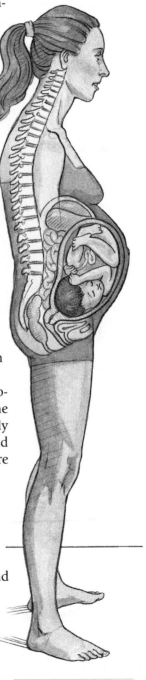

The female pelvis is designed to flare in the last weeks or days of pregnancy to tip the structure's bottom rim down and out of the way. Imagine a bowl being emptied—that's what's supposed to happen. But a pelvis in flexion doesn't flare and empty the bowl. The bottom rim is swinging upward.

The baby has a problem. In a functional pelvis, thanks to the flare, the baby's head is positioned more or less over the birth canal so gravity will help it drop. The uterus forms something of a chute, at roughly a sixty-five-degree angle, ascending from the front to the back of the mother's body. But a dysfunctional pelvis pulls the head forward and away from the birth canal, so it's riding up and forward on the rim of the bowl. Tucked up into a nice little bundle, the baby should be doing a slow-motion clockwise somersault into the canal. Instead it's cartwheeling in the opposite direction.

Here comes the cesarean knife, or hours of prolonged labor while the baby fights her way into the canal. Thirty years ago cesarean sections were relatively rare. Now they are fairly common. Major surgery and birth are becoming synonymous. That's a drastic cure for a nine-month illness.

Pregnancy in Older Women

I don't subscribe to the point of view that blames infertility, miscarriages, birth defects (like autism, the rate of which appears to be doubling every five years in the United States), premature births, and difficult labor on the baby-boom generation's preference for delaying pregnancy past the more traditional childbearing window of the late teens to late twenties. That's a little too easy, and it smacks of blaming women and their inherent "frailty."

No, the body does not have a fertility and childbearing on-off switch that's tied to a preordained timetable. Not even for menopause, which I'll focus on in Chapter 13. There are wide variations. Some women have difficulty at age twenty, while others make it look easy at forty. But isn't that true not just of the reproductive system, but of all our internal systems? A teenager may have a delicate stomach and digestive tract, while her seventy-year-old grandmother has a cast-iron belly. Age isn't relevant. The causal factors could range from genes to poor diet. This range of possibilities, other than age, could explain why some women have trouble conceiving and bearing children and others don't.

As modern women put off starting families until later in life, they do have more problems conceiving and difficult pregnancies. But the problem is not age as such. The fact is that after three or four decades of sedentary lifestyles, not to speak of a lack of development in childhood, they bring to the childbearing process a whole set of musculoskeletal system dysfunctions.

This is not an intractable situation, however, for someone interested in getting pregnant in her thirties or forties. A good place to start is the "Getting Pregnant and First-Trimester Menu." After a few weeks of following this menu, muscular disengagement, skeletal misalignment, and structural instability will begin to reverse. Give it four to six months prior to conception. A year is even better. While the body responds quickly to the correct stimulus, cumulative stimulus builds strength that locks in functions. It also helps establish the motion habit.

Pregnancy Prep

The E-cise menus ahead are designed to reposition the pelvis, strengthen the muscles, and stabilize other structures. The best time to undertake the program is before you are pregnant. It will take a month to six weeks to show results. But the E-cises are not strenuous, and if your obstetrician approves, you could start them as late as your seventh month. (But when you start, use the menu appropriate to the trimester that you're in.) If you've been doing the menu in the last chapter, switch over to these for the duration of your pregnancy. If you feel pain as you're doing any of the E-cises, drop it from the menu.

Remember, the idea is to correct your skeletal misalignment and boost your metabolism. That will take time. The more you move functionally according to design, the more you'll be able to move.

The first menu does double duty for women who are having trouble getting pregnant and for those in their first trimester of pregnancy. The reason for this is that we need to realign the skeleton and engage the proper muscles to facilitate conception in the first instance, and to realign the skeleton and engage proper muscles to facilitate gestation and deliver in the second. I'm using the same E-cises for both because the degree of difference in dysfunction and function between them is usually extremely narrow but just enough to have an impact on conception. The goal for heretofore "infertile" women is to gain sufficient musculoskeletal system function to allow an egg to be fertilized and the body to recognize that it is viable. And the goal for those who have achieved pregnancy is to build on the small extra measure of function that has allowed them to get to that point so that they'll have a better chance of going to full term.

▶ **FOOT CIRCLES and POINT/FLEXES
(Figure 10–4 a and b)**

PURPOSE This E-cise reminds your knees, ankles, and feet how to interact according to their designs.

Lie on your back with your left leg extended flat on the floor and the other leg bent toward your chest. For the Foot Circles, clasp your hands behind your bent knee to hold it in position while you circle your foot clockwise (a). The Foot Circles emanate from the ankle, not from the knee. Keep your knee still, and try to make full circles. (You may tend to make half circles; it will help to slow down and concentrate.) Meanwhile, keep the left foot pointed straight up toward the ceiling, with the left thigh muscles tight. Then reverse the direction and circle your right foot counterclockwise. For Point/Flexes, keep your legs in the same position. On the bent right leg, bring your toes back toward the shin to flex (a), then reverse the direction to point your toes (b). Switch legs and repeat both the Foot Circles and the Point/Flexes. Do a set of forty each (forty circles one way, forty the other, and forty Point/Flexes) with each foot.

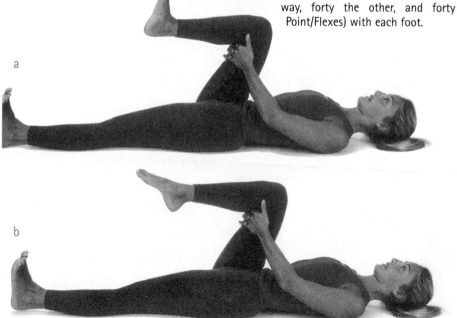

a

b

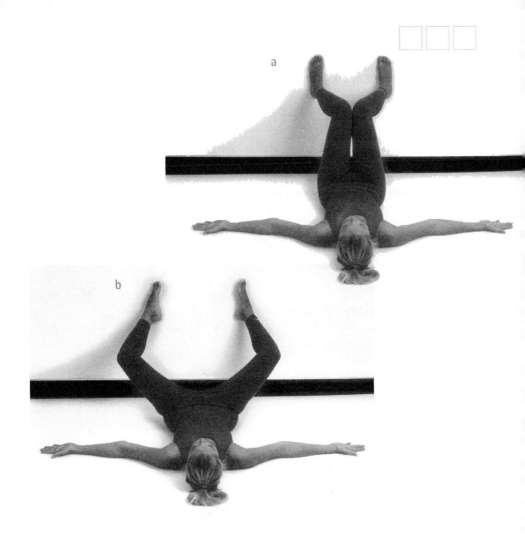

a

b

▸ ABDUCTION–ADDUCTION
(Figure 10–5 a and b)

PURPOSE This E-cise engages the muscles on the inside and outside of the thighs, which often interfere with muscle function on the front and rear of the thighs.

Lie on your back with your knees bent at ninety degrees and your feet on the wall. Set your feet parallel to each other on the wall, three or four inches wider than your hips, with your toes pointing up toward the ceiling. Now bring your knees together slowly (a), then move them apart so your feet roll laterally (b). As your feet roll, the bottoms of your feet will leave the wall while the outside edges remain on it. Keep your upper body relaxed. Do three sets of ten repetitions each.

▸ MODIFIED FLOOR BLOCK (MFB)
(Figure 10–6)

PURPOSE This E-cise puts the load-joints into the same plane.

Lie on your stomach with your forehead on the floor. Your feet should be pigeon-toed and your buttocks relaxed. Elevate your bent arms six inches by placing your forearms and elbows on whatever you are using as blocks. Breathe, and relax your upper body. Don't press your arms into the blocks. Let your stomach and chest fall into the floor, which will cause your hips to tilt forward. Hold for six minutes. Use this position as the starting point for the next two E-cises.

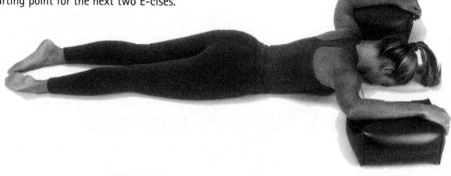

▸ MFB—PRONE ANKLE SQUEEZES
(Figure 10–7)

PURPOSE This E-cise retrains the buttock muscles (the "glutes") to operate without "help" from other muscles.

Stay in the Modified Floor Block position. Place a foam block or pillow between your ankles, and bend your knees to a ninety-degree angle. Without letting go, squeeze and release the block or pillow with your ankles, and feel the contraction in your buttocks. Do three sets of twenty repetitions each.

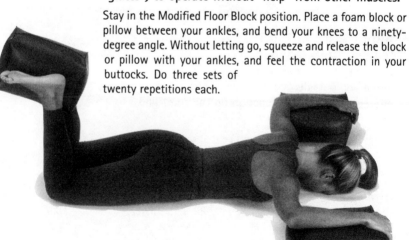

▶ MFB—PRONE HAMSTRING CURLS
(with a strap)
(Figure 10–8 a and b)

PURPOSE This E-cise makes the hamstrings work independently.

Stay in the Modified Floor Block position. With your feet hip-width apart, place a strap around your ankles, and press outward on the strap (a). While maintaining constant pressure on the strap, bring your feet up to your buttocks (b), and then lower them to the floor. Relax your upper body into the floor and control the motion. Do three sets of ten repetitions each.

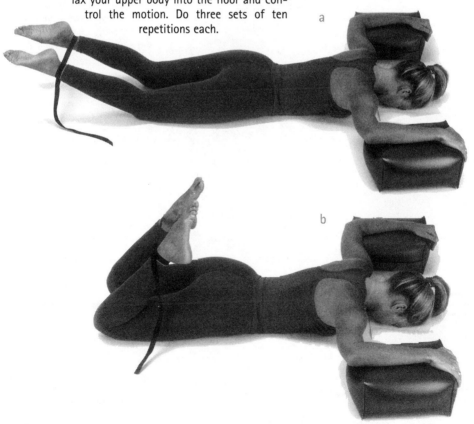

a

b

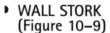

▶ WALL STORK
(Figure 10-9)

PURPOSE This E-cise levels the hips into a parallel position, under a load that's held in vertical alignment.

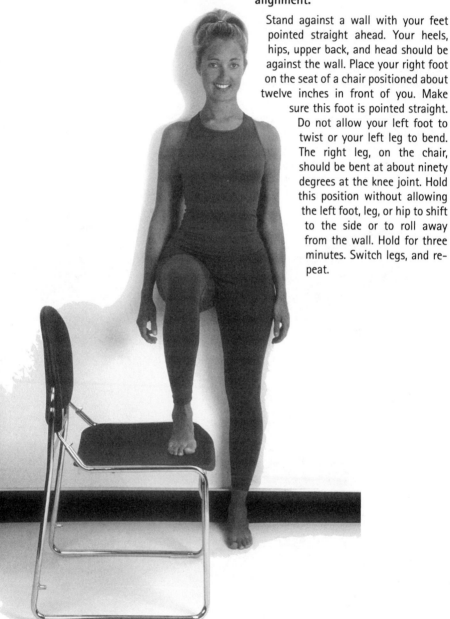

Stand against a wall with your feet pointed straight ahead. Your heels, hips, upper back, and head should be against the wall. Place your right foot on the seat of a chair positioned about twelve inches in front of you. Make sure this foot is pointed straight. Do not allow your left foot to twist or your left leg to bend. The right leg, on the chair, should be bent at about ninety degrees at the knee joint. Hold this position without allowing the left foot, leg, or hip to shift to the side or to roll away from the wall. Hold for three minutes. Switch legs, and repeat.

▸ HIP FLEXOR ABDOMINALS
(Figure 10–10 a and b)

PURPOSE This E-cise strengthens the hip flexor muscles.

Lie on your back with your knees bent, feet flat on the floor, and your hands clasped behind your head. Keep your elbows out to the side (a). Lift your knees, keeping them in line with the hips and bending them into the groin no more than ninety degrees. Simultaneously, lift your head and shoulders off the floor by about two inches, to perform an abdominal crunch (b). Do two sets of twenty-five repetitions each.

a

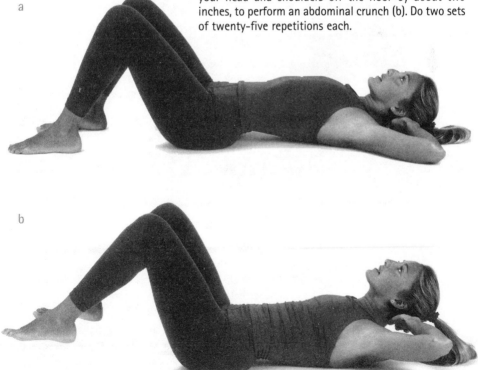

b

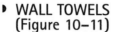

▶ WALL TOWELS
(Figure 10–11)

PURPOSE This E-cise reestablishes the lost S-curve of the spine. Holding the towels in place prevents the hips and shoulders from moving away from the wall.

Stand against a wall with your feet pointed straight ahead and hip-width apart. Your heels should be two to three inches from the wall. Your buttocks, upper back, and head should be against the wall. Place a rolled-up towel (about 3½ inches in diameter) behind your low back and another behind your neck. In this position you'll perform the following three E-cises.

▶ WALL TOWELS—GLUTEAL CONTRACTIONS (not illustrated)

PURPOSE This E-cise prevents the torso from rotating or getting the low back involved in the work of the buttock muscles.

In the Wall Towels position described above, keep your shoulders and upper back relaxed, and begin to squeeze and release your buttock muscles. Don't squeeze so hard that your buttocks come off the wall. Make sure your feet don't flare out. Squeeze simultaneously on both buttocks, not separately. Do three sets of twenty repetitions each.

▶ WALL TOWELS—SCAPULAR CONTRACTIONS (not illustrated)

PURPOSE This E-cise counteracts shoulder and hip rotation with the towels while engaging and activating the shoulder blades.

In the Wall Towels position, hold your arms against the wall at about a forty-degree angle, palms out. Slowly and evenly squeeze and release your shoulder blades. Do three sets of twenty repetitions each.

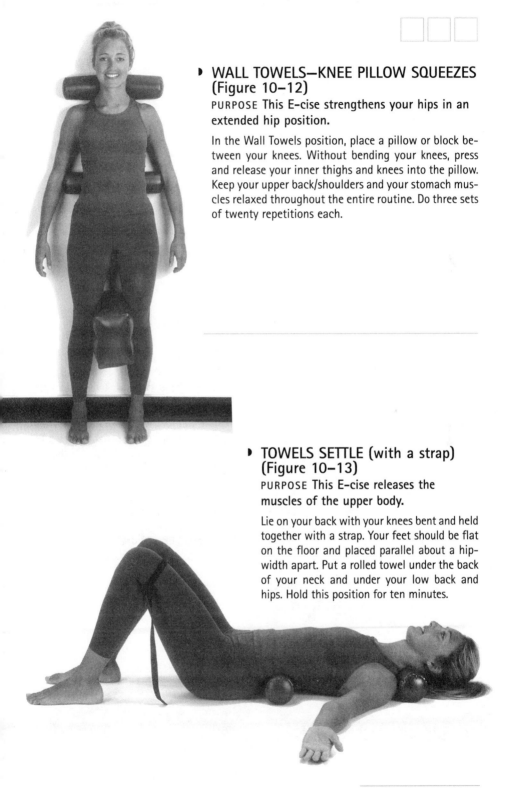

▸ WALL TOWELS—KNEE PILLOW SQUEEZES (Figure 10–12)

PURPOSE This E-cise strengthens your hips in an extended hip position.

In the Wall Towels position, place a pillow or block between your knees. Without bending your knees, press and release your inner thighs and knees into the pillow. Keep your upper back/shoulders and your stomach muscles relaxed throughout the entire routine. Do three sets of twenty repetitions each.

▸ TOWELS SETTLE (with a strap) (Figure 10–13)

PURPOSE This E-cise releases the muscles of the upper body.

Lie on your back with your knees bent and held together with a strap. Your feet should be flat on the floor and placed parallel about a hip-width apart. Put a rolled towel under the back of your neck and under your low back and hips. Hold this position for ten minutes.

▶ SUPINE GROIN—TOWELS
(Figure 10–14)

PURPOSE This E-cise disengages your groin muscles and those along the outside of your thighs, as the towels hold the hips level and keep your neck in a design position.

Lie on your back on the floor, with the right leg bent at a right angle and resting on a block, bench, or chair. The left leg extends straight out on the floor, with the foot propped on the outside to keep it pointing up. Extend your arms out to the side at forty-five-degree angles (resting on the floor). Place towels as you did in Towels Settle. Relax your upper body, your knees, and your feet. The longer you are in this position, the more your back will settle into the floor. Breathe from your diaphragm. Hold for fifteen minutes, switch sides, and repeat.

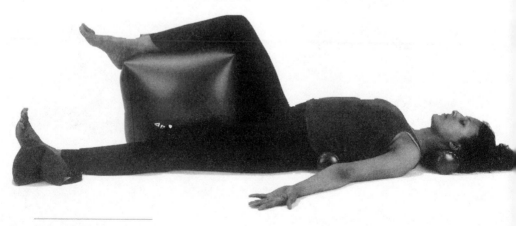

▶ STATIC EXTENSION
(Figure 10–15)

PURPOSE This E-cise tackles hip rotation. Hips that "rotate" are actually twisting to the right or left and disrupt knee and ankle function. If you look closely in the mirror, one hip will appear to be a little nearer to the mirror than the other.

Kneel on a large block (approximately three feet square) with your hands on the floor ahead of you. Keep your elbows straight and locked while you ease your hips in front of your knees. (Please refer to the photograph.) You don't want your knees and hips to align one atop the other, or for your hips to be behind your knees. The idea is to let the pelvis swing free and engage with the upper torso. Allow your low back to arch, with the movement coming from the tilt of your pelvis. Your shoulder blades should collapse together and form a distinct valley. Keep your elbows straight. Drop your head, and hold the position. If your low back begins to hurt, back your hips up toward your knees a bit. This will also make it easier on your arms. Hold this position for three minutes.

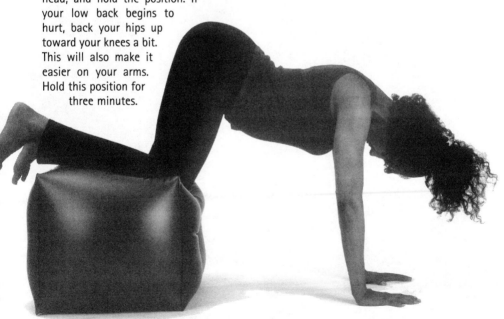

▸ **STAIR CRABS**
(Figure 10–16 a and b)
PURPOSE This E-cise strengthens and balances the hips.

Stand at the bottom of a flight of stairs. Bend over, and place the palms of both hands on the third step (a). Bring your right foot to the third step and place it outside your right hand (b). Do the same with the left foot. Don't lift your hands off the stairs. Repeat the procedure for the next step up and so on. Do two sets of ten repetitions each.

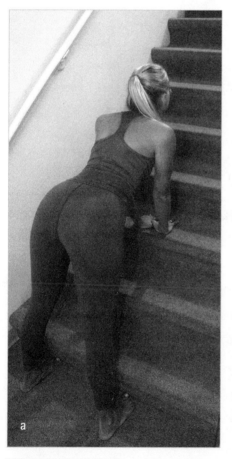

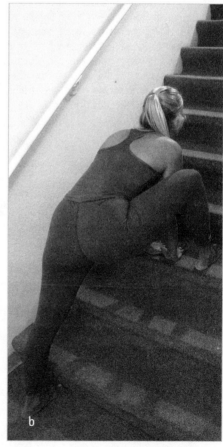

[Second-Trimester Pregnancy Menu]

▶ **STANDING ARM CIRCLES (with a pillow) (Figure 10-17)**

PURPOSE This E-cise strengthens the muscles of the upper back that are involved with the shoulders' ball and socket function. The pillow keeps the hips in place, instead of popping up or twisting laterally.

Stand facing a mirror with your feet pointed straight ahead and with a doubled-up pillow or a foam block held between your knees. The pillow should be six to eight inches thick. Don't scrunch it hard, just hold it in place. Loosely curl your fingertips into the pads of each palm (the fleshy area at the base of the fingers), and point your thumbs straight out, forming the "golfer's grip." Squeeze your shoulder blades together, and bring your arms out to your sides at shoulder level, elbows straight. With your palms facing down, circle up and forward for the repetitions specified. With your palms facing up, circle up and back for the desired repetitions. Remember to keep your feet straight and your shoulder blades squeezed together. Do two sets (one forward, one back) of forty repetitions each.

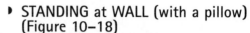

▸ STANDING at WALL (with a pillow) (Figure 10–18)

PURPOSE This E-cise reminds the body what an upright and truly vertical posture feels like.

Stand with your heels, buttocks, upper back, and head against a wall. If you cannot get your head against the wall without straining too hard, then place it in a comfortable and relaxed position. Relax your stomach muscles and your arms. Let your body settle into this new position. Place a doubled-up pillow or foam block (six or eight inches thick) between your knees. It should feel as though it's pushing your knees slightly apart. Do not squeeze or push in on it—we want it to trigger some of your hip muscles to help stabilize you in this position. Make sure that your feet remain pointed straight ahead for the entire E-cise and that your stomach is relaxed out. Hold this position for five minutes.

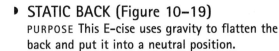

▶ STATIC BACK (Figure 10–19)

PURPOSE This E-cise uses gravity to flatten the back and put it into a neutral position.

Lie on your back, with both legs bent at right angles and resting on a chair, bench, or block. (The large blocks we use in the clinic are 20 inches high by 14 inches wide by 24 inches long.) Rest your hands palms up on the floor; your arms are at your sides below shoulder level. As you let your back settle into the floor, breathe from your diaphragm so your abdominal muscles rise as you inhale and fall as you exhale. Hold for five minutes.

▶ STATIC BACK—PULLOVER PRESSES (Figure 10–20)

PURPOSE This E-cise reminds the shoulders' ball and socket that it is not exclusively a hinge.

Stay in the Static Back position. Extend both arms straight back behind your head with your hands clasped, elbows locked. Press your clasped hands into a block or pillow, and release. Don't contract your abdominal muscles. Let your low back muscles react. Keep your feet parallel to each other. Do three sets of ten repetitions each.

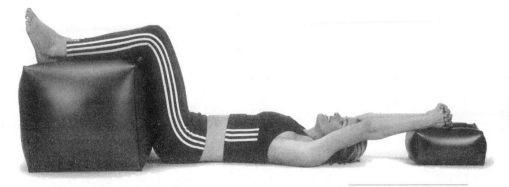

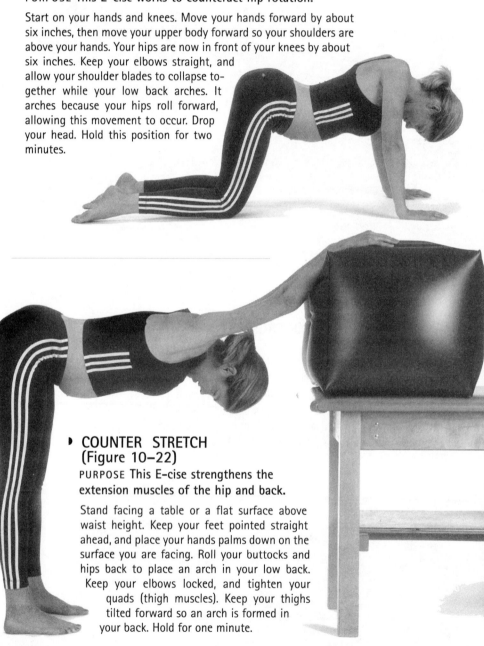

▸ STATIC EXTENSION POSITION
(Figure 10–21)

PURPOSE This E-cise works to counteract hip rotation.

Start on your hands and knees. Move your hands forward by about six inches, then move your upper body forward so your shoulders are above your hands. Your hips are now in front of your knees by about six inches. Keep your elbows straight, and allow your shoulder blades to collapse together while your low back arches. It arches because your hips roll forward, allowing this movement to occur. Drop your head. Hold this position for two minutes.

▸ COUNTER STRETCH
(Figure 10–22)

PURPOSE This E-cise strengthens the extension muscles of the hip and back.

Stand facing a table or a flat surface above waist height. Keep your feet pointed straight ahead, and place your hands palms down on the surface you are facing. Roll your buttocks and hips back to place an arch in your low back. Keep your elbows locked, and tighten your quads (thigh muscles). Keep your thighs tilted forward so an arch is formed in your back. Hold for one minute.

‣ DOWNWARD DOG
(Figure 10–23 a and b)

PURPOSE This E-cise reestablishes linkage from the wrists to the feet.

Assume the Cats and Dogs position. Curl your toes under, and push with your legs to raise your torso until you are off your knees (a).

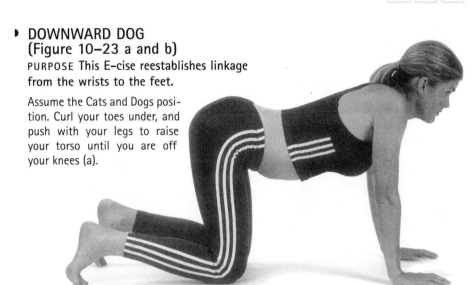

a

Keep pushing until your hips are higher than your shoulders and you have formed a tight, stable triangle with the floor. Your knees should be straight, your calves and thighs tight. Don't let the feet flare outward; keep them pointing straight ahead in line with your hands, which need to stay in place—no creeping forward! Your back should be flat, not bowed, as your hips push up and back into your heels (b). Breathe. If you cannot bring your heels flat onto the floor, get them as close as possible, but don't force them. It may take several sessions before they go all the way down. Hold for one minute.

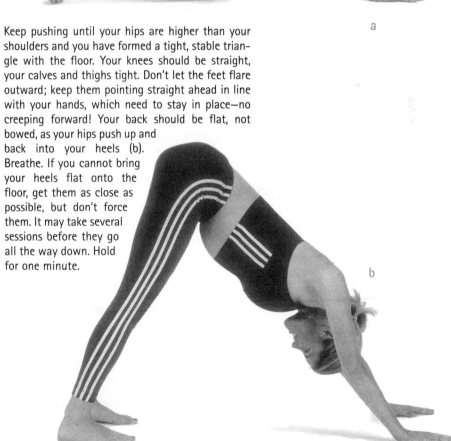

b

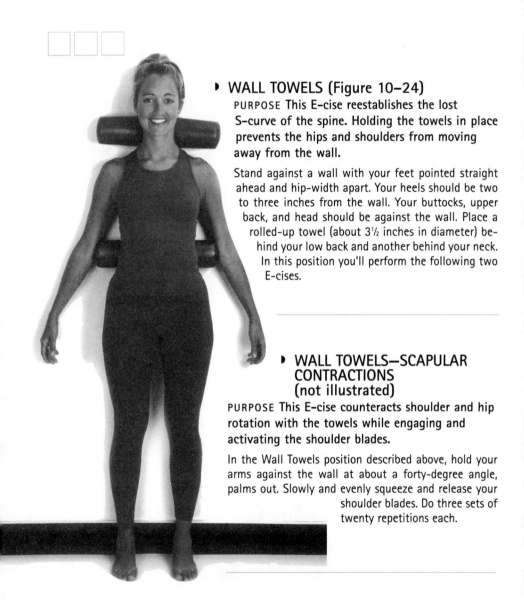

▶ **WALL TOWELS (Figure 10-24)**

PURPOSE This E-cise reestablishes the lost S-curve of the spine. Holding the towels in place prevents the hips and shoulders from moving away from the wall.

Stand against a wall with your feet pointed straight ahead and hip-width apart. Your heels should be two to three inches from the wall. Your buttocks, upper back, and head should be against the wall. Place a rolled-up towel (about 3½ inches in diameter) behind your low back and another behind your neck. In this position you'll perform the following two E-cises.

▶ **WALL TOWELS—SCAPULAR CONTRACTIONS**
(not illustrated)

PURPOSE This E-cise counteracts shoulder and hip rotation with the towels while engaging and activating the shoulder blades.

In the Wall Towels position described above, hold your arms against the wall at about a forty-degree angle, palms out. Slowly and evenly squeeze and release your shoulder blades. Do three sets of twenty repetitions each.

▶ **WALL TOWELS—GLUTEAL CONTRACTIONS**
(not illustrated)

PURPOSE This E-cise prevents the torso from rotating or getting the low back involved in the work of the buttock muscles.

In the Wall Towels position, keep your shoulders and upper back relaxed, and begin to squeeze and release your buttock muscles. Don't squeeze so hard your buttocks come off the wall. Make sure your feet don't flare out. Squeeze simultaneously on both buttocks, not separately. Do three sets of twenty repetitions each.

▶ SITTING STATIC ABDUCTOR PRESS (Figure 10–25)

PURPOSE This E-cise equalizes the strength of the abductor muscles of the thighs, requiring them to work without cheating by using gravity to swing the thigh from side to side.

Sit on a bench or the edge of a chair with your feet pointed straight ahead, a hip-width apart and directly under your knees. Place a strap around your legs just under your knees, and pull it taut so your knees are together. Relax your stomach, and put an arch in your low back by rolling your hips forward. Push out on the strap. Release. Make sure to keep the arch in your back throughout. Do one set, squeezing and releasing for five minutes.

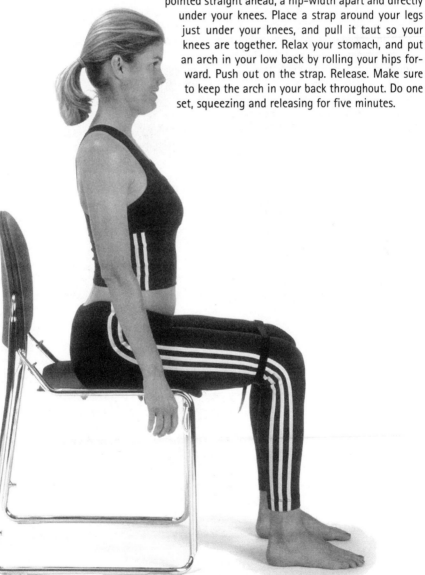

▶ CATS and DOGS
(Figure 10–26 a and b)

PURPOSE This E-cise works the hips, spine, shoulders, and neck in coordinated flexion and extension.

Get down on the floor on your hands and knees. Make a table by aligning your knees with your hips and your wrists with your shoulders. Your lower legs should be parallel with each other and with your hips. Your weight should be distributed evenly. For the Cat, smoothly round your back upward and let your head curl under, to create a curve that runs from your buttocks to your neck—like a cat with an arched back (a). For the Dog, smoothly sway your back down while bringing your head up (b). Make these two moves flow continuously back and forth. Exhale as you move into the Cat position; inhale during the Dog. Do one set of ten repetitions.

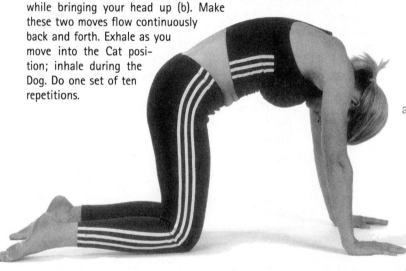

a

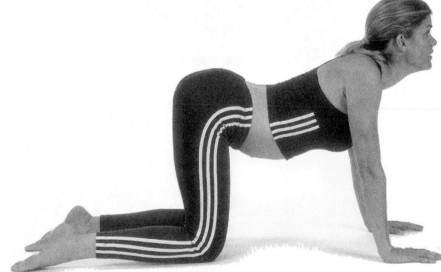

b

[Third-Trimester Pregnancy Menu]

▶ **SITTING KNEE PILLOW SQUEEZES**
(Figure 10–27)
PURPOSE This E-cise strengthens the hip-
stabilizer muscles.

Sit on the edge of a chair with a pillow or foam block
between your knees. (In the clinic our blocks are about
seven inches thick.) Roll your pelvis forward to
put an arch in your low back. Your feet should
point straight ahead, about a hip-width
apart, positioned under your knees. Squeeze
and release the pillow between your knees.
Remember to keep the arch in your low
back. Do three sets of twenty each.

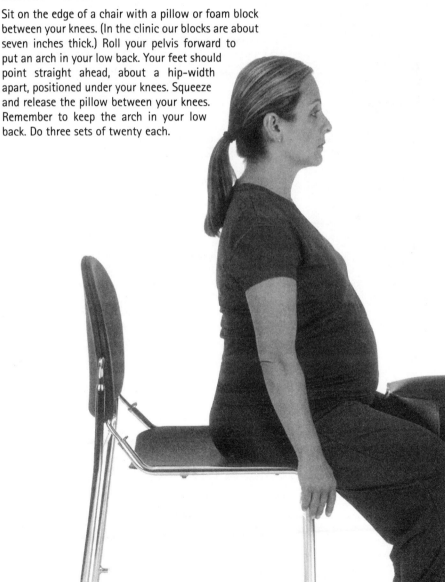

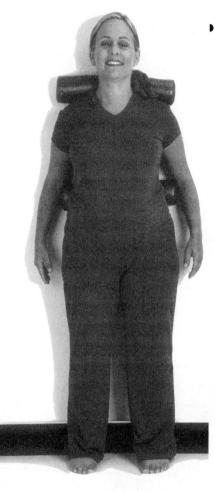

▸ WALL TOWELS
(Figure 10–28)

PURPOSE This E-cise reestablishes the lost S-curve of the spine. Holding the towels in place prevents the hips and shoulders from moving away from the wall.

Stand against a wall with your feet pointed straight ahead, a hip-width apart. Your heels should be two to three inches from the wall. Your buttocks, upper back, and head should be against the wall. Place a rolled-up towel (about 3½ inches in diameter) behind your low back and another behind your neck. In this position you'll perform the following three E-cises.

▸ WALL TOWELS—
GLUTEAL CONTRACTIONS
(not illustrated)

PURPOSE This E-cise prevents the torso from rotating or getting the low back involved in the work of the buttock muscles.

In the Wall Towels position described above, keep your shoulders and upper back relaxed, and begin to squeeze and release your buttock muscles. Don't squeeze so hard your buttocks come off the wall. Make sure your feet don't flare out. Squeeze simultaneously on both buttocks, not separately. Do three sets of twenty repetitions each.

▶ WALL TOWELS—
SCAPULAR CONTRACTIONS
(not illustrated)

PURPOSE This E-cise counteracts shoulder and hip rotation with the towels while engaging and activating the shoulder blades.

In the Wall Towels position, hold your arms against the wall at about a forty-degree angle, palms out. Slowly and evenly squeeze and release your shoulder blades. Do three sets of twenty repetitions each.

▶ WALL TOWELS—KNEE PILLOW SQUEEZES
(Figure 10–29)

PURPOSE This E-cise strengthens the hips in an extended hip position.

In the Wall Towels position, place a pillow or block between your knees. Press and release your inner thighs into the pillow without bending your knees. Keep your upper back/shoulders and your stomach muscles relaxed throughout the entire routine. Do three sets of twenty repetitions each.

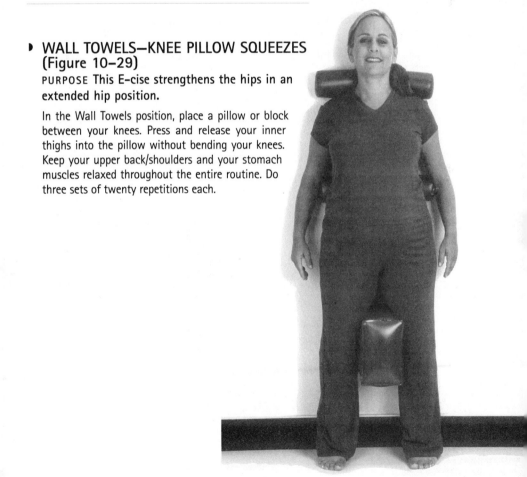

▶ STATIC EXTENSION POSITION
(Figure 10–30)

PURPOSE **This E-cise works to counteract hip rotation.**

Start on your hands and knees. Move your hands forward by about six inches, then move your upper body forward so that your shoulders are above your hands. Your hips are now in front of your knees by about six inches. Keep your elbows straight, and allow your shoulder blades to collapse together while your low back dips to form the tail of an S-curve. It dips because your hips roll forward, allowing this movement to occur. Drop your head. Hold this position for two minutes.

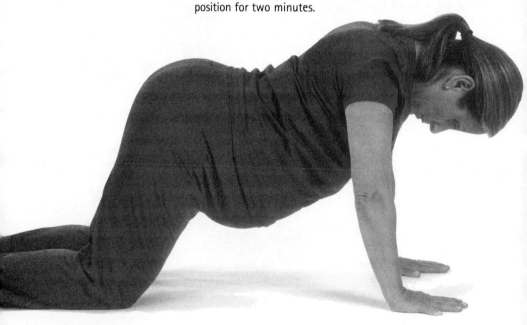

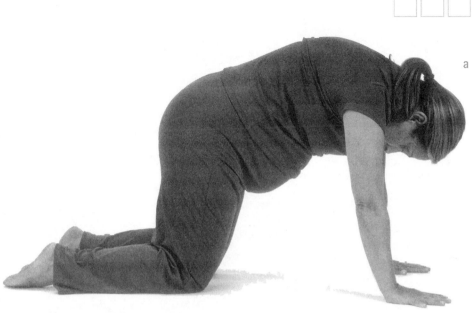

a

‣ CATS and DOGS
(Figure 10–31 a and b)

PURPOSE This E-cise works the hips, spine, shoulders, and neck in coordinated flexion and extension.

Get down on the floor on your hands and knees. Make a table by aligning your knees with your hips and your wrists with your shoulders. Your lower legs should be parallel with each other and with your hips. Your weight should be distributed evenly. For the Cat, smoothly round your back upward and let your head curl under, to create a curve that runs from your buttocks to your neck—like a cat with an arched back (a). For the Dog, smoothly sway your back down while bringing your head up (b). Make these two moves flow continuously back and forth. Exhale as you move into the Cat position; inhale during the Dog. Do one set of ten repetitions.

b

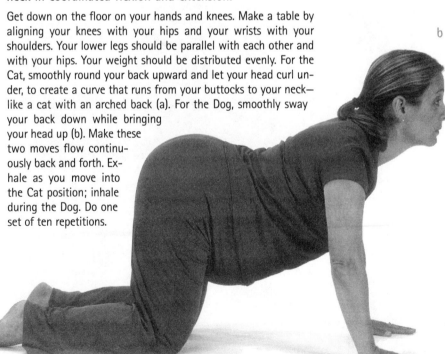

▸ SITTING KNEE PILLOW SQUEEZES (Figure 10–32)

Follow instructions that appear earlier in this menu.

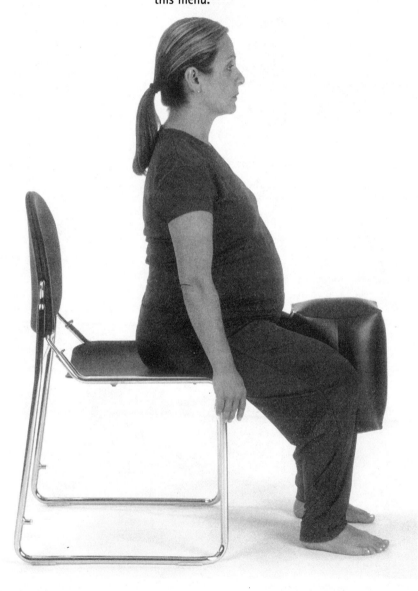

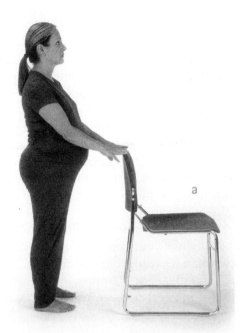

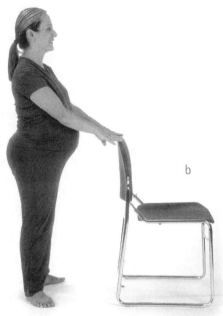

a

b

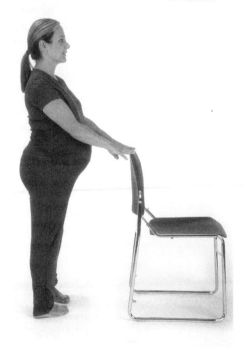

> **THREE-POSITION TOE RAISES**
> **(Figure 10–33 a, b, and c)**

PURPOSE This E-cise lets the feet and ankles know how it feels to go through their proper range of motion during flexion and extension without interference from hip and knee dysfunction.

For all three positions, stand with your head and shoulders back, with an arch in your low back. Face a pillar, doorjamb, or the back of a chair with your feet about a foot away. Hold on with both hands for support, but don't lean forward, and don't tense your shoulders.

Position 1: Place your feet about a hip-width apart with the toes pointed straight ahead (a). *Position 2:* The toes point outward (b). *Position 3:* Your toes point in (c). In each position rise up onto the balls of your feet and all five toes of each foot, then lower your heels back to the floor. Throughout, it is very important to keep your body aligned vertically so your hips remain over your heels. Don't rock. Do three sets (one at each position) of ten repetitions each.

What's next? Lots of diapers—and sheer magic. But after childbirth you'll need to work on restoring musculoskeletal function disrupted during pregnancy. The extent of the disruption will depend on how serious you were about doing your E-cise menus in this chapter and on how dysfunctional you were to begin with.

I've included a Postpregnancy Menu in the next chapter, with instructions on how to roll it out in three phases. If you went into pregnancy fully functional, after having done the menus in this chapter and Chapter 9, you may be able to cut the transition time between phases by about half. Take your time, though, and let your body tell you when it's ready to move ahead. Once the Phase III menu is under control, return to the menu in Chapter 9—and don't forget those baby E-cises in the Appendix.

Beating the Baby Blues

One last run at musculoskeletal system dysfunction and motherhood. Almost invariably, during the nine months from conception to delivery, pregnancy drains motion and movement out of your life. It's a good idea to undertake not only prepregnancy and pregnancy E-cise programs but the postpregnancy program as well. New mothers will find it helpful as a prelude to whatever fitness and/or eating program they plan to embark on once the hectic pace of the baby's arrival begins to settle down into a routine. Simply heading to the gym without working on musculoskeletal system dysfunctions first runs the risk that those dysfunctions will be such an obstacle to progress that you'll soon give in to discouragement.

My message and tone in this chapter have been purposely blunt, because it doesn't do women any favors to give them the impression that infertility, miscarriages, premature birth, and other problems of the kind are merely inconveniences or mistakes on the body's part that can be brushed aside by powerful drugs or surgery. But I'd hate to leave the impression that by adopting this tone, I'm blaming the victim. Far from it—I'm blaming the perpetrator. A woman who gets pregnant (or attempts to) knowing that her musculoskeletal system is dysfunctional, knowing the risks that that presents, and knowing she has other options (like becoming functional) is no victim. She is an informed adult who is making a deliberate decision. I'm not about to sugarcoat that message.

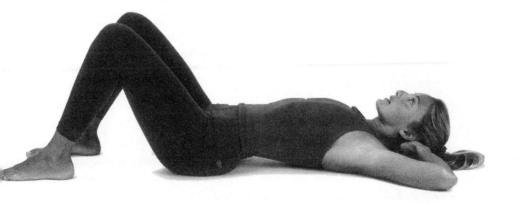

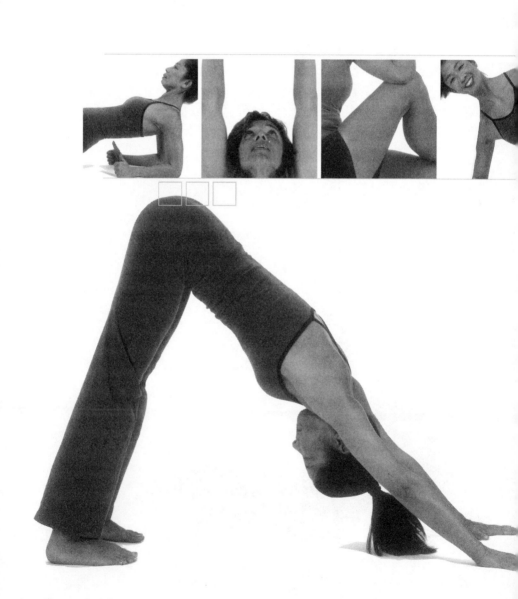

CHAPTER 11

S^3: stronger, smarter, sexier

Muscle and Bone Loss

Most researchers agree that women begin losing muscle mass in their mid-thirties. This finding is usually presented as just another "girl thing," but it's a guy thing too. Men and women alike can lose muscle mass in their mid-thirties—*and* in their mid-twenties *and* in their mid-teens. At any point in life, retention of muscle is about activity level and musculoskeletal function. The more you move—and move properly—the more muscle you will build and retain.

A teenager or twentysomething woman who doesn't develop adequate muscle mass in the first place is, for all practical purposes, losing muscle mass long before middle age sets in. The loss puts them behind the strength and metabolism curves for the rest of their lives. It may explain why illnesses and conditions associated with middle age such as diabetes, arthritis, and lupus are striking young adults more frequently.

Medical researchers also tell us that by the age of forty, the average woman is losing a half pound of muscle each year and that it is replaced by the same amount of fat. We could just shrug our shoulders and say *adios*, but let's not

I clustered the material on pregnancy in Chapter 10, so the twenty- and early-thirtysomething set would have access to the material sooner rather than later. That the biological clock ticks on into the forties and beyond does not change the musculoskeletal system's requirements. A mom is a mom is a mom.

give in to that temptation. For one thing, these averages—and *average* is one of my least favorite words and concepts—do not take function into account. I'd wager that the average fully functional woman adds muscle each year from forty to sixty and is holding her own from sixty on.

Don't get me wrong—for many women this conversion of muscle to fat does occur. But it doesn't have to. Young girls, teenage girls, and young women who have their musculoskeletal system function in place reach middle age powered by a healthy, vigorous metabolism. All they need to do is keep doing what they're doing. The same goes for men. For both genders, muscles and metabolism are inextricably linked. An absence of muscular development precludes full metabolic development, which in turn sets the stage for muscle loss later in life, which is itself accompanied by another turn in a downward spiral of metabolic activity. You've heard of feedback? This is *starveback*. One starves the other.

I can't write another paragraph on the topic without quoting author Natalie Angier: "Women need muscle, as much muscle as they can muster. They need muscle to shield their light bones, and they need muscle to weather illness." At thirty-five or forty a woman has another fifty years or more ahead of her. The prospect of losing roughly a third of your muscle mass by the time you are eighty should be a powerful incentive for you to develop into a bit of a muscle maniac. Your bones will thank you—and reward you—for it.

At thirty-five—just about the same time that muscle loss begins—the average woman starts losing about half a percent of her bone mass each year. For the time being, let's forget about estrogen levels and hormone shifts. The old "Use 'em or lose 'em" rule has a corollary: "Lose 'em and lose 'em." When muscles go, bones are right behind. Here again, it doesn't have to happen.

The muscle and bone partnership is a perfect example of supply and demand. The more you move, the more muscle you develop; the more muscle you have, the more bones you build to support it. As muscle size and density increase, so does bone size and density. We've talked about how the body thrives on stimulation. Muscular contraction directly stimulates bone growth and density. As we walk, run, twist, and jump, the impact also provides stimulation.

Whenever a client tells me that she has given up running because her joints can't handle the impact, I cringe. She's both right and wrong. Dysfunctional joints can't handle the impact, but functional joints can, and they pass along the impact to the bones to keep them healthy and growing. Riding a bike, swimming, or in-line skating don't provide the stimulation of impact.

Strong Medicine

Miriam E. Nelson, a distinguished Tufts University medical researcher, did women a great service when she wrote *Strong Women Stay Young* and the sequel, *Strong Women Stay Slim*. Dr. Nelson proved conclusively that by following a strength-training routine, women can prevent and/or reverse muscle and bone loss. A year after undergoing strength training twice a week, the women who participated in her original study were described as fifteen to twenty years more youthful.

It's worth buying a copy of Dr. Nelson's first book just to see the three CAT scans of cross-sections of thighbone and muscle that she presents. The first photograph, from the thigh of an active twenty-five-year-old woman, shows a slice of muscle that is large, fine-grained, and dense. It surrounds a thick disk of bone made up of substantial walls around a small bone marrow core area. They sit on what could be mistaken for a slightly larger, round dinner plate but is actually the thigh's fat tissue. The second photo, taken of the thigh of a sedentary fifty-eight-year-old woman, shows a dark bone marrow core three times larger, with the walls of the bone correspondingly reduced. The muscle surrounding the bone seems to be breaking up into chunks, losing density, and shrinking by about 25 percent. The "dinner plate" of fat is about twice as large. The few bits of free-floating muscle look like tiny islands that have drifted away. The third photo, from the thigh of a sixty-three-year-old woman who took part in the strength-training study, is almost identical to the twenty-five-year-old's cross-section of muscle and bone. The major differences are a slightly larger bone marrow core and reduced walls, a little less density in the muscle fiber, and perhaps a bit more overall mass and less fat. But it's impressive. You'd never guess that there is a thirty-eight-year age difference between the first and third photos.

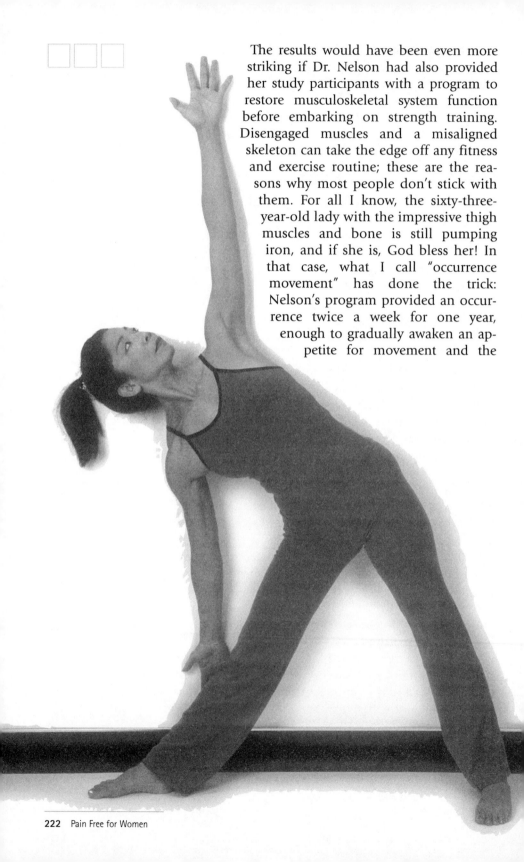

The results would have been even more striking if Dr. Nelson had also provided her study participants with a program to restore musculoskeletal system function before embarking on strength training. Disengaged muscles and a misaligned skeleton can take the edge off any fitness and exercise routine; these are the reasons why most people don't stick with them. For all I know, the sixty-three-year-old lady with the impressive thigh muscles and bone is still pumping iron, and if she is, God bless her! In that case, what I call "occurrence movement" has done the trick: Nelson's program provided an occurrence twice a week for one year, enough to gradually awaken an appetite for movement and the developing metabolism to support it. Occurrence by occurrence—some scheduled, some not—the woman rebuilt her functions from the ground up.

Unfortunately, that doesn't always happen in many exercise and strength-training programs. The workouts generate positive impact, like lowered blood pressure, weight loss, or building muscle and bone strength. But that's not enough. Entrenched dysfunctions are still more than ample to drain off metabolic capability to such an extent that it feels better to stop the activity and drop out than to continue.

Repetitive movement is the culprit. It crowds out the full range of spontaneous movement upon which the body depends for total function. A recurring pattern of motion in a favorite strength-training program or a workout on the treadmill or StairMaster accesses only the same few muscles and joints over and over again. Those get big and strong, but other bones and muscles are bypassed because of dysfunction and lose strength, density, and mass. A handful of buffed-up muscles will not have a substantial, long-term metabolic impact, particularly since the bypassed muscles are the crucial deep posture muscles, the ones that keep the spine erect and the pelvis stable.

These are the body's power generators. They allow us to defeat gravity by standing upright, and they are literally the movers and shakers. Peripheral and surface muscles tend to handle joint stabilization, torso orientation and positioning, and limb adjustment. They are the attention-getters because they shape the outer contours of the body. But a workout program that homes in on specific body parts or zones undermines balance and flexibility by overstimulating select muscles and structures. Once that process gets started, the stronger body parts continue to attract more and more stimulus because they're easier to move. That's why we start preferring certain pieces of exercise equipment and routines to others. But at the same time, neglected muscles and structures get harder to move. Before long, hard cancels out easy. And the excuse-making machine whirls into action: "I'm too busy to go to the gym," "I hate the instructor," "My shoulder hurts."

Every person who ever started and stopped an exercise program or sport had a *good* reason for doing so—it didn't feel good. I'm not trying to discourage you

Good Sports, Bad Sports

I've never met a sport, workout routine, or piece of gym equipment that I didn't like. It doesn't matter what your favorite physical activity is. If it's bungee jumping—okay. But make sure you come to the activity with a fully functional musculoskeletal system; otherwise the repetitive motion involved in the sport or workout will end up strengthening your dysfunctions and destabilizing your body.

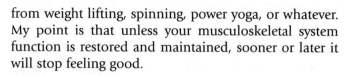

from weight lifting, spinning, power yoga, or whatever. My point is that unless your musculoskeletal system function is restored and maintained, sooner or later it will stop feeling good.

Easy as 1–2–3

The E-cise menus in this chapter, labeled "S³ Restoration and Postpregnancy," are presented in three phases. They're designed to allow women who have recently given birth to ease back into function gradually. They're also for any woman between the ages of thirty-five and fifty. For you, the goal is the same: full function. The only difference is how fast you'll get there.

If you are a new mother, you need extra time to recover from the rigors of pregnancy and childbirth. Phase I is an easy first step. I recommend taking six weeks to two months doing Phase I before moving to Phase II. Give Phase II another two months, and then move on to Phase III. There's no rush. If you are in pain, don't do the E-cises. Go to the doctor for an evaluation. If you were severely dysfunctional going into pregnancy, you're bound to be severely dysfunctional—and maybe worse—coming out. Pain is a message that mustn't be ignored.

If you are not in postpregnancy, then Phase I may take you only two weeks to feel comfortable before moving on to Phase II. In another month to six weeks, you'll be ready for Phase III. The key to the timing is to pay attention to what your body is telling you. An E-cise program becomes easier, almost boring, as dysfunctions are corrected. You'll know when it's time to switch to the next phase; your body will be eager for new challenges. When Phase III fully kicks in—after three to four months of daily workouts—you will be ready to alternate it with one of the Strength Menus in Chapter 12. The combination will serve as a maintenance menu for many, many years to come.

If you're a new mom, stay with Phase III for at least six months before moving to a Strength Menu.

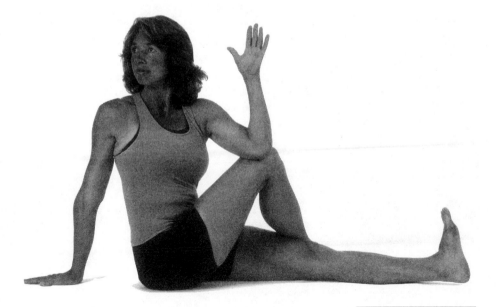

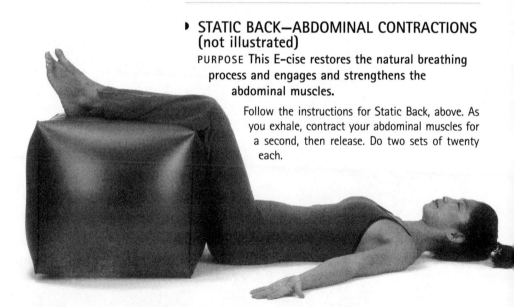

▶ **STATIC BACK**
(Figure 11–1)
PURPOSE This E-cise uses gravity to flatten the back
and put it in a neutral position.

Lie on your back, with both legs bent at right angles and
resting on a chair, bench, or block. (The large blocks we use
in the clinic are 20 inches high by 14 inches wide by 24
inches long.) Rest your hands on the floor, extended below
shoulder level, with the palms up. Let your back settle into
the floor. Breathe from your diaphragm, so your abdominal
muscles rise as you inhale and fall as you exhale. Hold this
position for five minutes.

▶ **STATIC BACK—ABDOMINAL CONTRACTIONS**
(not illustrated)
PURPOSE This E-cise restores the natural breathing
process and engages and strengthens the
abdominal muscles.

Follow the instructions for Static Back, above. As
you exhale, contract your abdominal muscles for
a second, then release. Do two sets of twenty
each.

▶ SUPINE GROIN PROGRESSIVE
(Figure 11–2 a and b)

PURPOSE This E-cise unlocks tight hip flexor muscles.

You'll need to improvise two pieces of apparatus to duplicate the large foam blocks and steps we use in the clinic. I recommend an armless chair or bench and a stepladder. Lie on your back with your right leg resting on the chair or bench, bent at a ninety-degree angle. Extend the left leg straight, placing the heel on the fifteen-inch rung of the ladder. Your foot should be pointed straight at the ceiling. Prop it against a book or another heavy object to keep it from flopping to the side. Make sure your feet, knees, hips, and shoulders are in alignment. Hold this position until your low back settles down into the floor (a), which will take ten to fifteen minutes. Then move your foot to the next step down, about ten inches, and hold it there until the back settles (b). Repeat on the five-inch level, and finally do it one last time on the floor. Always, always, repeat the entire cycle on the other side. This E-cise may take as long as an hour, but it's worth it. The more frequently you do this E-cise, the less time it will take for the hip flexors to let go. Eventually, a few minutes at each level will be enough.

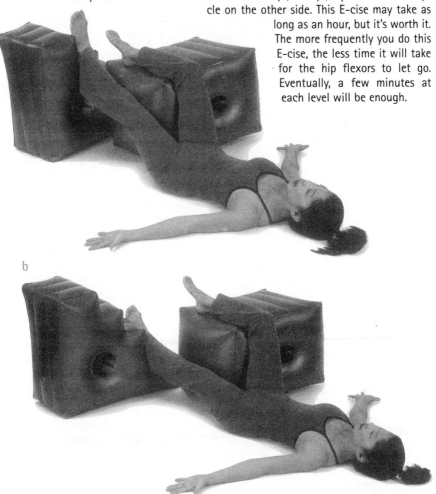

a

b

▸ CATS and DOGS
(Figure 11–3 a and b)

PURPOSE This E-cise works the hips, spine, shoulders, and neck in coordinated flexion and extension.

Get down on the floor on your hands and knees. Make a table by aligning your knees with your hips and your wrists with your shoulders. Your lower legs should be parallel with each other and with your hips. Your weight should be distributed evenly. For the Cat, smoothly round your back upward and let your head curl under, to create a curve that runs from your buttocks to your neck—like a cat with an arched back (a). For the Dog, smoothly sway your back down while bringing your head up (b). Make these two moves flow continuously back and forth. Exhale as you move into the Cat position; inhale during the Dog. Do one set of ten repetitions.

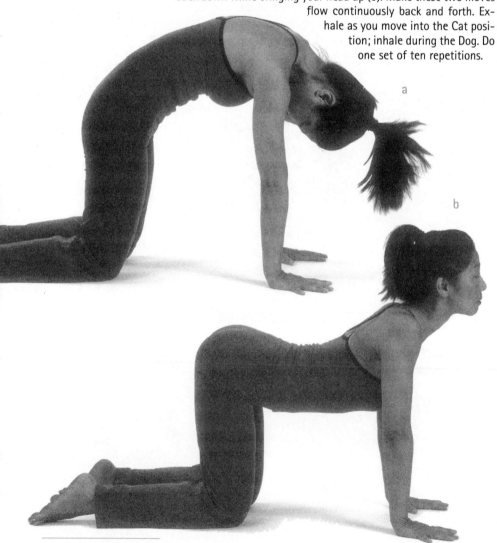

a

b

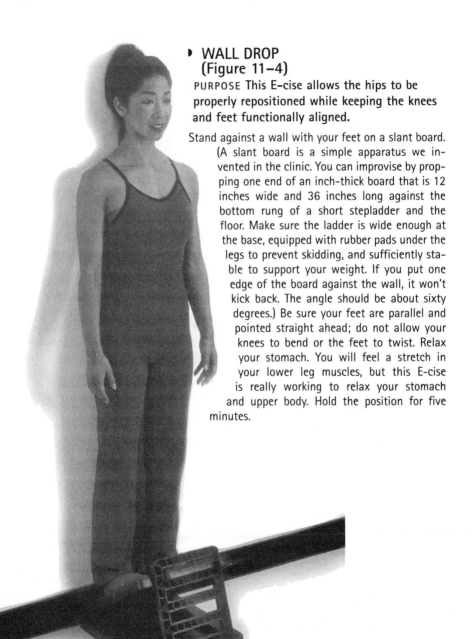

> ▸ **WALL DROP**
> **(Figure 11–4)**
> PURPOSE This E-cise allows the hips to be
> properly repositioned while keeping the knees
> and feet functionally aligned.

Stand against a wall with your feet on a slant board.
(A slant board is a simple apparatus we invented in the clinic. You can improvise by propping one end of an inch-thick board that is 12
inches wide and 36 inches long against the
bottom rung of a short stepladder and the
floor. Make sure the ladder is wide enough at
the base, equipped with rubber pads under the
legs to prevent skidding, and sufficiently stable to support your weight. If you put one
edge of the board against the wall, it won't
kick back. The angle should be about sixty
degrees.) Be sure your feet are parallel and
pointed straight ahead; do not allow your
knees to bend or the feet to twist. Relax
your stomach. You will feel a stretch in
your lower leg muscles, but this E-cise
is really working to relax your stomach
and upper body. Hold the position for five
minutes.

a

▸ SITTING ARM CIRCLES (with a pillow) (Figure 11–5 a and b)

PURPOSE This E-cise recognizes how much time we spend sitting down, by making sure the shoulders and hips are in alignment without help from the thighs, knees, lower legs, ankles, and feet. It puts the shoulders' ball and socket joints through a full range of motion.

Sit on the edge of a chair or bench that's not going to move or tip. Arch your back, and pull your head and shoulders back. Place your feet parallel on the floor about hip-width apart, pointing them straight ahead. Place a doubled-up pillow between your knees, and hold it there with knee pressure. Loosely curl your fingertips into the pads of each palm (the fleshy area at the base of the fingers), and point your thumbs straight out. This hand position, called the "golfer's grip," is imperative to the success of the E-cise. Squeeze your shoulder blades together, and bring your arms out to your sides at shoulder level, elbows straight. With your palms facing down, circle up and forward for forty repetitions (a). Now with your palms facing up, circle up and back for forty repetitions (b). Remember to keep your feet straight and your shoulder blades squeezed together. Do two sets, one forward, one back.

b

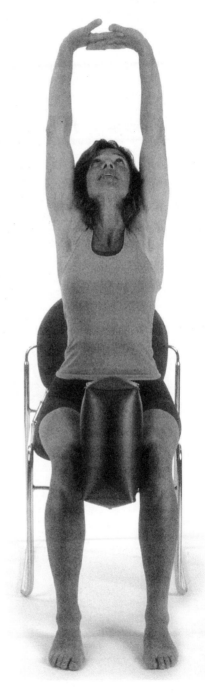

▶ SITTING OVERHEAD EXTENSION (Figure 11-6)

PURPOSE This E-cise opens up the thoracic back (upper back and neck) and the abdominal cavity, increases oxygen flow, and strengthens the back's extensor muscles.

Sit on the edge of a chair or bench. Place your feet flat and parallel on the floor, hip-width apart, pointing straight ahead. Make sure your shoulders and head are back, and that there is an arch in your lower back. Place a doubled-up pillow between your knees, and hold it there with knee pressure. Interlace your fingers, raise your arms and hands over your head, and roll your hands palm up. Look up at the backs of your hands. Your arms should be straight, on a line even with your ears, with elbows locked. Don't lean back; reach straight up. Keep your hands directly over your head, not in front of your head. Relax your stomach muscles, and remember to breathe. Hold this position for one minute.

▶ CATS and DOGS
(Figure 11–7 a and b)

PURPOSE This E-cise works the hips, spine, shoulders, and neck in coordinated flexion and extension.

Get down on the floor on your hands and knees. Make a table by aligning your knees with your hips and your wrists with your shoulders. Your lower legs should be parallel with each other and with your hips. Your weight should be distributed evenly. For the Cat, smoothly round your back upward and let your head curl under, to create a curve that runs from your buttocks to your neck—like a cat with an arched back (a). For the Dog, smoothly sway your back down while bringing your head up (b). Make these two moves flow continuously back and forth. Exhale as you move into the Cat position; inhale during the Dog. Do one set of ten repetitions.

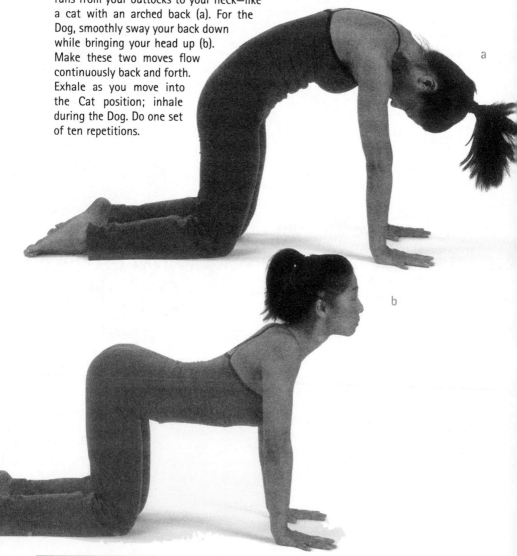

a

b

▶ DOWNWARD DOG
(Figure 11-8 a and b)

PURPOSE This E-cise reestablishes linkage from your wrists to your feet.

Assume the Cats and Dogs position (a). Curl your toes under, and push with your legs to raise your torso until you are off your knees and your weight is resting on your hands and feet. Keep pushing until your hips are higher than your shoulders and have formed a tight, stable triangle with the floor (b). Your knees should be straight, your calves and thighs tight. Don't let your feet flare outward; keep them pointing straight ahead in line with your hands, which need to stay in place—no creeping forward! Your back should be flat, not bowed, as your hips push up and back into the heels. Breathe. If you cannot bring your heels flat onto the floor, get them as close as possible. Don't force them. It may take several sessions before they go all the way down. Hold this position for one minute.

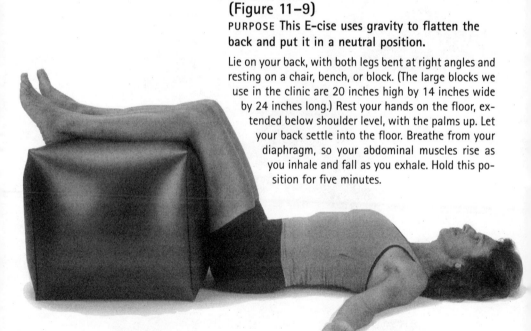

▸ STATIC BACK
(Figure 11–9)

PURPOSE This E-cise uses gravity to flatten the back and put it in a neutral position.

Lie on your back, with both legs bent at right angles and resting on a chair, bench, or block. (The large blocks we use in the clinic are 20 inches high by 14 inches wide by 24 inches long.) Rest your hands on the floor, extended below shoulder level, with the palms up. Let your back settle into the floor. Breathe from your diaphragm, so your abdominal muscles rise as you inhale and fall as you exhale. Hold this position for five minutes.

▸ SUPINE GROIN PROGRESSIVE
(Figure 11–10 a and b)

PURPOSE This E-cise unlocks tight hip flexor muscles.

You'll need to improvise two pieces of apparatus to duplicate the large foam blocks and steps we use in the clinic. I recommend an armless chair or bench and a stepladder. Lie on your back with your right leg resting on the chair or bench, bent at a ninety-degree angle. Extend the left leg straight, placing the heel on the fifteen-inch rung of the ladder. Your foot should be pointed straight at the ceiling. Prop it against a book or another heavy object to keep it from flopping to the side. Make sure your feet, knees, hips, and shoulders are in alignment. Hold this position until your low back settles down into the floor (a), which will take ten to fifteen minutes. Then move your foot to the next step down, about ten inches, and hold it there until the back settles (b). Repeat on the five-inch level, and finally do it one last time on the floor. Always, always, repeat the entire cycle on the other side. The E-cise may take as long as an hour, but it's worth it. The more frequently you do this E-cise, the less time it will take for the hip flexors to let go. Eventually, a few minutes at each level will be enough.

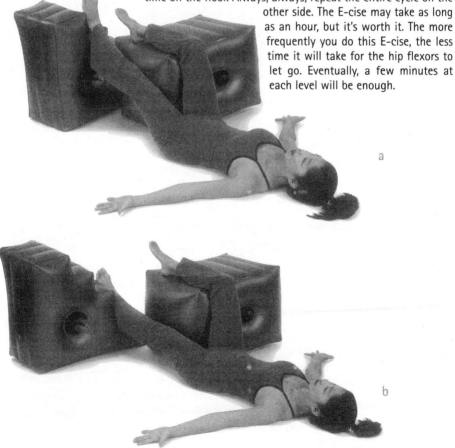

a

b

▶ PELVIC TILTS
(Figure 11–11 a and b)

PURPOSE This E-cise breaks the hips out of their flexion fixation, showing them how to move again from flexion to neutral to extension and back again.

a

b

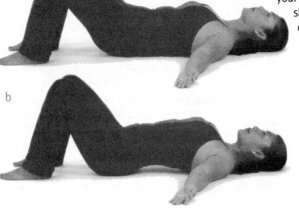

Lie on your back with your knees bent and feet on the floor, hip-width apart. Make sure your hips, feet, and knees are aligned. Roll your hips backward to flatten your back to the floor (a), then roll them forward to put an arch in your lower back (b). Keep your upper back relaxed and your arms out to your sides just below shoulder level, palms up. Do one set of ten repetitions.

[S³ Restoration and Postpregnancy Menu, Phase III]

▶ WALL STORK
(Figure 11–12)

PURPOSE This E-cise levels the hips into a parallel position, under a load that's held in vertical alignment.

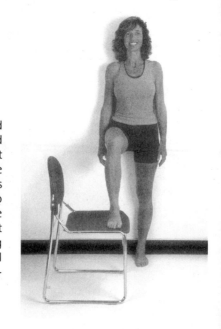

Stand against a wall with your feet pointed straight ahead. Your heels, hips, upper back, and head should be against the wall. Place your right foot on the seat of a chair positioned about twelve inches in front of you. Make sure this foot is pointed straight. Do not allow your left foot to twist or your left leg to bend. The right leg, on the chair, should be bent at about ninety degrees at the knee joint. Hold this position without allowing the left foot, leg, or hip to shift to the side or to roll away from the wall. Hold for three minutes. Reposition the chair, switch legs, and repeat.

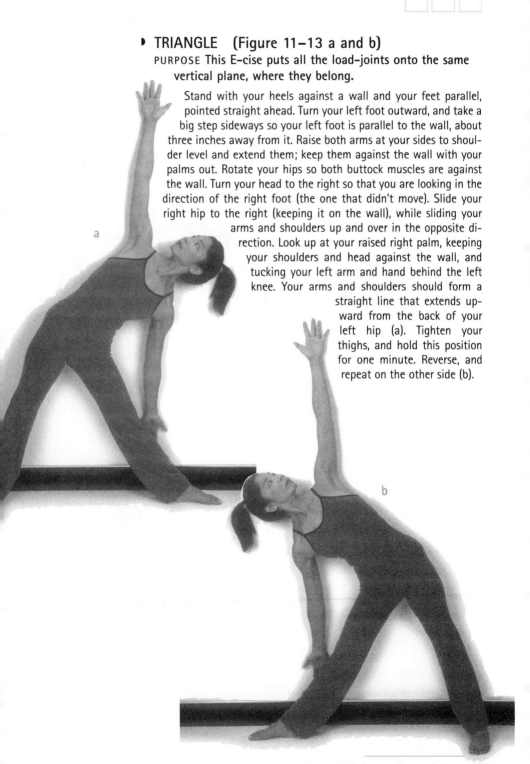

▶ TRIANGLE (Figure 11-13 a and b)

PURPOSE This E-cise puts all the load-joints onto the same vertical plane, where they belong.

Stand with your heels against a wall and your feet parallel, pointed straight ahead. Turn your left foot outward, and take a big step sideways so your left foot is parallel to the wall, about three inches away from it. Raise both arms at your sides to shoulder level and extend them; keep them against the wall with your palms out. Rotate your hips so both buttock muscles are against the wall. Turn your head to the right so that you are looking in the direction of the right foot (the one that didn't move). Slide your right hip to the right (keeping it on the wall), while sliding your arms and shoulders up and over in the opposite direction. Look up at your raised right palm, keeping your shoulders and head against the wall, and tucking your left arm and hand behind the left knee. Your arms and shoulders should form a straight line that extends upward from the back of your left hip (a). Tighten your thighs, and hold this position for one minute. Reverse, and repeat on the other side (b).

▶ CATS and DOGS
(Figure 11–14 a and b)
PURPOSE This E-cise works the hips, spine, shoulders, and neck in coordinated flexion and extension.

Get down on the floor on your hands and knees. Make a table by aligning your knees with your hips and your wrists with your shoulders. Your lower legs should be parallel with each other and with your hips. Your weight should be distributed evenly. For the Cat, smoothly round your back upward and let your head curl under, to create a curve that runs from your buttocks to your neck—like a cat with an arched back (a). For the Dog, smoothly sway your back down while bringing your head up (b). Make these two moves flow continuously back and forth. Exhale as you move into the Cat position; inhale during the Dog. Do one set of ten repetitions.

a

b

▶ CORE ABDOMINALS
(Figure 11–15 a, b, c, and d)
PURPOSE This four-position E-cise gives your deepest layer of abdominal muscles a workout.

Position 1: Lie on your stomach propped on your elbows; your chest is off the floor, and your head is up. Look straight ahead. Loosely curl your fingers inward on the palms, and extend your thumbs straight up. Pull your toes under, and bridge your body off the floor. Your weight is resting on your toes and elbows (a). Press down and outward on your forearms without moving your elbows. Roll your hands outward at the wrists, and let your shoulder blades collapse together. Hold for thirty seconds.

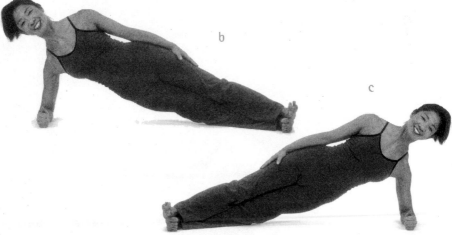

Positions 2 and 3: Lie on your right side propped up on your elbow, feet together, and legs straight. Keep your shoulders, hips, knees, and ankles in a straight line (b). Hold for thirty seconds. Switch sides, and hold for another thirty seconds (c).

Position 4: Lie on your back with your legs straight, your heels down and together. Prop your elbows under your shoulders, flex your toes, and lift your pelvis off the floor (d). Hold for thirty seconds.

▶ CATS and DOGS
(Figure 11–16 a and b)
Follow the instructions that appear earlier in this menu.

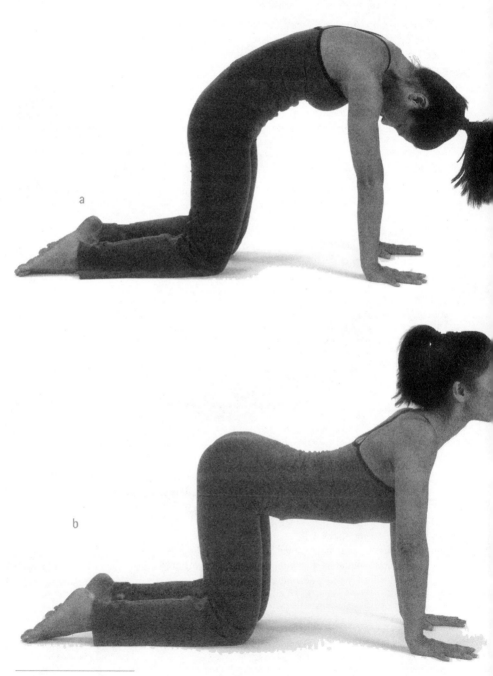

a

b

▶ **SITTING FLOOR TWIST**
(Figure 11–17 a and b)
PURPOSE This E-cise teaches the spine that it can rotate while the hips remain in place.

Sit on the floor with your legs extended straight in front. Bend your left leg, and cross it over the right, placing it flat on the floor just outside of and slightly below the right knee. Place your right elbow outside your left knee. Roll your hips forward to create an arch in the lower back. (Hold this arch throughout.) Now twist your upper body to the left, using your back muscles to rotate your spine. Turn your head to the left as you twist. Support yourself with your left hand on the floor off to the side and be-hind. Hold this position for one minute and breathe. Your straight leg should be tight, with the toes flexed toward your knee (a). Re-peat on the other side (b).

a

b

▶ PELVIC TILTS
(Figure 11–18 a and b)

PURPOSE This E-cise breaks the hips out of their flexion fixation and shows them how to move again from flexion to neutral to extension and back again.

Lie on your back with your knees bent and your feet flat on the floor hip-width apart. Keep your upper back relaxed and your arms out to your sides just below shoulder level, palms up. Make sure your hips, feet, and knees are aligned. Roll your hips backward toward your feet to flatten your back to the floor (a). Then roll them away to make an arch in your low back (b). Remember to breathe in concert with the hip movement—inhale up, exhale down. Do one set of ten repetitions.

a

b

▶ SITTING FEMUR ROTATIONS
(Figure 11–19 a and b)

PURPOSE This E-cise reintroduces full lateral movement of the knee and ankle via the hip socket.

Sit on the floor with both legs extended straight in front of you. Your feet should be eight to ten inches apart. For support, place your hands behind your hips, about four inches. Tighten your thigh muscles, flex your toes, and roll your hips forward to arch your back. Using your hips, rotate your knees and feet inward (a) and then outward (b). It's important to keep your hips rolled forward, thighs tight, and toes flexed. Do not lean too heavily on your hands; try to sit up straight with your head and shoulders back. Do three sets of twenty repetitions. (One rotation in and one out counts as one.)

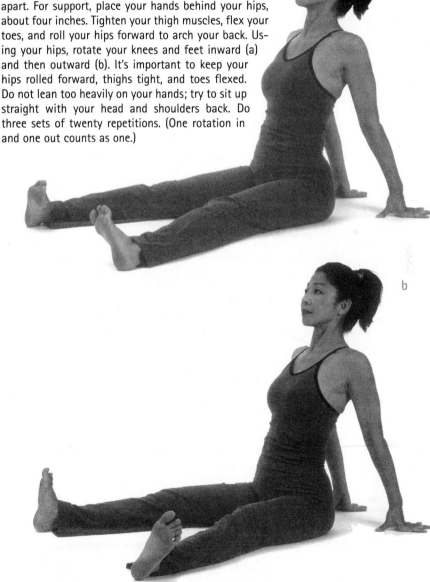

a

b

▸ FOOT CIRCLES and POINT/FLEXES (Figure 11–20 a, b, and c)

PURPOSE This E-cise reminds your knees, ankles, and feet how to interact according to their designs.

Lie on your back with your left leg extended flat on the floor and the right leg bent toward your chest. For the Foot Circles, clasp your hands behind your bent right knee to hold it in position while you circle your right foot clockwise (a). This motion emanates from the ankle, not from the knee. Keep your knee still, and try to make full circles with your foot. (You may tend to make half circles; it will help to slow down and concentrate.) Meanwhile, keep the left foot pointed straight up toward the ceiling, with the left thigh muscles tight. Do forty repetitions, and then reverse and circle in a counterclockwise direction (b). Do forty repetitions. For Point/Flexes, keep your legs in the same position while you flex your right toes back toward the shin. Then reverse the direction and point the toes (c). Do forty repetitions. Switch legs and repeat.

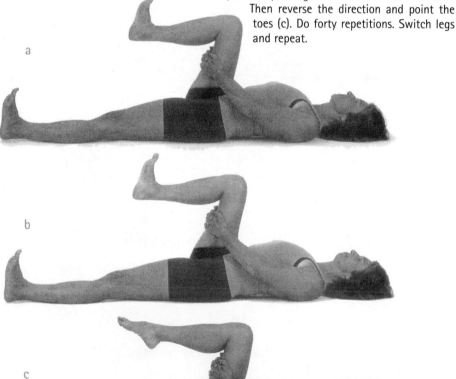

a

b

c

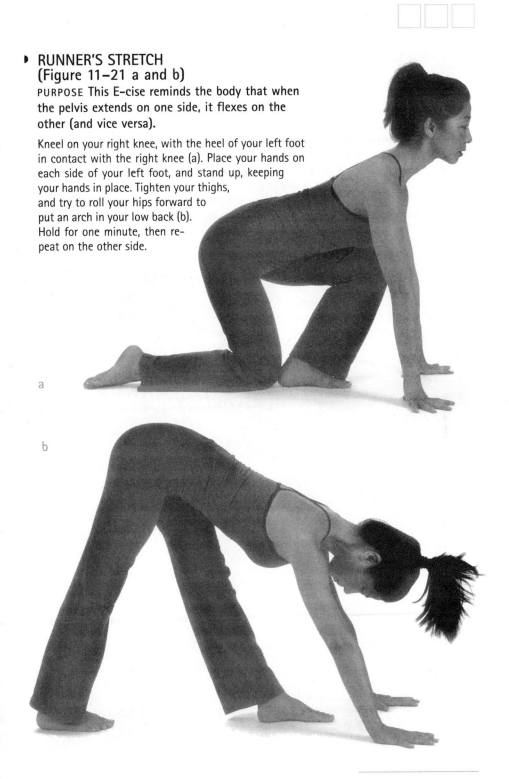

▶ RUNNER'S STRETCH
(Figure 11–21 a and b)

PURPOSE This E-cise reminds the body that when the pelvis extends on one side, it flexes on the other (and vice versa).

Kneel on your right knee, with the heel of your left foot in contact with the right knee (a). Place your hands on each side of your left foot, and stand up, keeping your hands in place. Tighten your thighs, and try to roll your hips forward to put an arch in your low back (b). Hold for one minute, then repeat on the other side.

a

b

▶ DOWNWARD DOG
(Figure 11–22 a and b)

PURPOSE This E-cise reestablishes linkage from the wrists to the feet.

Assume the Cats and Dogs position (a). Curl your toes under, and push with your legs to raise your torso until you are off your knees and your weight is resting on your hands and feet. Keep pushing until your hips are higher than your shoulders and have formed a tight, stable triangle with the floor (b). Your knees should be straight, your calves and thighs tight. Don't let your feet flare outward; keep them pointing straight ahead in line with your hands, which need to stay in place— no creeping forward! Your back should be flat, not bowed, as your hips push up and back into the heels. Breathe. If you cannot bring your heels flat onto the floor, get them as close as possible. Don't force them. It may take several sessions before they go all the way down. Hold this position for one minute.

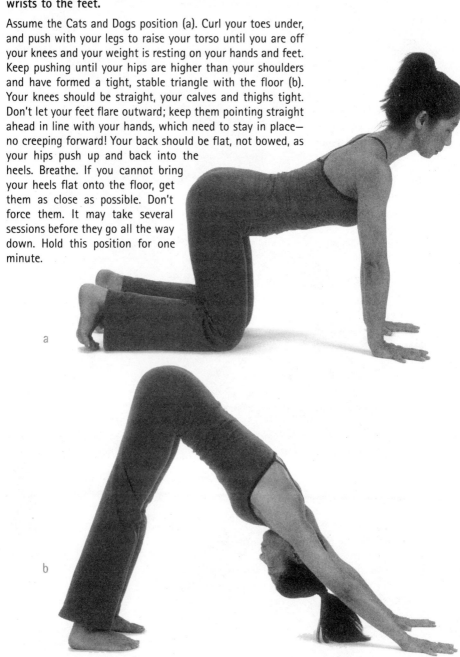

a

b

When I first wrote this chapter, I discovered that I had used the term *middle age* six or seven times. I erased many of those references and substituted S^3—stronger, smarter, sexier. We need a better way to measure our status as passengers on Space Ship Earth, the name Adlai Stevenson conjured up when he saw the first satellite photos of our planet. To voyagers aboard a craft that's cutting through infinity itself, counting the years and dividing them into an actuarial table to determine how much time is gone or left doesn't seem adequate.

My advice is to treat years as irrelevancies, as accounting gimmicks. They don't tell the whole truth about health or about the rewards that tomorrow can bring. As we move through time, the human body is designed to be capable of getting stronger and smarter.

So, Ms. S^3, where's the middle? The middle of what? Time doesn't have a middle.

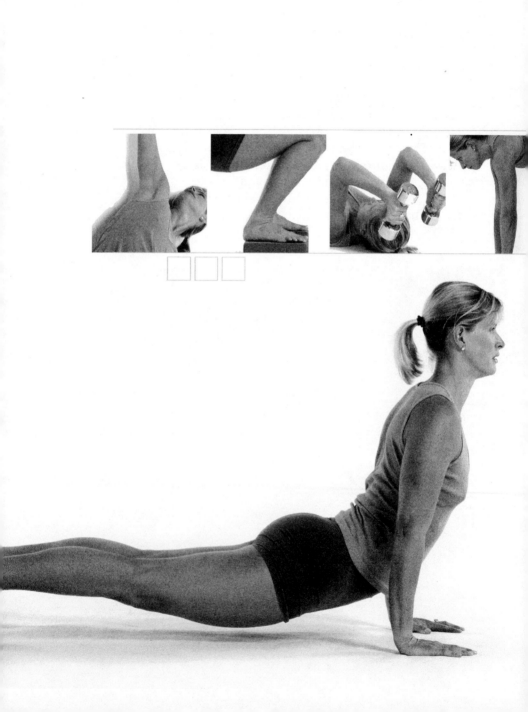

CHAPTER 12

body shop

☐☐☐

In Chapter 11 I discussed how musculoskeletal system dys-functions undermine the effectiveness of fitness and workout pro-grams. I've found that these dysfunctions also affect the efforts of millions of women who are trying to manage their weight. If losing or controlling your weight is your goal, I'll show you how to do it faster and easier than ever before. Here's how to take off unwanted and unhealthy pounds and keep them off, without a yo-yo effect.

Are you skeptical? You have a right to be. Most women who lose weight on diet programs regain those pounds within six months to a year. And it's no wonder. Food (amount and type), physi-cal activity, and function are all requirements for successful weight management.

That's so important I need to repeat it. Weight manage-ment depends on:

▶ The amount and type of food we consume;

▶ The work we do to utilize those calories; and

▶ The state of our musculoskeletal system function.

When you cut your total food intake and load up on pro-tein (as a Dr. Atkins devotee), or consume carbs or fat-free food (as a follower of other popular diet gurus), you're only one-third of the way there. Unless enough physical activity is accomplished by a fully functional musculoskeletal system, the conversion of food into energy is disrupted, and weight control is an uphill struggle.

I'm currently fighting in a crusade to break the automatic, unquestioned link between skinniness and health. The two words are not synonymous. I won't try to sell you on the notion that you can be fit and flabby—extreme obesity is a serious illness. But people who starve to death are skinny. It's possible to be big, beautiful, and in the best of health.

"Fat," a 1998 documentary by the PBS program *Frontline,* featured Dave Alexander, who is five feet eight inches tall and weighs 250 pounds, more than a hundred pounds over his so-called "ideal weight." At the time Alexander was training for a triathlon, so in a routine week he swam five miles, ran thirty miles, and biked two hundred. For Alexander, grueling triathlon competition is not just a passing whim dreamed up between pig-outs at Taco Bell—he has finished 264 of them. Even so, his weight raises red flags with physicians and insurance companies, since it puts him in the life-threatening category of "morbid obesity." And without his rigorous training regimen and pursuit of triathlon glory, he would indeed be in danger.

But Alexander is an excellent example of how fitness and fat can coexist. There's no way he could compete in the triathlon without significant muscle mass, and the principle is exactly the same for both sexes. Muscle mass means extra weight (since it's denser and holds more water than fat), and that weight gets counted toward the "morbid obesity" designation. Furthermore, whatever fat a woman is also carrying serves an important practical purpose. Fat is the original Meals on Wheels. Ounce for ounce, fat supplies twice the amount of energy available from any other source. This high-octane fuel is stored in handy fat cells that aren't involved in vital operational functions and therefore can afford to donate energy to those that are doing more important work. A female triathlon athlete can tap her energy resources hour after hour as she runs, swims, and bikes. When she draws down the available supply of energy from carbohydrates and protein, the fat is there in reserve. Without fat, as other fuel supplies approach empty, the body would begin breaking down muscle tissue for energy. A supply of fat also allows glucose from carbohydrates to be diverted to the central nervous system, which under normal circumstances does not utilize fuel from either fat or protein.

Mounting research evidence shows that people who are fit but *overweight* have lower death rates than those who are unfit and of *normal* weight. Additional studies show that most overweight women do not overeat—their problem is lack of physical activity, promoted and compounded by musculoskeletal system dysfunction. Therefore fat is not a cause of illness and death: it's a symptom. The real killer is inactivity.

It would be so simple to stop right here and say, "Toss out those diet books and get yourself a new pair of walking shoes." Go to a gym, hit the StairMaster, or run, run, run. But it's not so easy. Inactivity is itself a symptom. It starts as a reflection of our modern lifestyle and degenerates into musculoskeletal system dysfunction. Functional women are active women; they have the right stuff, and they use it. Dysfunctional women are not active—and it's not because they're lazy. They simply lack the musculoskeletal resources that would allow them to be active enough to control their weight. Functional women, thanks to a musculoskeletal system that is engaged and operating according to its design, may weigh more or less than "normal." But that's terrific, because they feel good and are racking up years of good health and good times.

Fat Facts

As words go, *diet* is another loser. Let's dump it in the same place where we disposed of *middle age*. A diet is a last resort, implying drudgery, discomfort, and sacrifice. But an *eating program* or *plan* carries none of that baggage. Since we eat to maintain our health and well-being, it only makes sense to take control of the process and manage it the way we manage projects at work or the crazy chaos associated with everyday family life. Furthermore, management is an ongoing affair. It takes place day in and day out. Consistent control is the objective.

There's a big difference between management and manipulation. Without being consciously aware of it, most people with weight problems are manipulators.

They aren't feeding themselves in order to fuel the 700 trillion cells of their bodies; they are, rather, eating to manipulate their blood chemistry and metabolism in order to feel good enough to get through another day.

Salt, sugar, caffeine, fats, starches, and all the other usual suspects are means to that end. Their actual nutritional value is of secondary importance, if it rates even that high. Up until about ten thousand years ago, we ingested carbohydrates a few berries or beans at a time. Then our ancestors began systemically cultivating cereal grains and refining them into bread, porridge, pasta, and other forms of highly concentrated, high glycemic "supercarbohydrates." Inadvertently, humankind started messing around with its blood chemistry by introducing massive doses of carbohydrates into a system that was unprepared by evolution to properly process them into fuel.

That's one theory anyway, which has been persuasively advanced by Barry Sears, the author of the best-selling diet and fitness books *The Zone* and *Enter the Zone*. He recommends carefully balancing the intake of carbohydrates and proteins (with a slight overweighting to the carbs). But that solution amounts to more manipulation. In fact, all the best-selling diet gurus are manipulators, not managers. Their solution to obesity is to encourage other forms of fiddling with blood chemistry to adjust the body's metabolism. Dr. Robert Atkins uses protein to pluck the strings. Dean Ornish tunes his cello to the pitch of low-fat foods. Joyce and Gene Daoust play the viola da gamba to the beat of fat-burning high-fiber carbohydrates—and so on.

All of them overlook the central question: why does our metabolism need such overt adjusting?

Sears, to be fair, does address the question, and he may be right that supercarbs precipitated the original blood chemistry problem. By releasing a rush of glucose into the bloodstream in concentrated form, these carbohydrates triggered outpourings of insulin to counteract it, which in turn provoked glycogen, which sopped up excess insulin. The seesaw went wild, and hormonal balance was forever lost. But I'm not sure he's entirely right, because there's yet another question hanging out there: why are some people seemingly immune to obesity?

Have they adapted to supercarbs? It's unlikely. Evolutionary changes in humans are rarely known to occur in a mere ten thousand years. Plus, the tide seems to be going in the opposite direction: we're getting fatter, not thinner. Yet significant numbers of us can consume and process refined and highly concentrated carbohydrates. Their diets are probably salty, sugary, fatty, and laced with caffeine to some extent as well. Yet they manage their weight. Why?

My answer to all these questions is: musculoskeletal system function. Those who are immune from obesity are functional. Their bodies are able to efficiently process whatever they eat and turn it into energy. They don't feel the need to fiddle with their blood chemistry, because thanks to a robust, muscle-driven metabolic process, it takes care of itself. They easily meet all three of the requirements for weight management:

- Overeating isn't a problem for them, because their metabolic burn rate and their intake of calories naturally converge. They feel no craving for salt, sugar, and excess fats and carbohydrates to make up for an imbalance.
- Since it's a pleasure for them to move, they have enough physical exercise to convert fuel into energy.
- They have full musculoskeletal system function, to keep the major muscle groups up and running.

Are all thin people functional? Not at all. You can starve yourself thin and in so doing trash your metabolic process. In fact, the strongest signs of metabolic deficiency are both obesity and hyperskinniness. Both cases often involve an extreme lack of engaged, working musculature. The obese person's bulk hides this crucial shortcoming, while the skinny ones are regarded as fashion model and movie star look-alikes. But the consequences are the same for both: peak metabolic efficiency is impossible to attain or maintain. And both types resort to metabolic manipulation. The obese hop on and off the latest diet fads (or give up entirely) and in the meantime generally feel lousy. The hyperskinny choke off their food intake to squeeze into thong bikinis and live on pills, cigarettes, and diet sodas—and generally feel lousy. A subcategory of the hyperskinny— those who eat like a horse, who never gain an ounce, and whose musculoskeletal systems are disaster areas—

are living off surplus metabolic resources that aren't being replaced and will eventually run out.

Is there a middle ground? You bet there is—musculoskeletal system function. Effective weight management starts with function and thereby ensures that we can achieve, not an ideal weight, but an ideal metabolism. When the musculoskeletal system is operating according to its design, this is what happens metabolically:

- What we eat can be easily broken down into fuel.
- That fuel is delivered to the body's cells to be converted into energy quickly, to allow the work of the head, hands, and heart to occur.
- The waste products of this vital inner bonfire are fully eliminated from the body.

Otherwise, we end up losing on each count:

- We struggle to manipulate a lackluster metabolism that is sluggish at breaking down food into fuel, which is in overall short supply.
- That fuel is haphazardly delivered to the cells, where it smolders instead of burning, making us tired, stressed out, and unhappy.
- Without sufficient heat and energy, waste products accumulate and grow toxic to our systems.

Muscles, motion, and metabolism are all linked, and function provides the nexus. The first step toward weight management, therefore, is to take two protective measures. First, bring your musculoskeletal system back to full function; and second, undertake a strength-training program. Here again I endorse Miriam E. Nelson and her books *Strong Women Stay Young* and *Strong Women Stay Slim*. Consider following the strength programs in both those books—but first take care of your musculoskeletal system function. Do the Restoration and Maintenance Menus that I laid out in Chapter 9 each day for at least a month before starting the Strength Menu that closes this chapter. Switch between them on alternating days for another month before beginning Nelson's programs. I recommend combining the Nelson and Egoscue programs into a three-pronged affair. On Day 1 do the Egoscue Restoration and Maintenance Menus; on Day 2 it's the Egoscue

Strength Menu; then on Day 3 work in one of Nelson's programs. Then start over.

Why the switch-off? Skeletal misalignment and muscular disengagement undermine the effects of strength training. The drawings in Figures 12–1a and 12–1b show a dysfunctional woman—let's call her Joyce—using free weights; and those in Figures 12–2a and 12–2b depict a fully functional women—Angie—doing the same. Compare the posture of the two women. Joyce

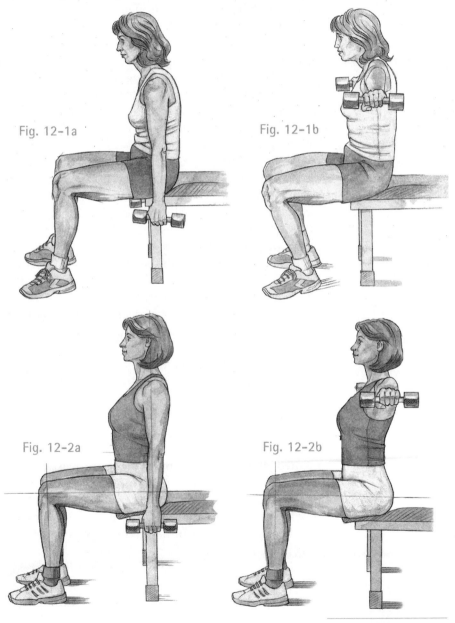

Fig. 12–1a

Fig. 12–1b

Fig. 12–2a

Fig. 12–2b

and Angie are both trying to shape and strengthen their upper arms and shoulders. But Joyce's hips are rolled forward into flexion, which flattens the S-curve of her spine and brings her shoulders, neck, and head forward. When she lifts the dumbbells, she is stressing her upper-back muscles and neck because they are not getting kinetic support for the hips and spinal erector muscles. Her shoulders are hinged forward, which shifts the work to the rotator cuffs, in the vicinity of the shoulder blades, rather than to the upper-arm muscles and the shoulders' ball-joint mechanism. By contrast, notice the S-curve in Angie's back and how her shoulders are squarely over her level hips. Her rotator cuffs are disengaged—as they should be—bringing the shoulders' ball-joints into play. From her hips to her head, her muscles are performing as a team. Meanwhile the deltoid and pectoralis major muscles are engaging fully instead of being bypassed or restricted.

Dysfunctional Joyce is unlikely to stick with the strength-training program. It won't make her feel good, permanently lose weight, or firm up. The muscles she is strengthening are actually making her more unstable and stiff. Those that are disengaged are liable, if she begins a weight-loss program, to get weaker.

Weaker? That's right. To fuel itself, if asked to choose between inactive muscles and energy-rich fat, the body is ready and willing to sacrifice muscle. That's why maintaining and building strength is particularly important when you're trying to lose weight. Take it from Lucy, our hominid poster girl from Chapter 1.

In the African grasslands from which our ancestors probably emerged, fat was a rare and delicious prize, usually the payoff for hard work, bravery, and ingenuity. Starchy, high-energy carbohydrates in the form of fruits and vegetables were everyday staples. To maintain and rebuild muscle and cell structure our ancestors supplemented them with plant protein, principally nuts, beans, grains, and other seeds. Animal protein—meat—was scarce, but humans need only a small amount: roughly 12 to 15 percent of the total food intake. A primitive galloping gourmand could get that by popping a few worms, lizards, or baby birds.

In terms of evolution, fat was a reward for success or at least good luck. It's so high in energy a little goes a long way, and as we have seen, any extra can be stored for use later. In hard times those who were fat had an energy advantage over the lean. Not only could they continue to hunt and forage more vigorously and endure privation longer, but their body's muscles were not being broken down and consumed as a last-resort energy source.

Faced with the sudden curtailment of carbohydrates and protein, the body goes into its famine-fighting mode. It does not know the difference between a trendy diet and starvation. Since its number-one priority is survival, it doesn't waste resources on muscles that are not being used, and it doesn't hesitate to convert all that good, easy-to-burn protein that's just sitting there. During a famine Lucy used her muscles (fueled by fat) as much or more than ever in search of new food supplies. The body does not lose what it uses. Except during the most severe and prolonged famines, any muscular breakdown for her was on the margins, and she and her male companion had far more muscle mass to begin with than the average modern woman and man. Their big posture and locomotor muscles allowed them to outwalk most local and regional food shortages. Today, without being fully functional, many dieters are reversing the Lucy paradigm. They use and retain their peripheral muscles to accomplish a limited range of physical activities, but they lose the core muscles that keep them erect and moving.

Use It and Lose It

A diet that is heavy in carbohydrates primes the body to burn the carbs first. The fuel from carbohydrates and protein—even after a huge meal—tends to be immediately available for energy expenditure and then, if unused, washes through the system and dissipates. That's why we must eat regularly, rather than stuffing ourselves on Monday and waiting a few days before eating again. Fat is our only major storage mechanism, and it is continually being rolled over and replenished with new fat. Somehow, like a conscientious bookkeeper, the body keeps track of the fat pluses and minuses and makes a deduction from the total only when it has to. In this case, the bottom line is indeed a bottom, which for millions of people is growing larger.

As I mentioned in the discussion of *The Zone*, humans are programmed by evolution to get their carbohydrate requirement from fruits and vegetables, not from heavily processed and concentrated grain-based products like bread, rice, and pasta. The main problem with these carbohydrates is that they quickly break down and load the bloodstream with a natural, simple form of sugar called glucose. In turn, the pancreas produces insulin to counteract the high blood sugar levels. Insulin signals the body to start absorbing the excess sugar generated by the carbs and at the same time puts the brakes on brain activity and energy levels. That's why we tend to feel sluggish and sleepy after a meal of pizza or pasta. But when the effects of insulin become too pronounced, its biochemical antidote, glycogen, is triggered. But with the next meal or snack, blood sugar will spike again, triggering another blast of insulin. By bombarding the system with sugars—both unrefined and refined—our munch-and-run habits aggravate the situation throughout the day. The resulting peak and valley fluctuations are a measure of the system's inability to smoothly handle heavily processed carbohydrates.

Muscle can come to the rescue. Strength training on a functional musculoskeletal system platform in conjunction with an eating plan will help the pancreas. Glucose that's efficiently and expeditiously utilized by the muscles is glucose that doesn't have to be neutralized by a heavy flood of insulin. The hormone is still secreted to launch the absorption process, but with the muscles active, the glucose is quickly consumed as fuel. The pancreas doesn't need to keep spraying insulin like a fire fighter hosing down a five-alarm fire—glucose in, glucose out.

In addition, active muscles burn more calories than fat tissue does, which is close to being inert. Having a few extra grams of muscle can make a big difference. Strength training also counteracts protein breakdown. Active, strengthening muscles are almost literally sending out a busy signal that forces the body to tap into its fat supplies once it's burned off all available carbs. For once, "Use it and lose it" becomes the rule: use muscle, lose fat.

Diets—and I'm deliberately resorting to the dirty word now—are a danger to women because research shows that 25 to 30 percent of the weight they drop is in the form of lost muscle, bone, other forms of lean tissue, and water. Strength-training programs can actually cancel that out and achieve weight-reduction goals.

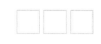

Miriam Nelson's study used two groups of volunteers: one diet-only, the other diet and strength training. The diet-only group lost 13 pounds, while the second group lost 14.2 pounds. That may not seem like much of a difference, but here's Dr. Nelson's take:

> *A dramatic difference occurred when we looked at body composition. Women in the diet-only group had lost an average of 2.8 pounds of lean tissue—mainly muscle—along with the fat. In contrast, the women who'd done strength training actually gained 1.4 pounds of lean tissue. So every ounce they lost was fat. Indeed, since the new muscle replaced fat, their total fat lost was 14.6 pounds. They lost 44 percent more fat than the diet-only group.*

Women who strength-train without any intention of losing weight report that they drop from one to three dress sizes. Muscles are more compact than fat, so by becoming stronger, these women aren't trading bulk for bulk. They are winding up more trim and toned. Plus the strength boosts their metabolism higher, which results in more calories being burned even when they are at rest.

Beneath the Surface

Spas are becoming fashionable again. Ads and articles featuring them conjure up inviting images of massages, saunas, carrot juice cocktails, facials, mud packs, and the like. There's nothing wrong with that. But spending a day or a week at the spa is nothing more than an attempt to use technical means—mud or massage, for instance—to work around and undo the effects of years of musculoskeletal system dysfunction, without bothering to directly address the central problem.

Just as weight management is profoundly influenced by the health of the musculoskeletal system, so too are complexion, skin tone, hair and nail quality, cellulite deposits, mood, and energy levels. The reason a massage feels so good is that the fingers and hands of the masseuse are stimulating muscles and other tissue that are otherwise disengaged and bypassed. For a half hour during the massage, blood with its precious cargo of nutrients and oxygen is flowing again. Also, a good massage practitioner is relieving constricted joints and muscles that are bearing the brunt of everyday dysfunctions. Likewise, facials and mud packs attempt to reen-

She did lots of long-distance running and other strength-building regimens during the rest of the day. When it was all over, Connie felt great, but when she weighed herself on the last day of camp, she found that she had picked up about six or eight pounds. Look out! Did I hear about that! But when Connie got back home and out of her shorts and T-shirts, she discovered that the clothes she wore to work at the law firm were baggy. She had dropped almost two dress sizes. Connie forgave me.

ergize, with minerals, nutrients, fluid, and oxygen, tissue that's no longer adequately served by the musculoskeletal system.

Years ago beauticians recommended that their clients stand on their heads, or at least spend time reclining with their feet higher than their heads, to promote blood flow to the face and scalp. More than a few balding men have tried this too. It's not a bad idea, but a better one is to actually eliminate what's restricting the flow of blood and oxygen in the first place. Take a look at Figures 12–1a and 12–2a, which show the difference between a dysfunctional and functional head position. Unconsciously, as the spine loses its S-curve, our heads come forward. Instead of being balanced on top of the spine like a pedestal supported by powerful erector muscles and vertebral disks, the head wants to topple downward under the influence of gravity. The muscles of the upper back, shoulders, and neck are trying to keep that from happening. To do so, they tend to stay in contraction, which impedes blood flow and diverts what's not being used by the brain and optic nerve away from the surface. In effect, your facial skin is being impoverished to keep the head on your shoulders.

Contracting muscles use up energy, and they have to get it from somewhere, which in addition to the face, includes the scalp, the gums, the eyes, and the ears.

Many of what are considered to be the cosmetic signs of aging are actually the effects of a system that's too busy and too stressed to worry about nonessentials like wrinkles, skin tone and color, hair texture, and brittle nails. When the entire head is signaling that it's apt to go south, the body stops messing with the small stuff. Sadly, it makes for a double loss. As the substance of health erodes, it takes with it the surface image of health. This crumbling process starts on the inside, not the outside. It is very important to keep that in mind.

Good posture has classically been associated with health, beauty, and a commanding presence, in part because its attributes have been self-evident and self-actualizing. Beauty is not skin deep. It's literally the product of inner strength, a projection of one's power and capabilities. Without that strength the body not only slumps, it loses the vitality and glow that are the genuine core of beauty, no matter what the season's fashion gurus have decreed is in or out, dazzling or dull.

I think that's why the American public has been falling in love with top-ranked female figure skaters, soccer players, and other athletes. They look strong, capable, confident, and happy. Their pure body language makes us feel good to watch them. Even from a distance we can see—and remember—the joy and power of what it means to stand up straight, run like the wind, turn on a dime, and reach for the stars.

Some people believe that if they look good, they'll feel good. But the truth of the matter is that if we feel good, we'll look good. That's what athletes are telling us: *We look like winners—because we have what it takes to win.*

Building Strength and Managing Weight

I'm presenting two Strength Menus here. The first one does not call for the use of free weights. The second one does and is therefore optional.

The body doesn't need dumbbells or other pieces of gym equipment to grow strong. I'm including the free-weight menu for folks who think they can't live without apparatus. But if you opt to use it, I want you to start by mastering the first Strength Menu, the one that doesn't use free weights. Don't move on to the free-weight menu until the first menu is a piece of cake.

Likewise, I suggest that if you want to use Dr. Miriam Nelson's strength-training programs, it's a good idea to become proficient with the first Strength Menu first, since the Nelson programs include free weights. Without musculoskeletal alignment and the strength to maintain it, dumbbells can actually aggravate misalignment. You end up strengthening dysfunctions and locking yourself in to misalignment. When you do an exercise/strength program without aligning and engaging your musculoskeletal system first, much of the benefit is lost.

This first Strength Menu is going to be challenging, but it's the quickest, most direct route to strength and dramatic aesthetic enhancement. If you want to drop down a few dress sizes, this is the way to go. You will have ample rewards for the effort. If the E-cises seem too hard at first, reduce the number of repetitions. Or if need be, assume the starting position and simply make an attempt to execute the sequence of moves. If you don't have enough strength, do what you can, stop, and relax for a moment. Then try again. If you still can't do it, that's all right. Try again the next day. Little by little you will gain the strength necessary to complete the moves. Keep at it, there's no rush.

On alternate days switch between the first Strength Menu and Phase III of the Postpregnancy Menu from Chapter 11, until you can fully perform the Strength Menu. At that point you can stop doing Phase III. There's no reason to give up your other favorite physical activities, like yoga, swimming, or workouts at the health club. Use the Strength Menu as a warm-up, and have fun!

Using the second Strength Menu is as easy as a walk in the park after using the first. But return to the first menu at least once a week to make sure you're keeping your alignment. Remember, pain and free weights don't mix. If something hurts, stop.

$$\left[\text{Strength Menu Without Free Weights} \right]$$

▸ FOOT CIRCLES and POINT/FLEXES
(Figure 12–3 a, b, and c)

PURPOSE This E-cise reminds the knees, ankles, and feet how to interact according to their designs.

Lie on your back with your right leg extended flat on the floor and your left leg bent toward your chest. For the Foot Circles, clasp your hands behind your bent knee to hold it in position while you circle your left foot clockwise (a). The Foot Circles emanate from the ankle, not from the knee. Keep your knee still, and try to make full circles. (You may tend to make half circles; it will help to slow down and concentrate.) Meanwhile, keep the right foot pointed straight up toward the ceiling, with the right thigh muscles tight. Do forty repetitions. Then reverse direction and circle your left foot counterclockwise. Repeat forty times. For the Point/Flexes, keep your legs in the same position. On the bent left leg, bring your toes back toward the shin to flex (b), then reverse the direction to point your toes (c). Do this twenty times. Switch legs and do forty repetitions of Foot Circles and twenty Point/Flexes with the other foot.

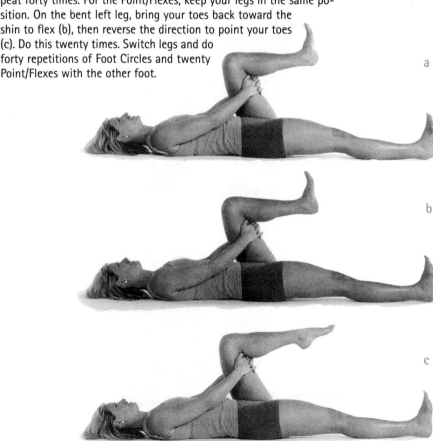

a

b

c

▸ STANDING ARM CIRCLES
(Figure 12–4 a and b)

PURPOSE This E-cise strengthens the muscles of the upper back that are involved with the shoulders' ball and socket function.

Stand facing a mirror with your feet parallel about a hip-width apart, your arms at your sides. Curl your fingertips into the pads of each palm (the fleshy area at the base of the fingers) and point your thumbs straight out. This hand position, called the "golfer's grip," is imperative to the success of the E-cise. Squeeze your shoulder blades together, and bring your arms out to your sides at shoulder level, elbows straight. With your palms facing down, thumbs pointing forward, circle up and forward for forty repetitions (a). Now with your palms facing up, circle up and back for forty repetitions (b). Remember to keep your wrists and elbows straight and your shoulder blades squeezed together—the circles must come from the shoulders.

a

b

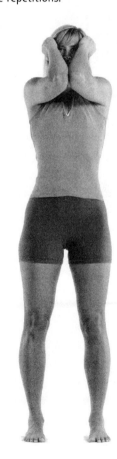

▸ STANDING ELBOW CURLS
(Figure 12–5 a and b)
PURPOSE This E-cise reminds the shoulder's "hinge" what full flexion and extension feel like.

Stand with your heels, buttocks, upper back, and head against a wall. Your feet, pointed straight ahead, are about a hip-width apart. Raise your hands in the "golfer's grip" (see Standing Arm Circles), placing your knuckles along your temples, thumbs extended down your cheeks (a). Bring your elbows together to meet in front (b). Make sure your elbows meet in the middle of your body (and are not skewed to the left or right, which would mean that one shoulder is flexing more than the other). Then pull your elbows back even with your shoulders to touch the wall. Your head should remain still, and your knuckles should not lift off your temples. Do one set of twenty-five repetitions.

a

b

▶ TRIANGLE
(Figure 12–6 a and b)

PURPOSE This E-cise puts all the load-joints onto the same vertical plane, where they belong.

Stand with your heels against a wall and your feet parallel, pointed straight ahead. Turn your left foot outward, and take a big step sideways so your left foot is parallel to the wall, about three inches away from it. Raise both arms at your sides to shoulder level and extend them; keep them against the wall with your palms out. Rotate your hips so both buttock muscles are against the wall. Turn your head to the right so that you are looking in the direction of the right foot (the one that didn't move) (a). Slide your right hip to the right (keeping it on the wall), while sliding your arms and shoulders up and over in the opposite direction. Look up at your raised right palm, keeping your shoulders and head against the wall, and tucking your left arm and hand behind the left knee. Your arms and shoulders should form a straight line that extends upward from the back of your left hip (b). Tighten your thighs, and hold this position for one minute. Reverse and repeat on the other side.

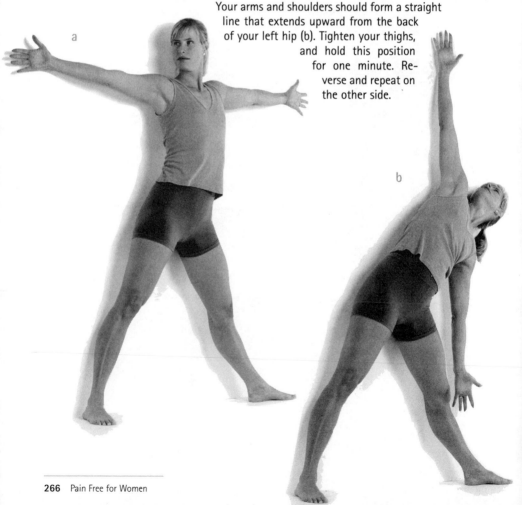

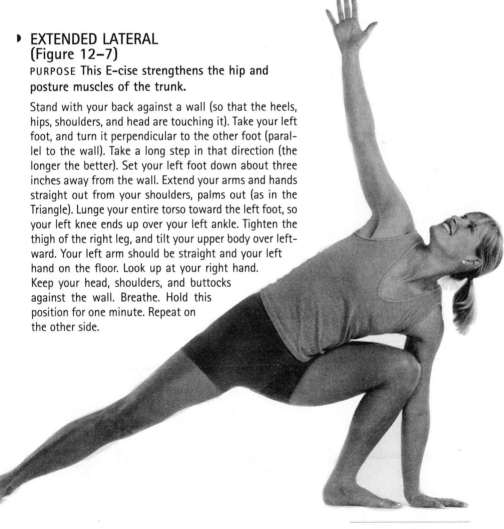

▸ EXTENDED LATERAL
(Figure 12-7)

PURPOSE This E-cise strengthens the hip and posture muscles of the trunk.

Stand with your back against a wall (so that the heels, hips, shoulders, and head are touching it). Take your left foot, and turn it perpendicular to the other foot (parallel to the wall). Take a long step in that direction (the longer the better). Set your left foot down about three inches away from the wall. Extend your arms and hands straight out from your shoulders, palms out (as in the Triangle). Lunge your entire torso toward the left foot, so your left knee ends up over your left ankle. Tighten the thigh of the right leg, and tilt your upper body over leftward. Your left arm should be straight and your left hand on the floor. Look up at your right hand. Keep your head, shoulders, and buttocks against the wall. Breathe. Hold this position for one minute. Repeat on the other side.

▸ CATS and DOGS
(Figure 12–8 a and b)

PURPOSE This E-cise works the hips, spine, shoulders, and neck in coordinated flexion and extension.

Get down on the floor on your hands and knees. Make a table by aligning your knees with your hips and your wrists with your shoulders. Your lower legs should be parallel with each other and with your hips. Your weight should be distributed evenly. For the Cat, smoothly round your back upward and let your head curl under, to create a curve that runs from your buttocks to your neck—like a cat with an arched back (a). For the Dog, smoothly sway your back down while bringing your head up (b). Make these two moves flow continuously back and forth. Exhale as you move into the Cat position; inhale during the Dog. Do one set of ten repetitions.

a

b

▶ CORE ABDOMINALS
(Figure 12-9 a, b, c, and d)
PURPOSE This E-cise gives your deepest layer of abdominal muscles a workout.

Position 1: Lie on your stomach propped on your elbows; your chest is off the floor, and your head is up. Look straight ahead. Loosely curl your fingers inward on the palms, and extend your thumbs straight up. Pull your toes under, and bridge your body off the floor. Your weight is resting on your toes and elbows (a). Press down and outward on your forearms without moving your elbows. Roll your hands outward at the wrists, and let your shoulder blades collapse together. Hold for thirty seconds.

Positions 2 and 3: Lie on your right side propped up on your elbow, with your arm resting atop your hip and thigh, your feet together, and legs straight. Keep your shoulders, hips, knees, and ankles in a straight line (b). Hold for thirty seconds. Switch sides, and hold for another thirty seconds (c).

Position 4: Lie on your back with your legs straight, your heels down and together. Prop your elbows under your shoulders, flex your toes, and lift your pelvis off the floor (d). Hold for thirty seconds.

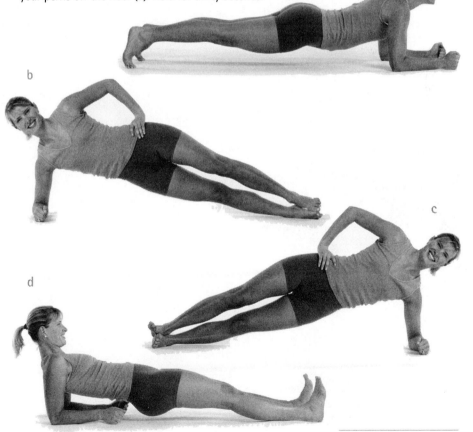

a

b

c

d

▶ WIDE ELEVATED SQUATS
(Figure 12–10)

PURPOSE This E-cise develops hip and leg strength.

Place two sturdy elevated objects (three to four inches high; metal or wooden footstools will do) about thirty inches apart. (Adjust this according to your height.) Stand on them with your feet parallel and pointed straight ahead. Arch your lower back. Extend your arms and hands straight out from your shoulders, with palms down. Now bend your knees, and lower your body until your knees and hips are parallel. Make sure your torso remains vertical and your feet stay straight. Hold for one minute.

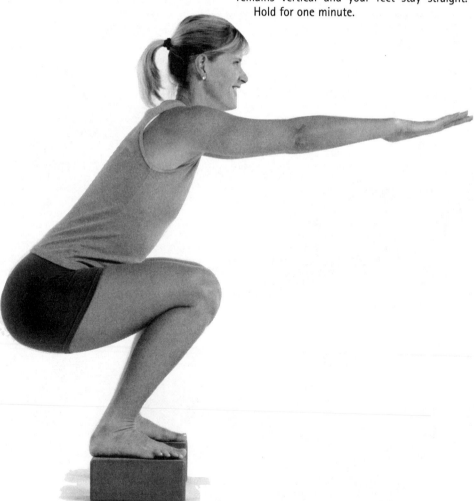

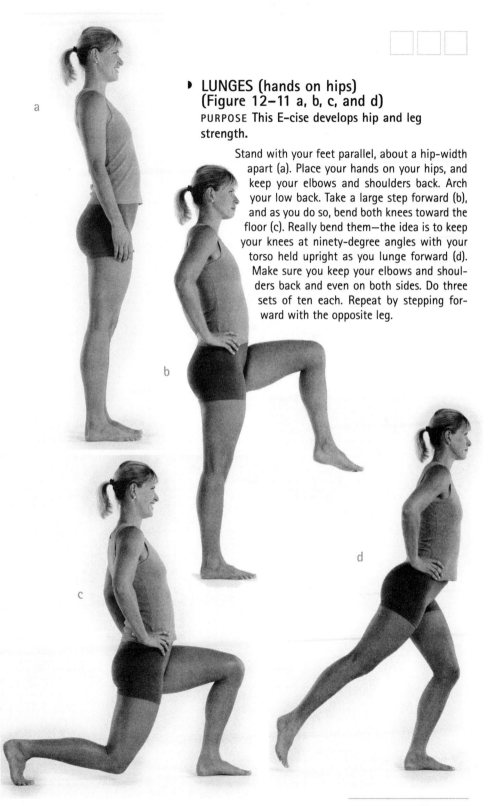

▸ LUNGES (hands on hips)
(Figure 12–11 a, b, c, and d)

PURPOSE This E-cise develops hip and leg strength.

Stand with your feet parallel, about a hip-width apart (a). Place your hands on your hips, and keep your elbows and shoulders back. Arch your low back. Take a large step forward (b), and as you do so, bend both knees toward the floor (c). Really bend them—the idea is to keep your knees at ninety-degree angles with your torso held upright as you lunge forward (d). Make sure you keep your elbows and shoulders back and even on both sides. Do three sets of ten each. Repeat by stepping forward with the opposite leg.

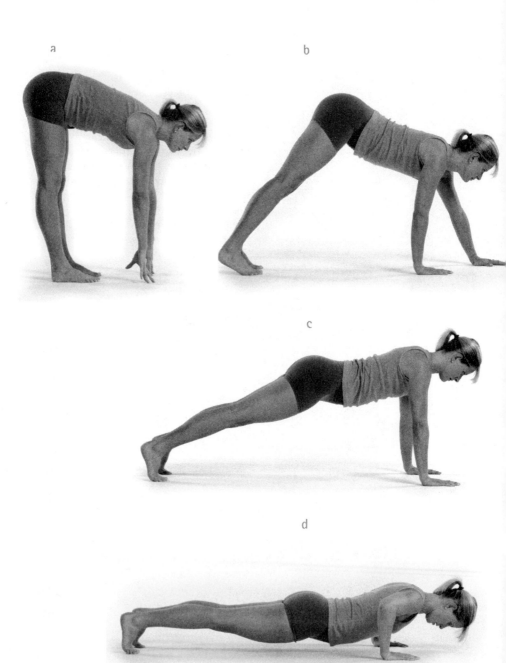

a

b

c

d

▸ WALK-OUTS
(Figure 12–12 a, b, c, d, e, f, and g)

PURPOSE This E-cise provides total body strength in a cardiovascular environment.

Bend over, and touch the floor in front of your toes (a), keeping your knees straight. "Walk" your hands out (b) until your body is in a classic starting push-up position (c). Lower your chest to the floor by bending your elbows (d). Straighten your elbows to return to the starting push-up position (e), and "walk" your hands back (f) to the starting point (g). Do one Walk-out (and back).

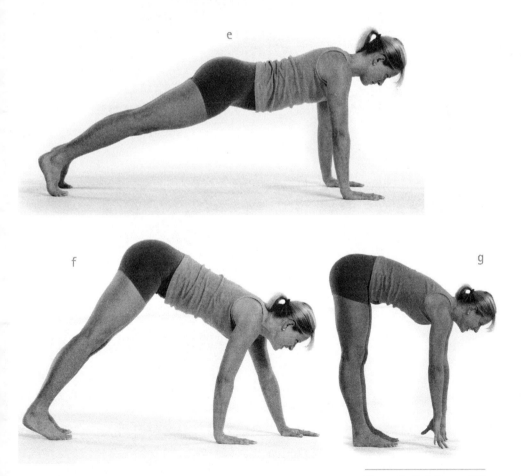

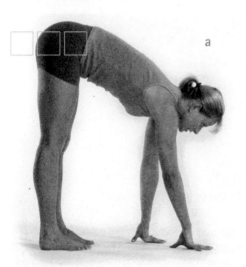

a

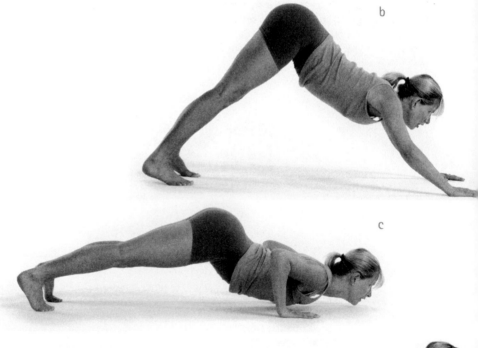

b

c

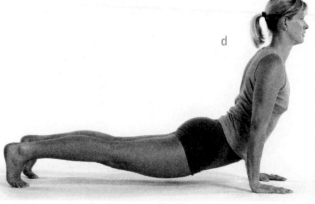

d

▶ ROLLER COASTERS
(Figure 12–13 a, b, c, d, e, and f)
PURPOSE This E-cise provides total body strength in a cardiovascular environment.

Stand with your feet pointed straight ahead, a hip-width apart. Bend over at the waist (knees straight!) and touch the floor in front of your toes (a). Walk your hands out far enough to put your body in a piked position (b). (Instead of having your back, buttocks, and legs on the same plane, as in a push-up, your hips and buttocks are higher than your shoulders and legs.) Lower your chest toward the floor by allowing your elbows to bend (c). The idea is for your chin, chest, and hips to just skim the floor before you straighten your elbows, raise your head, and arch your back without descending all the way to the floor (d). Reverse (e) and return to the piked position (inverted V) (f). Repeat. Do two sets of ten repetitions each.

e

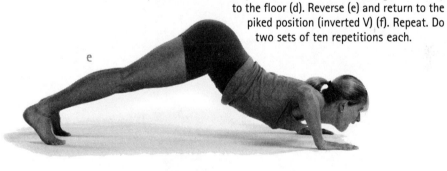

f

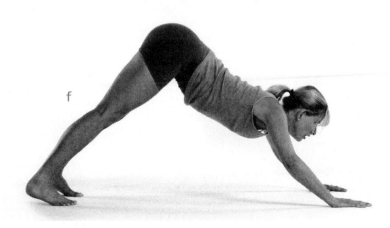

▸ FULL BRIDGE
(Figure 12–14 a and b)

PURPOSE This E-cise provides total body strength in a cardiovascular environment.

Lie on your back with your knees bent and your feet pointed straight ahead. Place your hands just above your shoulders with palms down (a), so that you can "bridge" by lifting up on your hands and feet (b). Try to keep your elbows locked out straight, and don't let your knees come together. Hold for one minute. If this E-cise proves difficult, come as close as you can each time. Keep trying and eventually a half bridge will evolve to a full bridge.

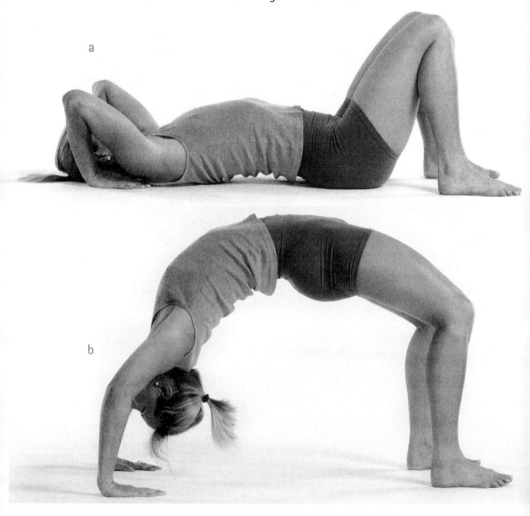

▸ BENCH HOPS
(Figure 12–15 a, b, c, and d)

PURPOSE This E-cise provides total body strength in a cardiovascular environment.

Stand sideways beside a sturdy bench. Place both hands on the bench for support (a), and hop to the other side by swinging both your legs up and over (b). Tuck your knees up into your chest as you make the hop. Then hop back (c and d). Keep your hands in the same position on the bench for each hop, and do not favor either side by hopping and then turning around to hop back, which some people will do if they sense that one side is "stronger" and more functional than the other. Do three sets of ten repetitions each. (Count each hop as one.)

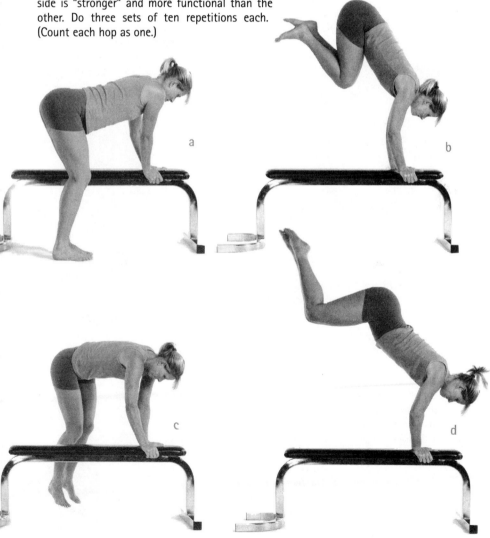

▸ AIR BENCH
(Figure 12–16)

PURPOSE This E-cise promotes lower leg, thigh, and hip strength, and it relaxes the muscles of the torso.

Stand against a wall with your feet pointing straight ahead, parallel, a hip-width apart. Walk your feet away from the wall approximately 2 to 2½ feet, as you bend your knees and slide your back down the wall. Stop sliding and walking when your thighs and hips form approximately a ninety-degree angle. Your knees should be over your ankles, not your toes. If you feel pain in your kneecaps, raise your body up the wall to relieve the pressure. Keep your weight on your heels. Hold this position for two minutes.

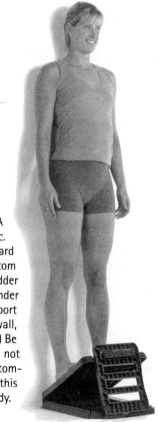

▸ WALL DROP
(Figure 12–17)

PURPOSE This E-cise synchronizes the feet, ankles, knees, and hips while under load and proper alignment.

Stand against a wall with your feet on a slant board. (A slant board is a simple apparatus we invented in the clinic. You can improvise by propping one end of an inch-thick board that is 12 inches wide and 36 inches long against the bottom rung of a short stepladder and the floor. Make sure the ladder is wide enough at the base, equipped with rubber pads under the legs to prevent skidding, and sufficiently stable to support your weight. If you put one edge of the board against the wall, it won't kick back. The angle should be about sixty degrees.) Be sure your feet are parallel and pointed straight ahead; do not allow your knees to bend or the feet to twist. Relax your stomach. You will feel a stretch in your lower leg muscles, but this E-cise is really working to relax your stomach and upper body. Hold the position for five minutes.

▶ STATIC BACK
(Figure 12–18)

PURPOSE This E-cise uses gravity to flatten the back and put it in a neutral position.

Lie on your back, with both legs bent at right angles and resting on a chair, bench, or block. (The large blocks we use in the clinic are 20 inches high by 14 inches wide by 24 inches long.) Rest your hands on the floor, extended below shoulder level, with the palms up. Let your back settle in to the floor. Breathe from your diaphragm, so your abdominal muscles rise as you inhale and fall as you exhale. Hold this position for five minutes.

[Strength Menu with Free Weights]

▸ **STANDING SHOULDER ROLLS**
(Figure 12–19 a, b, c, and d)
PURPOSE This E-cise strengthens the ball and socket function of the shoulders.

Stand in front of a mirror with your feet parallel and about a hip-width apart with a five-pound weight in each hand. Let your arms hang at your sides with your elbows straight. Keep your head back and shoulders square. Circle your shoulders by pulling them up (a), forward, and down (b). Do ten repetitions. Reverse by pulling them up (c), back, and down (d) for ten more circles in that direction. Do three sets; ten forward and ten back constitutes one set.

a b c d

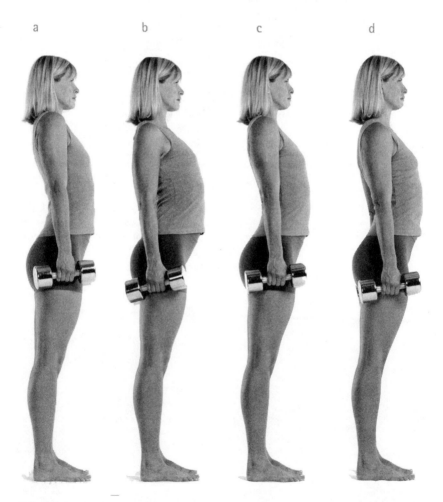

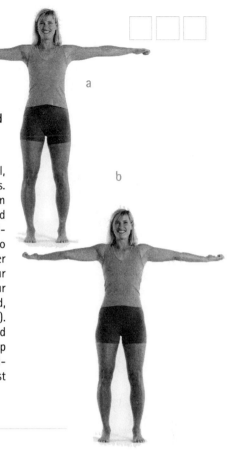

▶ STANDING ARM CIRCLES
(Figure 12–20 a and b)

PURPOSE This E-cise strengthens the muscles of the upper back that are involved with the shoulders' ball and socket function.

Stand facing a mirror with your feet parallel, about a hip-width apart, your arms at your sides. Curl your fingertips into the pads of each palm (the fleshy area at the base of the fingers), and point your thumbs straight out. This hand position, called the "golfer's grip," is imperative to the success of the E-cise. Squeeze your shoulder blades together, and bring your arms out to your sides at shoulder level, elbows straight. With your palms facing down, thumbs pointing forward, circle up and forward for forty repetitions (a). Now with your palms facing up, circle up and back for forty repetitions (b). Remember to keep your wrists and elbows straight and your shoulder blades squeezed together—the circles must come from the shoulders.

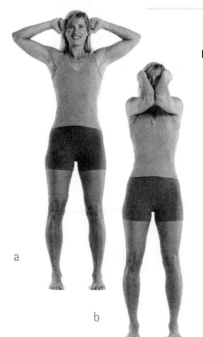

▶ STANDING ELBOW CURLS
(Figure 12–21 a and b)

PURPOSE This E-cise reminds the shoulder's "hinge" what full flexion and extension feel like.

Stand with your heels, buttocks, upper back, and head against a wall. Your feet, pointed straight ahead, are about a hip-width apart. Raise your hands in the "golfer's grip" (see Standing Arm Circles), placing your knuckles along your temples, thumbs extended down your cheeks (a). Bring your elbows together to meet in front (b). Make sure your elbows meet in the middle of your body (and are not skewed to the left or right, which would mean that one shoulder is flexing more than the other). Then pull your elbows back even with your shoulders to touch the wall. Your head should remain still, and your knuckles should not lift off your temples. Do one set of twenty-five repetitions.

a

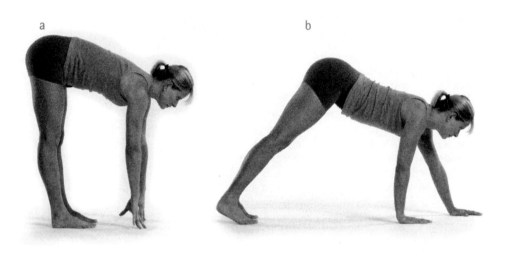

b

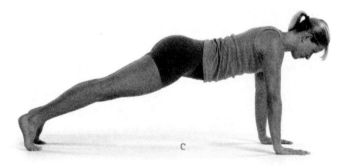

c

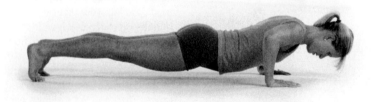

d

▸ WALK-OUTS
(Figure 12–22 a, b, c, d, e, f, and g)

PURPOSE This E-cise provides total body strength in a cardiovascular environment.

Bend over, and touch the floor in front of your toes (a), keeping your knees straight. "Walk" your hands out (b) until your body is in a classic starting push-up position (c). Lower your chest to the floor by bending your elbows (d). Straighten your elbows to return to the starting push-up position (e), and "walk" your hands back (f) to the starting point (g). Do one Walk-out (and back).

e

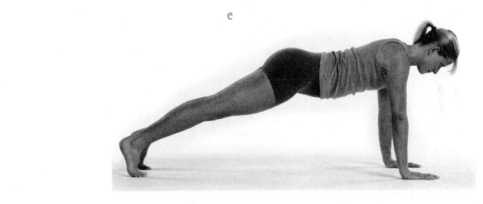

f

g

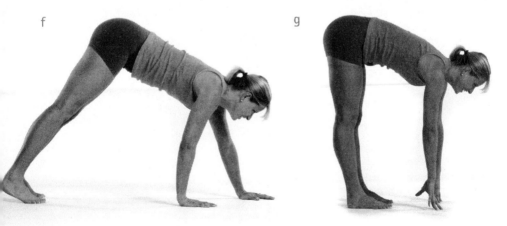

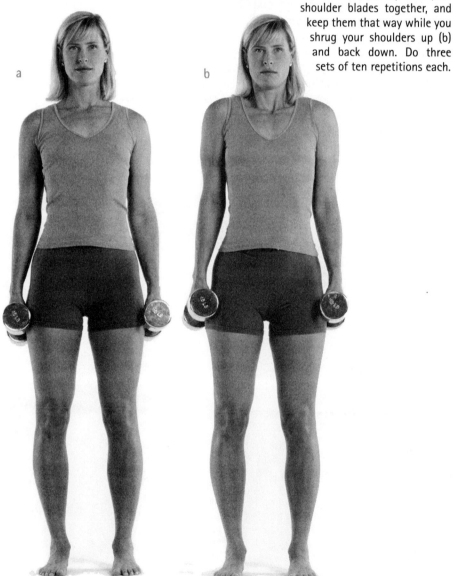

▸ STANDING SHOULDER SHRUGS (Figure 12–23 a and b)

PURPOSE This E-cise strengthens a shoulder function that is often lost when the shoulders are allowed to roll forward and stay there.

Stand in front of a mirror with your feet parallel, about a hip-width apart. Hold a five-pound weight in each hand with your arms at your sides (a). Squeeze your shoulder blades together, and keep them that way while you shrug your shoulders up (b) and back down. Do three sets of ten repetitions each.

a

b

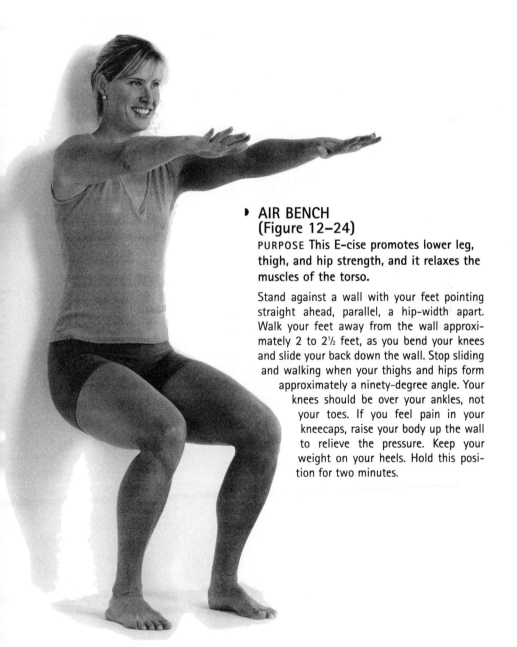

▸ AIR BENCH
(Figure 12–24)

PURPOSE This E-cise promotes lower leg, thigh, and hip strength, and it relaxes the muscles of the torso.

Stand against a wall with your feet pointing straight ahead, parallel, a hip-width apart. Walk your feet away from the wall approximately 2 to 2½ feet, as you bend your knees and slide your back down the wall. Stop sliding and walking when your thighs and hips form approximately a ninety-degree angle. Your knees should be over your ankles, not your toes. If you feel pain in your kneecaps, raise your body up the wall to relieve the pressure. Keep your weight on your heels. Hold this position for two minutes.

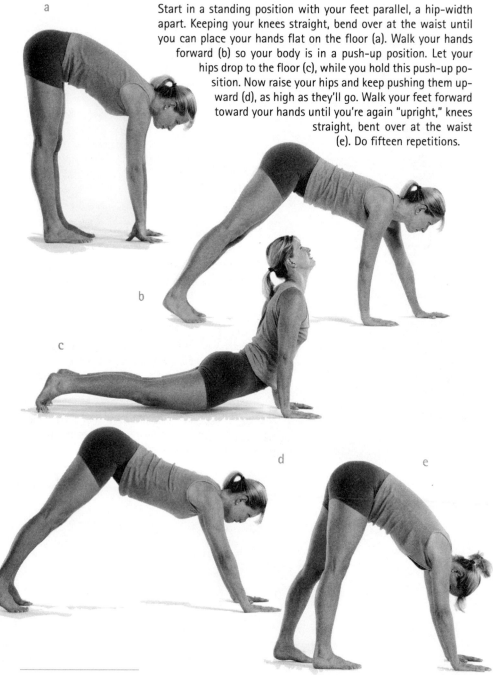

▶ INCH WORMS (Figure 12–25 a, b, c, d, and e)

PURPOSE This E-cise stabilizes and strengthens core muscles.

Start in a standing position with your feet parallel, a hip-width apart. Keeping your knees straight, bend over at the waist until you can place your hands flat on the floor (a). Walk your hands forward (b) so your body is in a push-up position. Let your hips drop to the floor (c), while you hold this push-up position. Now raise your hips and keep pushing them upward (d), as high as they'll go. Walk your feet forward toward your hands until you're again "upright," knees straight, bent over at the waist (e). Do fifteen repetitions.

a

b

c

d

e

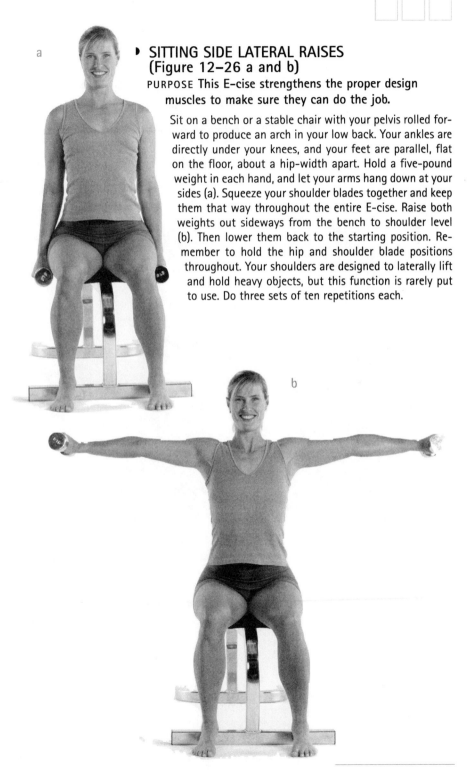

a

▶ SITTING SIDE LATERAL RAISES
(Figure 12–26 a and b)

PURPOSE This E-cise strengthens the proper design muscles to make sure they can do the job.

Sit on a bench or a stable chair with your pelvis rolled forward to produce an arch in your low back. Your ankles are directly under your knees, and your feet are parallel, flat on the floor, about a hip-width apart. Hold a five-pound weight in each hand, and let your arms hang down at your sides (a). Squeeze your shoulder blades together and keep them that way throughout the entire E-cise. Raise both weights out sideways from the bench to shoulder level (b). Then lower them back to the starting position. Remember to hold the hip and shoulder blade positions throughout. Your shoulders are designed to laterally lift and hold heavy objects, but this function is rarely put to use. Do three sets of ten repetitions each.

b

‣ BICEP CURLS
(Figure 12–27 a and b)
PURPOSE This E-cise strengthens the biceps.

Stand against a wall, but leave a little space between its surface and the back of your heels. Hold a five-pound weight in each hand, with the back of your hands toward the wall (a). Squeeze your shoulder blades together, and place your elbows against the wall. Curl the weights up toward your shoulders by bending the elbows (b) to lift your forearms, both at the same time. Do three sets of ten repetitions each.

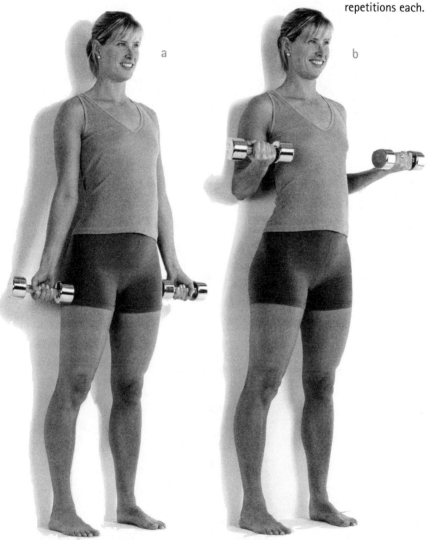

a b

▸ SUPINE TRICEP EXTENSIONS
(Figure 12–28 a, b, and c)

PURPOSE This E-cise strengthens the triceps.

Lie on your back with both legs bent at right angles and resting on a chair, bench, or block. Hold a pair of five-pound weights. Begin by lightly squeezing your shoulder blades together. Place your hands (holding the weights) beside your ears so that your elbows are pointing straight up (a). Without moving the elbow position, press the weights straight up and into the air above your head (b). Your elbows will straighten as they lift, but they are not to flare in or out or shift toward your feet. Now lower the weights back to the starting position beside your ears (c). Do three sets of ten repetitions each.

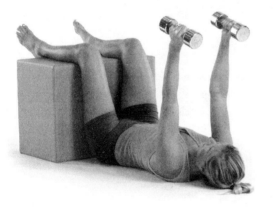

a

b

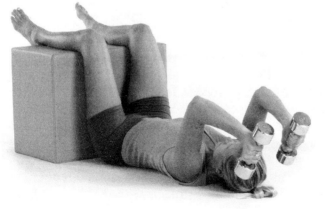

c

Anti-Aging

Brace yourself: I'm going to ask a profoundly philosophical question. Do you believe the glass is half empty or half full?

As trite as this cliché is, it neatly frames an issue that every person who reaches S^3 must confront. If life, like the glass, is seen as half empty, then the other half is bound to run dry as well. But while all life comes to an end eventually, it is far more renewable than we realize. In that sense at S^3, life really is half full, and we can choose to fill the glass or to continue to drain it off.

Chronic musculoskeletal pain is symptomatic not of advancing and accumulating years, but of advancing and accumulating dysfunctions. Bad backs and sore knees, aching shoulders and painful wrists, stiff necks, weak ankles, and tender feet have nothing to do with calendars or clocks. If they did, all forty-year-olds would have heel spurs, all forty-five-year-olds tennis elbow, and all fiftysomethings trick knees. Because many maladies seem to cluster around chronological mileposts, we conclude that age causes illness and makes accidents happen.

The idea of turning forty, not to mention the horror of fifty, haunts many people who assume that at those ages decline is inevitable and hot on their heels. But decline has already been going, in many cases, for years— years of overeating and underactivity, years of restricted and repetitive motion, years of dehydration, metabolic inefficiency, and immune system stress. We know how to tell time, but the body doesn't. It only measures damage and then tries its damndest to fix it.

The single most effective anti-aging tool available to us is a completely engaged, fully functional musculoskeletal system. Research study after research study tells us that increased levels of physical activity have beneficial effects on everything from helping an asthmatic breathe to ensuring that a zygote turns into a viable embryo and then a fetus. That influence occurs even when the research subjects remain dysfunctional, which they are since they are randomly drawn from the general population. The results would be dramatic indeed with fully functional participants. The body could then focus its entire resources on repair and restoration without having to also struggle with the consequences of disengaged or weak muscles, deteriorating bones, and frazzled joints.

In the next chapter we'll turn our attention to metabolic suppression and how it leads to chronic disease. Successful prevention of these diseases, and treatment if they occur, are hard work that requires the power of strong muscles, bones, and joints.

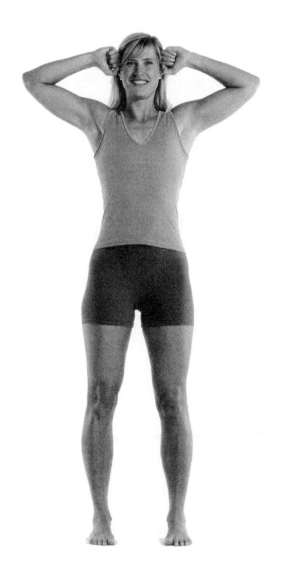

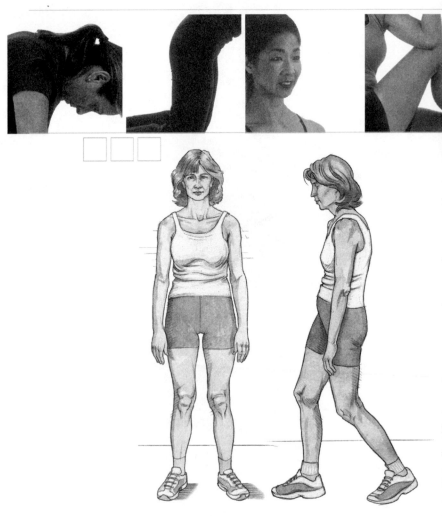

Fig. 13-1   Fig. 13-2

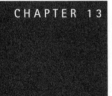

stoking the
metabolic bonfire

This chapter is about fighting disease with a powerful weapon—
posture. First let me introduce Tina, who is losing the fight.

She's in Figures 13–1 and 13–2. Notice her hips; they're tipped
forward in flexion, that classic symptom of dysfunction. Functional
hips are able to move smoothly from a neutral position (Figure
13–3a) into flexion (Figure 13–3b), back to neutral, and into extension (Figure 13–3c). Although the hip frozen in flexion is dysfunctional, it indicates that at least some muscles are strong enough

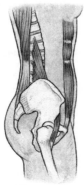

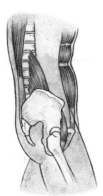

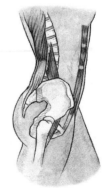

Fig. 13-3a   Fig. 13-3b   Fig. 13-3c

to contract and pull the hip over and down and keep it there. But Tina's muscles are so weak that they can't really achieve much flexion or extension. Her hips just wobble between the two. As a result, she is extremely weak and structurally unstable.

Remember, the pelvic muscles are among the body's most powerful, but in Tina's case they're probably providing only 10 or 20 percent of their capacity, just enough to keep her semi-upright and ambulatory. But that's not much. Check out her knees and feet. Both are turned outward because of the hip position. And her thigh and calf muscles are weak and atrophied. Above the waist Tina's spinal S-curve has flattened, her shoulders are slumped, and her head is jutting forward.

I suggest you try to duplicate this posture. Stand with your feet slightly splayed, and roll your hips back and under by tightening the muscles in your low back and buttocks. Let your shoulders slump, and hang your head. Try to take a reasonably deep breath in that position.

It feels awful, doesn't it? Seeing someone else in that posture is bad enough, but feeling it yourself is a shock. For Tina, that feeling permeates the entire ecology of her body. Every system, every scrap of tissue, every cell, and every molecule is saturated with that feeling of instability, ineffectualness, and insecurity. This posture used to be relatively rare. Today it's more and more common.

Now straighten your feet so they're parallel and about a hip-width apart. Arch your back, and pull your head and shoulders back. Relax and breathe. Do you notice the difference? In an instant you've changed your outward appearance—you have improved stability, better muscular engagement, more blood and oxygen flow—and your inner monitoring system knows that and is broadcasting the good news from head to foot.

For Tina, the bad news has been rolling in for years as her dysfunctions have deepened. Her body has been valiantly battling the consequences all along, but it's been at a serious disadvantage. Her posture tells us that too: it's the posture of metabolic collapse. Take another look. She has hardly any muscle mass. Without major thigh, hip, trunk, and shoulder muscle strength, Tina has only minor peripheral muscles to stoke the bonfire of her metabolism. Some blaze! It's more like a few embers and some smoke. Intensely active muscles can provide up to forty times the heat generated by the rest of the body. This requires (and helps ignite) an enormous metabolic capacity that not only services muscle contraction and relaxation but is available to every organ and system. And when these active muscles are at rest, the metabolic system has so much extra capacity that it can easily meet whatever other demands the body throws at it.

Unilateral Disarmament

What's so important about heat? It's a by-product of work, of energy expenditure and creation. The body's myriad chemical reactions require heat in order to break molecular bonds and reglue them into new compounds that keep us growing and going. Tina's body has not nearly enough heat and energy to generate this body-wide cellular burn rate. And without it she is susceptible to disease.

All of us are under constant siege by microbes. The immune system keeps them at bay, but only as long as it has adequate metabolic resources. To withstand an invasion of foreign bodies, bugs, and bacteria, the immune system must create millions and millions of B and T cells to act as the infantry and artillery. These cells must sheathe each invading body in membrane, and doing so requires a metabolic blast furnace to break down fat and gain the necessary lipids. Tina, however, is flirting with unilateral disarmament. Her ability to field an immuno-fighting force is seriously compromised by her dysfunctions. She's been fighting and losing this war of attrition for years. That's why she's so tired, irritable, and prone to colds, flu, and infections. She doesn't sleep well, she craves sugar, salt, and caffeine, and she has agonizing migraines.

Even in dysfunctional individuals, cell propagation is constantly taking place at an astronomically high rate. Therefore it's probable that the human body regularly produces aggressive misfit cells with genetic flaws—that is, cancer cells. (This is one widely held theory of the origin of cancer.) A healthy immune system immediately picks off those cells before they can dig in, mutate, and spread. Tina's immune system, however, is far from healthy. Her metabolism cannot generate enough energy to manufacture B and T cells in sufficient numbers to handle even an everyday invasion—a gust of pollen, for instance, or a run-in with common viruses—let alone effectively police 100 percent of the emerging cancer cells. Inevitably a few get through. Over time potentially deadly clusters may be established.

Once that happens the immune system turns into a leaky rowboat. It can't be rowed safely to shore because all hands are needed to bail, but unless someone mans the oars, the incoming waves threaten to sink the craft. As already limited and hard-pressed B and T cells are mobilized to combat the spreading cancer, fewer defender cells are available for duty elsewhere. They bail, but they don't row. More and more cancer cells go unchallenged. The predators multiply and start moving in from every direction.

The dire predicament is exacerbated by the way the immune system cuts its losses: it goes from zero tolerance of pathogens and toxins to accepting *manageable* pathogens and *low-level* toxins. It lets enough of them through to relieve the pressure on B and T cells so they can concentrate on the most immediately dangerous interlopers. In theory it's a sound strategy: deal with your biggest problem, then go back and mop up the secondary stuff. But that strategy assumes big problems won't keep cropping up. Unfortunately they do. Eventually the pressure builds again, and the immune system must lower its standards another notch and redefine what constitutes manageable pathogens and low-level toxins. In effect, yesterday's dangerous predator is given parole because the prison is too crowded. With each round, disease comes closer to gaining the upper hand.

For Tina this pattern of escalation and retreat is compounded by the fact that she has no quick way to boost her immune system, since she lacks the three essential M's: motion, muscle, and metabolism. If she had a fully functional musculoskeletal system, she would start with a higher metabolic rate and sufficient energy production to immediately mobilize a full army of B and T cells. She might not even get behind the curve in the first place. Even if she did, as more and more B and T cells were created and sent into battle, her stronger and engaged muscles would be there to meet the extra energy demand.

But instead Tina quickly runs out of energy. The effects of her illness will slow her down. She'll rest more, avoid stress, and conserve energy. Unfortunately, her metabolism will slow down too. It's a pure supply-demand system: as the motion-muscle demand for energy drops off, the supply is curtailed as well; overall capacity falls off too. This instinct to rest and recuperate is sound, but it's predicated on having sufficient muscular underpinning to the metabolic process to allow its resting rate to be several degrees higher than the bare minimum. When Tina is at rest, she's already in metabolic deficit. That's one reason she sleeps so fitfully at night. Her metabolism is nearly flatlining, which prompts the body to jolt her awake in order to trigger whatever metabolic activity can be gained when she rolls over or gets out of bed. Tina simply does not have the extra metabolic power to spare to support a lean, mean, immuno-fighting machine.

Transforming Tina into Tanya

Compare Tina and her cousin Tanya. They are basically the same age, size, and shape. The difference between Tina and Tanya is that Tanya's musculoskeletal system is fully functional and strong—she can whip through the two Strength Menus in Chapter 12. But Tina can't even motivate herself to give them a try.

But I'm not about to write Tina off. Her body—like yours and mine—will quickly start to recover lost functions (they're not really lost, just suspended) if small changes are made in demand. The following E-cise menu will do that slowly, over the course of about six months.

▶ **SITTING STATIC ABDUCTOR PRESS**
(Figure 13–4)

PURPOSE This E-cise equalizes the engaged and strength of the abductor muscles of the thighs, requiring them to work without cheating by using gravity to swing the thigh from side to side.

Sit on a bench or the edge of a chair with your feet pointed straight ahead, a hip-width apart and directly under your knees. Place a strap around your legs just under your knees, and pull it taut so that your knees are together. Relax your stomach, and put an arch in your low back by rolling your hips forward. Push out on the strap. Release. Make sure to keep the arch in your back throughout. Do one set, squeezing and releasing for five minutes.

▶ **STATIC EXTENSION POSITION**
(Figure 13–5)

PURPOSE This E-cise works to counteract hip rotation.

Start on your hands and knees. Move your hands forward by about six inches, then move your upper body forward so that your shoulders are above your hands. Your hips are now in front of your knees by about six inches. Keep your elbows straight, and allow your shoulder blades to collapse together while your low back dips to form the tail of an S-curve. It arches because your hips roll forward, allowing this movement to occur. Drop your head. Hold this position for two minutes.

▸ SITTING FLOOR TWIST
(Figure 13-6 a and b)
Purpose This E-cise forces the hip rotators to behave bilaterally and to function in cooperation with the shoulders.

Sit on the floor with your legs extended straight in front. Bend your left leg, and cross it over the right, placing it flat on the floor just outside (and slightly below) the right knee. Place your right elbow outside your left knee. Roll your hips forward to create an arch in the lower back. (Hold this arch throughout.) Now twist your upper body to the left, using your back muscles to rotate your spine. Turn your head to the left as you twist. Support yourself with your left hand on the floor off to the side and behind. Hold this position for one minute and breathe. Your straight leg should be tight, with the toes flexed toward your knee (a). Repeat on the other side (b).

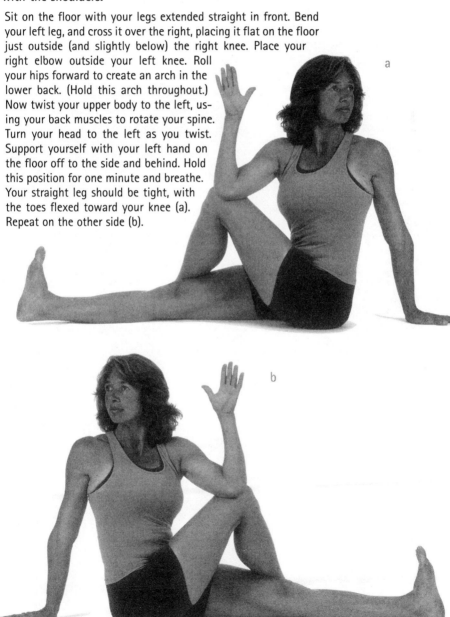

a

b

▶ CATS and DOGS
(Figure 13-7 a and b)

PURPOSE This E-cise works the hips, spine, shoulders, and neck in coordinated flexion and extension.

Get down on the floor on your hands and knees. Make a table by aligning your knees with your hips and your wrists with your shoulders. Your lower legs should be parallel with each other and with your hips. Your weight should be distributed evenly. For the Cat, smoothly round your back upward and let your head curl under, to create a curve that runs from your buttocks to your neck—like a cat with an arched back (a). For the Dog, smoothly sway your back down while bringing your head up (b). Make these two moves flow continuously back and forth. Exhale as you move into the Cat position; inhale during the Dog. Do one set of ten repetitions.

a

b

▸ WALL DROP
(Figure 13–8)

PURPOSE This E-cise allows the hips to be properly repositioned while keeping the knees and feet functionally aligned.

Stand against a wall with your feet on a slant board. (A slant board is a simple apparatus we invented in the clinic. You can improvise by propping one end of an inch-thick board that is 12 inches wide and 36 inches long against the bottom rung of a short stepladder and the floor. Make sure the ladder is wide enough at the base, equipped with rubber pads under the legs to prevent skidding, and sufficiently stable to support your weight. If you put one edge of the board against the wall, it won't kick back. The angle should be about sixty degrees.) Be sure your feet are parallel and pointed straight ahead. Relax your stomach and do not allow your knees to bend or the feet to twist. You will feel a stretch in your lower leg muscles, but this E-cise is really mainly to relax your stomach and upper body. Hold the position for five minutes.

Give this menu plenty of time to work its magic, about six months. You'll know that you are making progress when you get off the slant board and feel a noticeable surge of energy. We're also looking for a baseline metabolic response. Over the course of the six months, look for a gradual improvement in your appetite, mood, energy level, and sleep patterns. As soon as you feel up to it, add a twenty-minute walk each day (after completing the day's menu). The idea is to graduate to the Strength Menus in Chapter 12. Work your way through the Strength Menus, doing as many of the E-cises as you can in the order they appear. Those that are too difficult, do as much as you can, even if that's only to assume the starting position and hold it for a few seconds. Try to do a bit more each day.

Baby, It's Cold Inside

When it comes to personal health, what you don't know *can* hurt you. And most people don't know nearly enough about how important the metabolic process is to preventing illness, so they fail to spot signs of trouble in time to head them off.

Consider Tina's situation (before she became Tanya). She was so dysfunctional that she couldn't sleep at night. That's not unusual—many symptoms of illness become more pronounced at night because the metabolism is in a postabsorptive state—that is, it has ceased to actively digest and burn the nutrients consumed at the evening meal. Starting roughly four hours after eating, the body must rely on stored sources of energy. For a person with inefficient metabolism, this switch-over from absorption to postabsorption is like driving a car into a pothole. They wake up with night sweats, heart palpitations, heartburn, cramps, and many other conditions.

Much of what's going on is the body's struggle to maintain internal body temperature in the absence of an outside supply of fuel. Breaking down stored fat and protein reserves requires more energy expenditure than absorbing a stomach full of Domino's Pizza or a Big Mac and fries. If you are already metabolically challenged, the transition to the more demanding postabsorptive state is a rough one. When it happens during the day—in the late morning and midafternoon, once breakfast and lunch have been digested—some people become irritable, lose concentration, and get sluggish. But those are relatively mild symptoms: migraines, nausea, asthma attacks, menstrual difficulties, cardiac arrhythmia, chronic fatigue syndrome, and a host of other maladies can also result. Research showing a high incidence of heart attacks in the early morning hours confirms the potential danger of this metabolic transition. Struggling hard to come up with the needed energy supplies, the body overburdens the heart by asking it to do too much work with too little fuel. Just the extra demand of getting out of bed and moving around can be a metabolic load the heart can't handle.

The absence of muscle mass is a huge contributing factor to maintaining internal temperature. Twenty to 30 percent of the internal temperature is provided by resting skeletal muscles. This percentage presumably falls off in inverse relationship to the musculoskeletal system dysfunction, forcing the heart, liver, brain, and endocrine system—the body's main heat generators— to take up the slack. The bulkier the individual, the higher the danger, since the heat-generating requirement is that much greater. (There's more mass to heat, plus the increased surface area fosters cooling through the skin.)

As I noted earlier, intensely active muscles can produce up to forty times more heat than the rest of the body. A temperature rise of one degree Centigrade increases chemical reactions in the body by 10 percent. Thus the muscles act as something of a Bunsen burner: turn it off, and the body's chemistry is profoundly influenced. Either essential chemical reactions are curtailed, or other processes must take up the slack. In the latter case, again, a flood of hormones is released to manipulate the metabolism as a substitute for an engaged and strong musculoskeletal system. (Chapter 7 discussed this problem in relation to puberty.)

This is another instance of a secondary system being drafted into service when a primary system is disabled. What if the metabolic process were suddenly overwhelmed by a freak accident? Let's say a nine-year-old child falls through the ice into a Minnesota lake in mid-January. Her musculoskeletal system isn't powerful or developed enough to fire up the metabolism to handle the crisis on its own. Therefore nature uses her thyroid gland as a backup. The brain's hypothalamus and the pituitary gland release TSH, or thyroid-stimulating hormone, chemically revving up cellular metabolism and quickly raising body temperature.

Theoretically, adults who live in cold climates don't need rushes of TSH; their muscle-powered metabolism should be strong enough to raise the body's internal temperature by clambering out of the icy water and running home, stomping their feet, and shivering. In fact, shivering is a nonhormonal means of raising the temperature by activating the stretch reflexes of the muscles. Have you seen children shivering at the beach on a cold day? They don't have enough muscle mass to do the job. Shivering doesn't warm them enough, and that's why TSH is available.

But many adults are so dysfunctional, they never outgrow the need for TSH fixes. Slight dips in ambient temperature send their body heat crashing, and the hypothalamus and pituitary gland—aware that the musculature and metabolism are inadequate—kick in with a blast of hormonal antifreeze. Stress also apparently leads to the secretion of TSH, as the body tries to jump-start metabolic energy production that otherwise would be readily available to functional muscles.

I believe that researchers will one day demonstrate that hyperthyroidism—the extreme elevation of metabolism by way of excess thyroid hormones—is caused by the overstimulation of the thyroid gland to routinely regulate metabolism in the absence of muscular engagement. The thyroid would last a lifetime if it had only its real job to do—regulating growth, stimulating carbohydrate absorption, helping with fat oxidation by the cells, and standing by to jolt the nervous system in an emergency. It was not designed to permanently do heavy metabolic lifting.

From Hypo to Hyper

Isn't it interesting that just a few generations back the most common form of thyroid disorder involved an underactive thyroid gland? The availability of iodized salt has long since helped eliminate endemic goiter (thyroid gland enlargement). But the thyroid may be telling us important information about the deteriorating state of our metabolic health. Grandma and Grandpa may well have had enough musculoskeletal system function to drive their metabolism without the need for hormonal additives.

A section of the thyroid, called the parathyroid, releases a hormone, PTH, that is involved in calcium breakdown from the bones and its absorption into the bloodstream. The loss of bone mass from musculoskeletal system dysfunction is probably having a detrimental impact on the parathyroid in that it raises the calcium levels in the blood and shuts off the PTH flow by triggering another hormone that acts to inhibit calcium breakdown from the bones. Those two hormones work at opposite purposes, and such a conflict can't be helpful in managing proper calcium balance, which is needed for many essential purposes, among them muscle contraction—including the heart—and the operation of the central nervous system.

It's complicated, but the composition of this hormonal bouillabaisse has a profound influence on our health. We may be changing it for the worse by allowing our musculoskeletal system to deteriorate. But there's no reason why we can't fix it, and every reason why we must. Hormones aren't easy to manage, but fortunately our musculoskeletal system is.

Menopause: Light to Dispel a Dark Shadow

What do you think of when you see the words *hormones* and *calcium loss* in a book on health issues for women between the ages of thirty-five and fifty?

Chances are pretty good that you think "Menopause." The falloff in estrogen production and the potential for serious bone loss have in recent years become almost synonymous with menopause or perimenopause (*peri* means "about the time of"). As a result, some women regard this condition with dread. But menopause is not an illness; nor is it necessarily the onset of a personal health crisis.

Many characteristics of perimenopause and menopause closely resemble the symptoms of metabolic suppression and related musculoskeletal system dysfunction. As I've said, the body cannot tell time. It does not look at a calendar and decree, "Oh, she's about to turn forty-nine. Time to shut down ovulation and the rest of menses." But what the body can do—and does do—is monitor its systems and determine whether they are functioning properly or are in need of adjustment.

A Transition

I'm introducing the discussion of menopause in this chapter rather than the next because this event can occur any time from the mid-forties to the late fifties. And even citing that range is dicey, since premature menopause can develop prior to age forty, while there are instances of women in their seventies who have not gone through menopause. It's also confusing because the most noticeable signs of menopause—menstrual irregularities, PMS, hot flashes, and the like—can be experienced in the run-up to menopause as the monthly ovulatory cycle gradually shuts down.

Monthly ovulation is part of a sequence intended to lead to fertilization of an egg, implantation of a zygote in the uterine lining, development of an embryo into a fetus, and the birth of a child nine months after conception. It is a complicated and arduous process. The body will not allow it to happen without the proper resources—and that includes the mother's strength.

What we regard as menopause is simply the point at which the body determines that the woman can no longer bring a baby to full term without harming herself in the process. The estrogen supply as well as the overall hormonal flow and mix are included in this evaluation. Estrogen is almost a form of fertilizer, in that it promotes growth in a wide variety of different cells. Author Natalie Angier notes that the women of ancient Greece soaked barley seeds in their urine to test for pregnancy; they were thought to be with child if the seeds sprouted faster than normal.

Expectant mothers are awash in estrogen because they are being called on to facilitate explosive cell growth in the embryo and fetus. But a woman whose metabolism is weak probably won't be able to do that—and if she does, it's a risky business. Her own cell growth is lagging, not producing enough cells for the maintenance and renewal of bones, red blood cell propagation, immune system activity, and the tissues of every vital organ. That kind of cellular construction is constant and requires major league metabolic energy creation and consumption. If it's not happening, the body is hardly likely to keep the estrogen factory going full tilt. Why generate a jeroboam's worth of estrogen when a thimbleful will do? Again, supply and demand are at work: the estrogen supply falls, or never rises enough to support a viable embryo, because of lack of metabolic demand.

Menopause is a metabolically triggered event, a sophisticated and straightforward form of birth control. That's why it happens anywhere from the late thirties to the mid-sixties. Women in their seventies have been known to ovulate, and they're not freaks—they just have a good metabolism. The body sees no reason to put them out of the baby-making business. Nor does it see a reason to destroy their bones, give them breast cancer, or kill them with a heart attack.

These dire consequences are commonly cited as the

rationale for menopausal women to undergo hormone replacement therapy (HRT). Apparently HRT is most successful for women who are overweight, smoke, have high blood pressure, and present other markers for heart disease. In other words, it helps the most metabolically challenged women. But it does so only in the short run. Over time the reduction in heart attacks is statistically neutralized by an increase in breast cancer. After ten years of HRT the risk of breast cancer is actually 50 percent higher. And the heart-attack-prevention benefits, if any, may also turn out to be a mirage, since a study released in early 2000 found indications of a slight increase in heart attack rates as well.

I'll leave it to you to decide, but to me it sounds like hormone replacement therapy is treating symptoms, not the problem.

Old Enemies, New Diseases

It seems like every few weeks, the science and health media report the discovery of a new plague, epidemic, or outbreak of a heretofore rare disease. If it's not a new strain of TB, or an antibiotic-resistant virus, it's Lyme disease, West Nile fever, or the Ebola virus. For the last fifteen years or so, ever since AIDS exploded on the scene with such devastating consequences, we have had a panicky sense that we are under siege.

But why would the world suddenly become a far more dangerous place? Because of climatic change and global warming? Maybe. Pollution? Perhaps. The depletion of the ozone layer? Possibly. A sudden onset of human frailty? No. It's probably my incurable optimism, but I think these *new* diseases, including AIDS, have their origins in old organisms that have been around all along.

What's changed is our resistance to them. By adopting lifestyles that suppress the metabolic process, we have hammered our immune systems and other innate disease-fighting mechanisms and sapped our overall resilience and strength. The controversy over childhood immunization is an example. There is no credible evidence that the vaccine supply is tainted. The delivery methodology is basically unchanged from what it was thirty to fifty years ago. Yet more and more parents are now convinced that their children's health is being undermined by immunizations for serious diseases like mumps, measles, and rubella.

More likely, today's children may not be able to process the antigens to which they're being exposed. When a child is vaccinated, her body, instead of triggering antibodies that lead to the development of immunity, misreads the vaccination and issues an inappropriate and sometimes devastating response. To me, this looks like another case of the immune system being weakened by metabolic inefficiency. Relatively inactive children without fully functional musculoskeletal systems do not possess the metabolic capacity to fire up the immune system to meet normal requirements, let alone deal with the sudden invasion of foreign antigens from the vaccine.

During pregnancy a fetus receives immune system sustenance from the mother's placenta, and after birth the infant gets more helpings of it from breast milk. But if Mom's immune system is in trouble, the baby's is likely to be compromised as well. Everything's okay as long as no exotic bugs show up. Then along comes a vaccination, which by definition is swarming with bugs, and that's too much for the child's body to handle.

Likewise, metabolic suppression is a common denominator among AIDS victims. The virus actually attacks the immune system itself and infects helper T cells, which normally stimulate the formation of the invasion-fighting B and T cells. But why does this predator attack the immune system? One theory is that the virus has more different variations than the immune system can cope with, but that sounds like a lot of work for a lazy predator. But a system that's already badly stressed by intravenous drug use—and if ever there was a metabolic crusher, that's it—and by a lifestyle associated with risky sexual practices with multiple partners, is a perfect target for infection.

From the Heart

Heart disease is the number-one killer of women, and it kills more women than men. Even so, heart attacks are still considered by many to be a "guy thing." It's patently and statistically not true. But the myth persists, I believe, because at one time it was a reality. Before accurate medical record-keeping came along in this century, women died in childbirth, of childhood diseases or of blood poisoning, infections, pneumonia, and many other conditions, but heart attacks and heart disease were not as common. That's why we have this folklore about men and heart attacks.

My theory is that women were once too busy to have heart attacks—and too functional. Confronted by a wide variety of environmental stimuli, from farm chores to nursing duties, from scrubbing floors to gutting fish, and from chasing kids around to swinging a rivet gun on a B-29 assembly line, they built and maintained robust metabolisms. They gave their hearts enough fuel and musculoskeletal system support to keep pumping and stay healthy.

The heart is a muscle. It's closer kin to skeletal muscle, in terms of its composition, than any other nonskeletal muscle in the body. Like any living tissue, it requires fuel. But since it beats (contracts and relaxes) constantly, its fuel bill is that much greater. If metabolism is suppressed, all the users of its fuel and energy output are put on reduced rations. Yet the heart must go on beating. Unlike the hip muscles, it doesn't have the luxury of taking a semipermanent vacation.

Nor is the heart able to hand off its responsibilities, the way many of our major muscles do, by relying on peripheral and stabilizer muscles. These secondary systems keep us semi-upright and moving, but in some ways they cheat the heart out of the help it could otherwise derive from the blood-pumping action of major muscles on arteries and veins. In a functional musculoskeletal system, the heart has 666 heart helpers (the approximate number of skeletal muscles).

Lacking this assistance, the heart meets heavier-than-normal demands by working harder and getting booster shots of insulin, adrenaline, and other hormones to rev it up. "Normal" is a dicey concept, though. In our sedentary culture, *normal* demands are those that involve limited, repetitive movement. The heart can adjust to that demand and meet those demands without obvious strain. But outside of normal parameters, when motion stops being limited and

The Role of Estrogen and Heart Health

I'm a contrarian on estrogen. It may protect against heart attacks, but only because the body's primary protective system—a supercharged metabolic process—has been undermined by musculoskeletal system dysfunction. Hormones frequently act as back-ups and boosters when primary systems can't handle the job. As the estrogen supply tapers off after forty, the loss of the primary and secondary protective mechanisms has serious consequences. The possible link between estrogen replacement and breast cancer may arise from the body's inability to assimilate estrogen due to metabolic weakness.

repetitive, the heart is suddenly put under tremendous strain. It's asked to provide "abnormal" amounts of blood and oxygen. Like any flabby, underutilized muscle, it is not in condition to obey.

Make a tight fist with your right hand. Imagine that you are holding a water-filled balloon, and give it a good, hard, long squeeze. What happens to the water? Right—in one squeeze it's pumped out of the fist-chamber.

Now make a loose fist. The water-filled balloon is still there. Give it many fast, little squeezes without fully clenching the fist. What happens? Moving the same amount of water takes much more work.

When the heart muscle is deconditioned by inactivity, musculoskeletal system dysfunction, and metabolic suppression, it starts to resemble the loose fist. Interestingly enough, when the body senses it's not pumping enough volume, the heart will grow larger. It substitutes capacity for power. Amazing! The body has a huge bag of tricks, and every one of them is brilliant—but they have a limit.

I've argued for years with a prominent aerobic researcher who relies on treadmill tests to determine people's heart condition. Many people fall in the normal range—but as I've explained to him, normal is really subnormal. They can pass with flying colors, but it's by using secondary peripheral muscles in place of their major movers. Get them off the treadmill and climbing a set of steep stairs, where those compensating muscles can't engage and where the dormant major movers are needed, and the heart may be in serious overload. Only in that case the person isn't attached to an EKG machine, so we have no data other than a 911 call. *But she was fine on the treadmill.* Yeah, fine and "normal."

"Normal" is a case of double jeopardy. One, the heart doesn't have adequate metabolic support; and two, it is not being backed up by engaged and strong muscles performing according to their design specifications. Heart attacks are killing women, but not because they are approaching menopause or for other reasons relating to their gender and their "frailty." Rather, the high mortality rate is caused by musculoskeletal system dysfunction. The heart muscle is suffering the same fate as the hip muscles. I don't call that normal. I call it premature, preventable death.

Keeping It Simple

What do we do about it? The E-cise menus featured in Chapters 10 and 11 will directly benefit your metabolism's ability to prevent disease, as will the Tina/Tanya Menu in this chapter.

I realize our discussion of metabolism has been rough going at times. But for all of its mind-numbing complexity, the metabolic process actually yields to an extremely simple question: What am I doing to my metabolism?

You're doing something important right now. So am I. Are we enhancing the trillions of chemical reactions that are taking place or suppressing them? By recognizing our own power to regulate the metabolic process through determining the "inputs"—food, fluid, sleep, stress, motion—we gain an enormous advantage. It's a form of liberation, really. Health stops being another version of the lottery. We're in charge. We can choose, and act on those choices.

I hope by this point that your first choice will be to engage and strengthen your musculoskeletal system. There isn't a better place to start. But it's your decision. Thanks to metabolism, it's that simple.

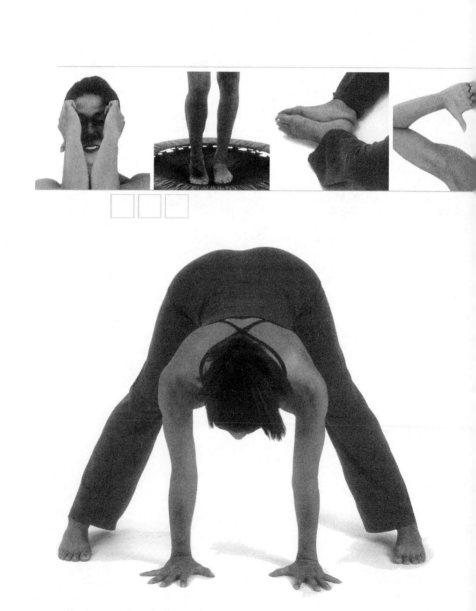

a fighting chance

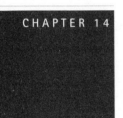

Breast cancer is the second most frequently diagnosed cancer among women. (Skin cancer is number one.) According to the American Cancer Society, there were an estimated 182,800 new cases of breast cancer in the year 2000 and 40,800 deaths from the disease. That means roughly that one woman died from the disease every thirteen minutes.

The two E-cise menus included in this chapter have a specialized anti–breast cancer mission. The first one is for women who have been diagnosed with breast cancer and are awaiting surgery or are undergoing nonsurgical treatment, such as radiation or chemotherapy. Under the circumstances, it is important to get your metabolism up to speed, and that's what the first menu endeavors to do.

The second menu is for those who have had breast cancer surgery, either a lumpectomy or a mastectomy. These E-cises take into account the physical trauma involved, while working both to increase the metabolism needed for recovery and to restore musculoskeletal system functions that have been compromised.

Frankly, I almost did not include this chapter at all. Once

I start offering E-cise menus keyed to specific diseases, I thought, where do I stop? The answer must be—I stop with these two menus. Why include breast cancer but no other disease? At the Egoscue Method Clinic, I see far more women who are facing breast cancer than those facing other serious illnesses. Almost every client is there for musculoskeletal system–related issues, like a bad back or sore knees. But those with breast cancer form the largest subgroup because the conventional treatment regimen can have such drastic effects on upper-body mobility, comfort, and function. The Egoscue Method has a good track record in easing pain and restoring mobility and function. That's why they come to us.

Furthermore, we believe—I'm using the authorial *we* here to include my coauthor, Roger Gittines—that a sound, robust metabolism is an essential precondition to the prevention and treatment of breast cancer and to full recovery from surgery. Roger's mother died of breast cancer in 1970 at the age of fifty-four, seven years after undergoing a radical mastectomy. The initial surgery shattered her spirit, and her health never recovered. Her lifestyle, both before and after the operation, amounted to a paradigm of metabolic suppression and abuse— from heavy smoking (she loved Kents) to a virtual addiction to soft drinks (especially Pepsi), a lack of exercise (never walking when she could drive), and musculoskeletal system dysfunction. She was an unhappy woman before the diagnosis and desperately unhappy after. With a strong metabolism she would have had a fighting chance to survive to see her grandchildren grow up. What happened to Miriam Gittines didn't have to happen in 1970; nor should it have to happen to women more than thirty years later.

Motion and metabolism are inextricably linked, and we have to get women in this predicament moving and functional again. If that's you, consult with your physician, and together please consider putting the appropriate program to work on your behalf. It's not a substitute for anything you're already doing; it's a valuable supplement.

[Breast Cancer Menu: Diagnosis and Nonsurgical Treatment]

▸ STANDING ARM CIRCLES
(Figure 14–1 a and b)

PURPOSE This E-cise strengthens the muscles of the upper back that are involved with the shoulders' ball and socket function.

Stand facing a mirror with your feet parallel about a hip-width apart, your arms at your sides. Curl your fingertips into the pads of each palm (the fleshy area at the base of the fingers), and point your thumbs straight out. This hand position, called the "golfer's grip," is imperative to the success of the E-cise. Squeeze your shoulder blades together, and bring your arms out to your sides at shoulder level, elbows straight. With your palms facing down, thumbs pointing forward, circle up and forward for forty repetitions (a). Now with your palms facing up, circle up and back for forty repetitions (b). Remember to keep your wrists and elbows straight and your shoulder blades squeezed together—the circles must come from the shoulders.

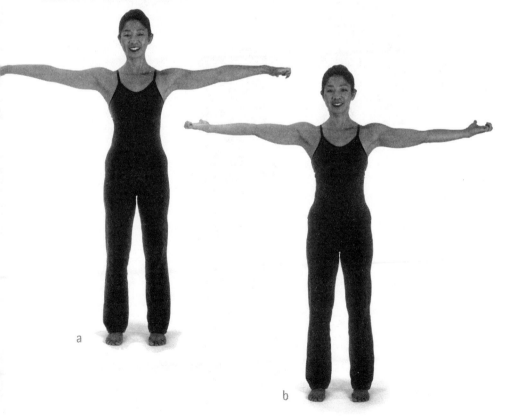

a

b

▶ STANDING ELBOW CURLS
(Figure 14–2 a and b)

PURPOSE This E-cise reminds the shoulder's "hinge" what full flexion and extension feel like.

Stand with your heels, buttocks, upper back, and head against a wall. Your feet, pointed straight ahead, are about a hip-width apart. Raise your hands in the "golfer's grip" (see Standing Arm Circles), placing your knuckles along your temples, thumbs extended down your cheeks (a). Bring your elbows together to meet in front (b). Make sure your elbows meet in the middle of your body (and are not skewed to the left or right, which would mean that one shoulder is flexing more than the other). Then pull your elbows back even with your shoulders to touch the wall. Your head should remain still, and your knuckles should not lift off your temples. Do one set of twenty-five repetitions.

a

b

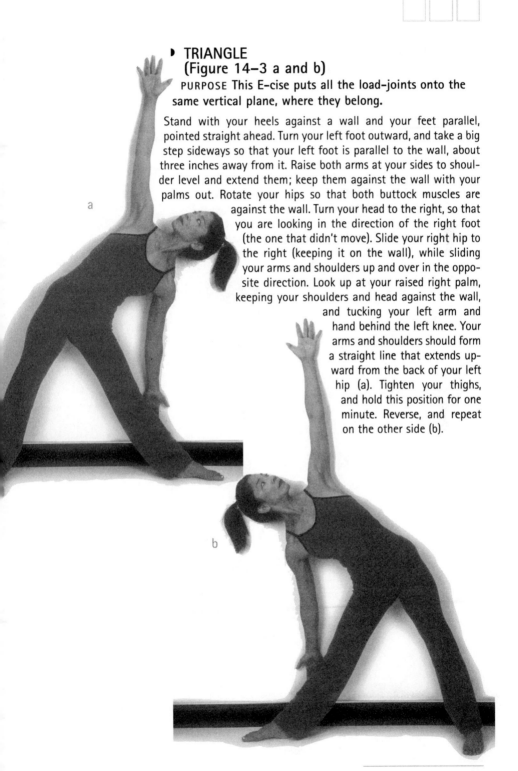

▸ TRIANGLE
(Figure 14–3 a and b)

PURPOSE This E-cise puts all the load-joints onto the same vertical plane, where they belong.

Stand with your heels against a wall and your feet parallel, pointed straight ahead. Turn your left foot outward, and take a big step sideways so that your left foot is parallel to the wall, about three inches away from it. Raise both arms at your sides to shoulder level and extend them; keep them against the wall with your palms out. Rotate your hips so that both buttock muscles are against the wall. Turn your head to the right, so that you are looking in the direction of the right foot (the one that didn't move). Slide your right hip to the right (keeping it on the wall), while sliding your arms and shoulders up and over in the opposite direction. Look up at your raised right palm, keeping your shoulders and head against the wall, and tucking your left arm and hand behind the left knee. Your arms and shoulders should form a straight line that extends upward from the back of your left hip (a). Tighten your thighs, and hold this position for one minute. Reverse, and repeat on the other side (b).

a

b

▶ CATS and DOGS
(Figure 14–4 a and b)

PURPOSE This E-cise works the hips, spine, shoulders, and neck in coordinated flexion and extension.

Get down on the floor on your hands and knees. Make a table by aligning your knees with your hips and your wrists with your shoulders. Your lower legs should be parallel with each other and with your hips. Your weight should be distributed evenly. For the Cat, smoothly round your back upward and let your head curl under, to create a curve that runs from your buttocks to your neck—like a cat with an arched back (a). For the Dog, smoothly sway your back down while bringing your head up (b). Make these two moves flow continuously back and forth. Exhale as you move into the Cat position; inhale during the Dog. Do one set of ten repetitions.

a

b

▸ SPREAD FOOT FORWARD BEND
(Figure 14–5 a, b, c, and d)

PURPOSE This E-cise puts your hips into a neutral position and allows your prime movers to do their jobs without secondary muscles getting in the way.

Stand with your legs spread about as far as they will go without your feet flaring out. Go to the limit on this one. Bending forward at the hips will help you get into the stretch.

Position 1: Bend forward at the hips, and with both hands touch the floor in front of you (a). If this is too difficult, use a small block or book for elevation. Tighten your thighs, and relax your torso toward the floor. Hold this position for one minute.

Position 2: Without straightening up, slide your hands in front of your left foot, keeping both thighs tight and the torso relaxed (b). Hold one minute.

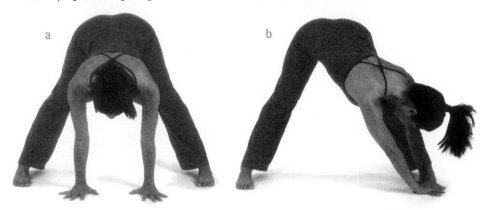

Position 3: Move your hands back to the starting center position briefly, then slide them in front of the right foot, keeping the thighs tight and torso relaxed (c). Hold for one minute.

Position 4: Slide your hands back to the center starting position, keeping the thighs tight and torso relaxed (d). Hold for one minute.

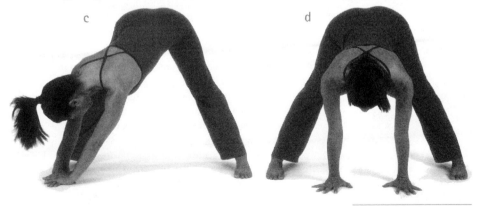

▸ TRAMPOLINE
(Figure 14–6)

PURPOSE This E-cise helps lymph system movement and increases balance and metabolic stamina.

Invest in a small five-foot-diameter trampoline (sold in sporting goods stores), the kind that is raised off the ground only a couple of feet. Stand in the middle of the trampoline with your feet a hip-width apart. Make sure they are parallel and pointing straight ahead. Walk in place by lifting your heels, keeping your toes in contact with the trampoline's surface. Bend your knees and put bounce in each step. Make sure your head is up and level, with your shoulders back and square. Without hunching your shoulders, place the first three fingers of each hand at points midway on a line between your clavicle and the nipples of the breasts. Press gently as you walk in place. (These are release points for the lymph system's "valves.")

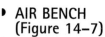

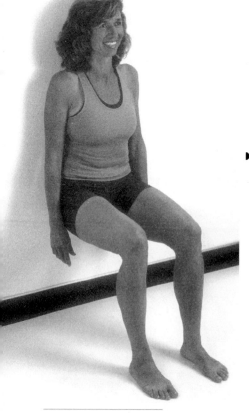

▸ AIR BENCH
(Figure 14–7)

PURPOSE This E-cise promotes lower leg, thigh, and hip strength, and it relaxes the muscles of the torso.

Stand against a wall with your feet pointing straight ahead, parallel, a hip-width apart. Walk your feet away from the wall approximately 2 to 2½ feet, as you bend your knees and slide your back down the wall. Stop sliding and walking when your thighs and hips form approximately a ninety-degree angle. Your knees should be over your ankles, not your toes. If you feel pain in your kneecaps, raise your body up the wall to relieve the pressure. Keep your weight on your heels. Hold this position for two minutes.

▶ STATIC BACK
(Figure 14-8)

PURPOSE This E-cise uses gravity to flatten the back and put it in a neutral position.

Lie on your back, with both legs bent at right angles and resting on a chair, bench, or block. (The large blocks we use in the clinic are 20 inches high by 14 inches wide by 24 inches long.) Rest your hands on the floor, extended below shoulder level, with palms up. Let your back settle into the floor. Breathe from your diaphragm, so your abdominal muscles rise as you inhale and fall as you exhale. Hold this position for five minutes.

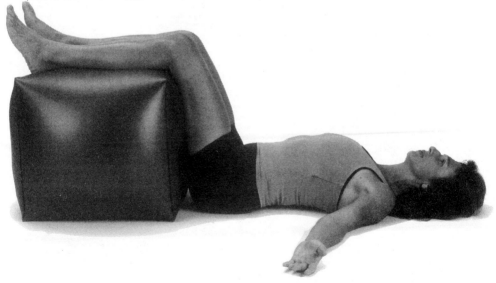

▸ SUPINE GROIN PROGRESSIVE (Figure 14-9 a and b)

PURPOSE This E-cise unlocks tight hip flexor muscles.

You'll need to improvise two pieces of apparatus to duplicate the large foam blocks and steps we use in the clinic. I recommend an armless chair or bench and a stepladder. Lie on your back with your right leg resting on the chair or bench, bent at a ninety-degree angle. Extend the left leg straight, placing the heel on the fifteen-inch rung of the ladder. Your foot should be pointed straight at the ceiling. Prop it against a book or another heavy object to keep it from flopping to the side. Make sure your feet, knees, hips, and shoulders are in alignment. Hold this position until your low back settles down into the floor (a), which will take ten or fifteen minutes. Then move your foot to the next step down, about ten inches, and hold it there until the back settles (b). Repeat on the five-inch level, and finally do it one last time on the floor. Always, always, repeat the entire cycle on the other side. This E-cise may take as long as an hour, but it's worth it. The more frequently you do this E-cise the less time it will take for the hip flexors to let go. Eventually, a few minutes at each level will be enough.

a

b

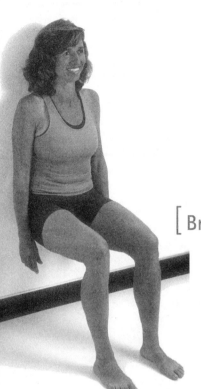

▸ **AIR BENCH**
(Figure 14-10)
Follow the instructions for this E-cise earlier in this menu.

[Breast Cancer Menu: Postsurgery]

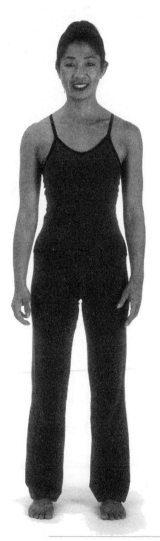

▸ **STANDING GLUTEAL CONTRACTIONS**
(Figure 14-11)
PURPOSE This E-cise stabilizes the pelvis in a loaded posterior position and strengthens the gluteal muscles in that position.

Stand with your feet about a hip-width apart and slightly turned out. Contract and release your buttock muscles, on both sides and at the same time. Don't contract your stomach or thigh muscles. Relax your upper body, stomach, and thighs. Putting your hands on your buttocks will make it easier to feel and control the contractions. Do three sets of twenty repetitions each. If this position seems too difficult, turn your feet out to an angle of forty-five degrees for one set of twenty repetitions, and then straighten your feet and do the next two sets.

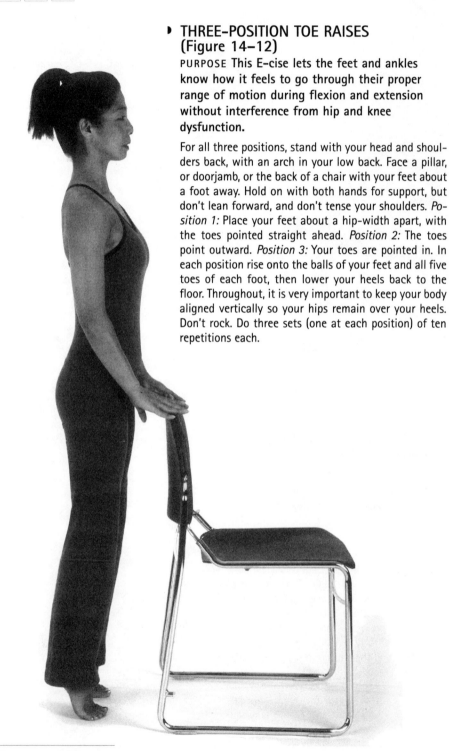

▶ THREE-POSITION TOE RAISES
(Figure 14–12)

PURPOSE This E-cise lets the feet and ankles know how it feels to go through their proper range of motion during flexion and extension without interference from hip and knee dysfunction.

For all three positions, stand with your head and shoulders back, with an arch in your low back. Face a pillar, or doorjamb, or the back of a chair with your feet about a foot away. Hold on with both hands for support, but don't lean forward, and don't tense your shoulders. *Position 1:* Place your feet about a hip-width apart, with the toes pointed straight ahead. *Position 2:* The toes point outward. *Position 3:* Your toes are pointed in. In each position rise onto the balls of your feet and all five toes of each foot, then lower your heels back to the floor. Throughout, it is very important to keep your body aligned vertically so your hips remain over your heels. Don't rock. Do three sets (one at each position) of ten repetitions each.

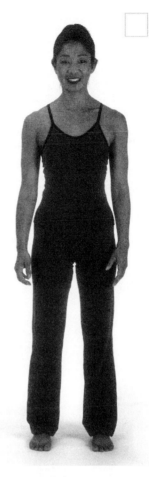

▶ STANDING GLUTEAL CONTRACTIONS
(Figure 14–13)
Follow the instructions for this E-cise earlier in this menu.

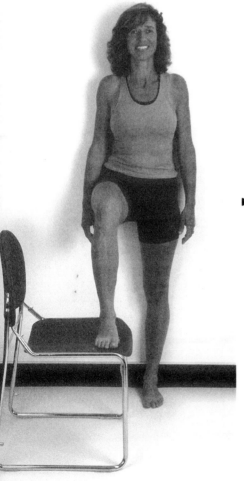

▶ WALL STORK
(Figure 14–14)
PURPOSE This E-cise levels the hips into a parallel position, under a load that's held in vertical alignment.

Stand against a wall with your feet pointed straight ahead. Your heels, hips, upper back, and head should be against the wall. Place your right foot on the seat of a chair positioned about twelve inches in front of you. Make sure this foot is pointed straight. Do not allow your left foot to twist or your left leg to bend. The right leg, on the chair, should be bent at about ninety degrees at the knee joint. Hold this position without allowing the left foot, leg, or hip to shift to the side or to roll away from the wall. Hold for three minutes. Switch legs, and repeat.

▶ SITTING KNEE PILLOW SQUEEZES (Figure 14–15)

PURPOSE This E-cise strengthens the hip-stabilizer muscles.

Sit on the edge of a chair with a pillow or foam block between your knees. (In the clinic, our blocks are about seven inches thick.) Roll your pelvis forward to put an arch in your lower back. Your feet should point straight ahead, about a hip-width apart, positioned under your knees. Squeeze and release the pillow between your knees. Remember to keep the arch in your lower back. Do three sets of twenty each.

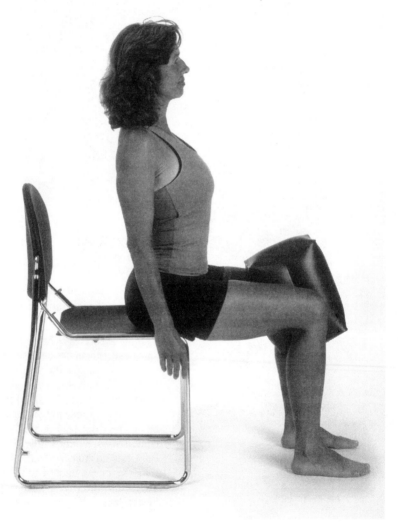

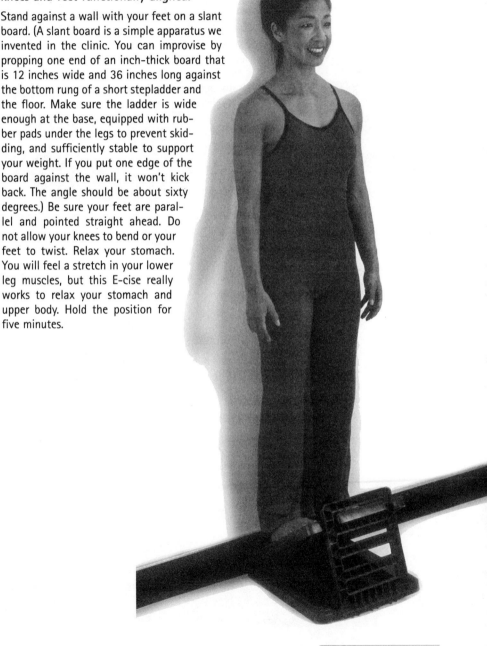

▸ WALL DROP
(Figure 14–16)

PURPOSE This E-cise allows the hips to be properly repositioned while keeping the knees and feet functionally aligned.

Stand against a wall with your feet on a slant board. (A slant board is a simple apparatus we invented in the clinic. You can improvise by propping one end of an inch-thick board that is 12 inches wide and 36 inches long against the bottom rung of a short stepladder and the floor. Make sure the ladder is wide enough at the base, equipped with rubber pads under the legs to prevent skidding, and sufficiently stable to support your weight. If you put one edge of the board against the wall, it won't kick back. The angle should be about sixty degrees.) Be sure your feet are parallel and pointed straight ahead. Do not allow your knees to bend or your feet to twist. Relax your stomach. You will feel a stretch in your lower leg muscles, but this E-cise really works to relax your stomach and upper body. Hold the position for five minutes.

▶ STATIC BACK
(Figure 14–17)
PURPOSE This E-cise uses gravity to flatten your back and put it in a neutral position.

Lie on your back, with both legs bent at right angles and resting on a chair, bench, or block. (The large blocks we use in the clinic are 20 inches high by 14 inches wide by 24 inches long.) Rest your hands on the floor, extended below shoulder level, with the palms up. Let your back settle into the floor. Breathe from your diaphragm, so your abdominal muscles rise as you inhale and fall as you exhale. Hold this position for five minutes.

▶ STATIC BACK—REVERSE PRESSES
(Figure 14–18)
PURPOSE This E-cise causes scapular retraction and releases the thoracic erector muscles.

Stay in the Static Back position, with your legs up and over a large block, bench, or chair. Position your elbows on the floor straight out from your shoulders, with your forearms and hands, clenched lightly, pointing up toward the ceiling. Squeeze your shoulder blades together, and release. The squeeze is downward into the floor, not toward your neck and head. Relax your stomach muscles. Do not try just to push your elbows into the floor; the point is to get your shoulder blades engaged. Do three sets of ten repetitions each.

► FROG
(Figure 14–19)

PURPOSE This E-cise positions the pelvis symmetrically left to right.

Lie on your back with your knees bent. Make sure your feet are centered in the middle of your body, and then let your knees and legs fall away to the sides. Put the soles of your feet together. Your lower back does not need to be flat on the floor, and in fact, there may be an arch due to the hip changing its position. Relax. Don't press the thighs out and down. Feel the stretch in the inner thighs and groin. Hold this position for two minutes.

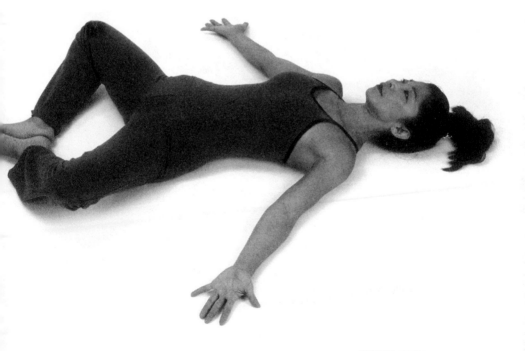

▶ SUPINE GROIN PROGRESSIVE
(Figure 14–20)

PURPOSE This E-cise unlocks tight hip flexor muscles.

You'll need to improvise two pieces of apparatus to duplicate the large foam blocks and steps we use in the clinic. I recommend an armless chair or bench and a stepladder. Lie on your back with your right leg resting on the chair or bench, bent at a ninety-degree angle. Extend the left leg straight, placing the heel on the fifteen-inch rung of the ladder. Your foot should be pointed straight at the ceiling. Prop it against a book or another heavy object to keep it from flopping to the side. Make sure your feet, knees, hips, and shoulders are in alignment. Hold this position until your low back settles down into the floor (a), which will take ten or fifteen minutes. Then move your foot to the next step down, about ten inches, and hold it there until the back settles (b). Repeat on the five-inch level, and finally do it one last time on the floor. Always, always, repeat the entire cycle on the other side. This E-cise may take as long as an hour, but it's worth it. The more frequently you do this E-cise the less time it will take for the hip flexors to let go. Eventually, a few minutes at each level will be enough.

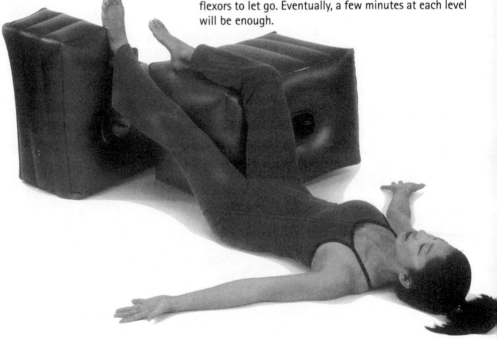

▶ PELVIC TILTS
(Figure 14–21 a and b)

PURPOSE This E-cise breaks the hips out of their flexion fixation and shows them how to move again from flexion to neutral to extension and back again.

Lie on your back with your knees bent and feet on the floor, a hip-width apart. Make sure your hips, feet, and knees are aligned. Roll your hips backward to flatten your back to the floor (a), then roll them forward to put an arch in your low back (b). Keep your upper back relaxed and your arms out to your sides just below shoulder level, palms up. Do one set of ten repetitions.

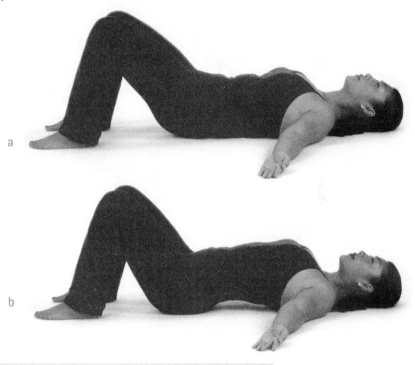

a

b

When you're ready—it's likely to be after three to six months—switch to the Postpregnancy Menus in Chapter 11, which is designed for musculoskeletal system restoration after a stressful experience. Work through all three phases, then move on to the Strength Menus in Chapter 12. I won't wish you good luck. Luck has nothing to do with it. I'll wish you good metabolism.

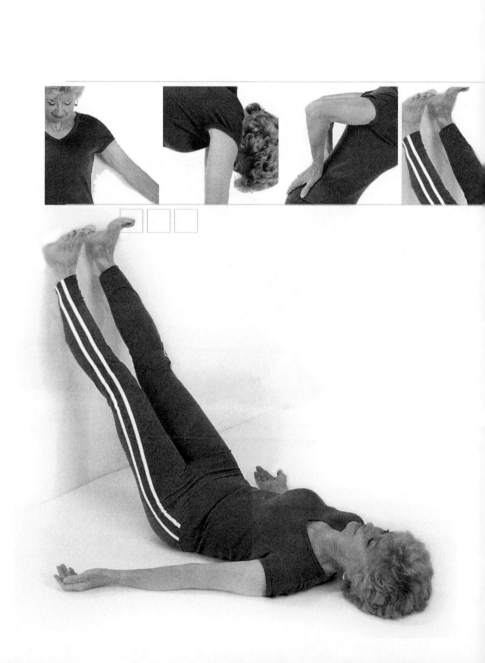

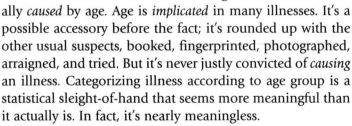

[PART SIX]

the vintage years: fifty and beyond

CHAPTER 15

season of mists and mellow fruitfulness

Oscar Wilde once famously quipped: "One should never trust a woman who tells one her real age. A woman who would tell one that, would tell one anything." While his humor seems a little dated these days—women aren't quite so reluctant to own up to their years as they apparently once were—the custom of women being *ageless* is actually worth retaining.

Age may indeed measure experience, wisdom, or folly, but assessing your health and well-being by counting years is a mistake. As for "age-related illness," I don't know of a single disease that's actually *caused* by age. Age is *implicated* in many illnesses. It's a possible accessory before the fact; it's rounded up with the other usual suspects, booked, fingerprinted, photographed, arraigned, and tried. But it's never justly convicted of *causing* an illness. Categorizing illness according to age group is a statistical sleight-of-hand that seems more meaningful than it actually is. In fact, it's nearly meaningless.

Statistics tell us that more sixty-five-year-olds have symptoms of arthritis than twenty-five-year-olds. But not all sixty-five-year-olds suffer from arthritis; nor is the disease entirely unknown among twenty-five-year-olds. Arthritis strikes all ages. If age causes arthritis, then young people and those of middle age should be immune.

Hmmm. Maybe age causes arthritis when you're old, and something else causes it when you're young? No, that doesn't hack it. It doesn't address the problem of why millions of older people never develop arthritis at all. Maybe they do develop it but are not aware of it. No, a stealth disease that never makes itself known doesn't seem like much of a disease. How do we square the numbers without being swamped by generalities?

It might seem safe to say that age increases our chances of developing arthritis. Okay, but in that case age becomes just another variable, among other variables of diet, occupation, smoking, activity levels, family medical history, and the like. One variable may cancel out another, and the cause of arthritis is still a mystery. All we've really done is correlate two sets of big numbers and make the assumption that one of them—the number of years a person has lived—is telling us something significant about arthritis or some other condition.

Assigning importance to a variable is the problem, and it's very tricky.

Is the number of right-handed arthritis sufferers versus lefties significant?

Is the number of blue-eyed arthritis sufferers versus brown-eyed significant?

Italians versus Irish?

Sports fans versus classical music buffs?

Disease by disease, we could construct a minutely detailed profile of the most likely victims—which would serve the sole purpose of scaring the hell out of all ambidextrous vegetarian oboists of Icelandic descent who avidly read murder mysteries written by female British authors. *Look out, you're probably going to come down with terrible malady X—and there's nothing you can do about it. Nothing.*

By linking age and illness, this is exactly what we're doing. Since age is unavoidable and incurable—and it is—we're saying that the illness is incurable and unavoidable. As a result, many women give up on their health without a fight. The age-illness link is present every time I hear someone say, "My [fill in the blank] hurts, but what do I expect? I'm seventy-two" or, "I used to love to [fill in the blank], but it got too much for me when I hit sixty."

I'm going to show you how to break that link. It's the next best thing to turning back the clock.

Play It Again

Let's transform the age-illness monologue into the kind of dialogue that occurs almost every day at the Egoscue Method Clinic.

"How's your hip feeling today, Ann, after the E-cises and your morning walk?"

"Fine. No pain at all."

"I thought you told me yesterday, and I quote, 'My right hip hurts, but what do I expect? I'm seventy-two.' Now you're seventy-two plus one more day."

"That's true."

"The dynamic of cause and effect is pretty inflexible, Ann. The greater the cause, the greater the effect. You're older by one whole day. You should be feeling more pain, not no pain. What do you suppose is going on?"

Ann thinks about it for a moment. "My sore hip doesn't have anything to do with age." I smile.

In another part of the clinic, this conversation is under way: "I used to play a lot of doubles tennis, but I gave it up when I hit sixty."

"Do you miss it, Pat?"

"Definitely."

"Would you like to play again?"

"I'm two years older."

"So what?"

"You can do that for me?"

"No, I can't. But you can do it for yourself."

Both Ann and Pat were still skeptical, but they were willing to let their own "show me" common sense challenge the age-illness linkage. And I don't think they would have been in the clinic in the first place if they truly believed their problems were caused by age. Despite our cultural predisposition to blame our ills on age, millions of people over the age of fifty or sixty still routinely undergo major surgery. Why? Because of hope? Sure. Because they wish to squeeze out a few more years? That too. But I think it's even more intuitive. We feel an inner certainty that we were intended to live longer than that arbitrary threescore and ten.

Negative Capability

We need a new definition of aging. The one we have now amounts to a self-fulfilling prophecy, to wit: as the years roll by, humans lose strength and physiological capabilities until they fall prey to disease, which hastens the decline and eventually kills them. Right on schedule, give or take a few years, we will all end up dead.

Presumably time is the enemy. But look at time from a different angle. What if, over the course of time, humans were gaining strength and physiological capabilities instead of losing them? What if, as hours, days, weeks, months, and years passed, they became ever more efficient, powerful, and adept? What if the passage of time measured, not decline, but growth? Time, in that case, would be an ally. The more of it we had, the better off we'd be. Better? That's an understatement—we'd be superhuman.

In fact, we are superhuman—until the age of about twenty-five or thirty. But time-related growth (as opposed to time-related illness) is intended to happen to us from birth onward for many, many decades—not for a mere two or three. We stop being superhuman because we start being mere adults. Our behavior settles into patterns that are not broken by youthful exuberance and unpredictability. The randomness goes out of our lives. We don't have time to waste in frivolous things like dancing, running, jumping—*playing*.

The fact that the crossover into physiological decline occurs almost simultaneously with mounting career and family responsibilities is treated as a coincidence. But it's not a coincidence. Apart from this pronounced change in lifestyle, from one that is rich in stimulus to one that is not, there are no other apparent biological reasons why we humans shouldn't continue to add to our physiological capabilities for many more years, or at least achieve a balance that makes full use of our innate potential commensurate with the amount of time and resources that have gone into creating it. Otherwise, given our complexity and relatively long maturation process, we are entirely overbuilt and front-loaded, all granite foundation and flimsy cardboard structure. Nature tends not to waste precious assets and effort that way. Or at least if it does, it admits the mistakes and lets extinction erase them.

We may be headed for that fate, but if so, the mistake

will be ours. We have taught ourselves how to prematurely age and die. To unlearn that lesson, it's necessary only to look to young children. They don't know any better—all they do is spend their waking hours push, push, pushing against their limits and limitations. Starting off virtually immobile and defenseless, they grasp, reach, roll over, crawl, stand, walk, climb stairs, run, and quickly gain an incredible array of physical skills and an elaborate inner support system to confront and master their environment.

Out of this need to overcome life-threatening limitations, they manufacture themselves. In a way, it's pure negative capability: if you don't crawl, you'll never stand (or never stand with confidence, strength, and stability); if you don't stand, you'll never walk; if you don't walk, you'll never run; if you don't run, you'll never be president of the United States. It's a building process. The more they struggle and succeed, the more they are created. As with supply and demand, one feeds the other.

Humans produce trillions and trillions of cells, and kids start off producing them 24/7 to keep themselves healthy, happy, and growing. But this vast output is not automatic, as is sadly, tragically demonstrated by the increasingly common interruptions in early childhood development. Cells, be they brain, muscle, blood, organ, or any tissue, are produced *on demand*. They are organized and set to function *on demand* as well. About the only thing that humans are hardwired for is to respond in this way to the varied stimuli of the environment. Without such stimuli, trapped in an unchallenging bubble where only a relatively few demands are made and those are repeated over and over again, the child's physical and mental capabilities can never come close to full potential.

The magic of our *on demand* development dynamic is that first we change ourselves in response to the environment: we get bigger, stronger, smarter. Then we change the environment. Push leads to shove—that's why a once-lonely planet is now teeming with human life.

Most children are bombarded with environmental stimuli, and so they grow. Most modern adults are not, and so they stop growing and start aging long before their time.

I consider aging to be a loss of physical and physiological capability that stems from the body's inability to replace damaged and destroyed cells. The body, in other words, starts running a cellular deficit, by consuming more cells than it produces. It can happen at any age. Chronology is irrelevant. The shortfall adversely impacts every internal process, including metabolism. As metabolism falters, the ability to build replacement cells declines notch by notch. The body simply doesn't have enough fuel and fire to drive its myriad biochemical reactions. When that happens, it doesn't matter whether you're four or forty; cell production is getting ready to go south. All too soon the plant is cold, dark, and empty.

Counting the Rings, Not the Years

Many age-related symptoms of illness would more accurately be described as *ring-related symptoms.* No matter what your age, the route that leads to these symptoms involves traversing eight zones or rings of muscu-

Fig. 15-1

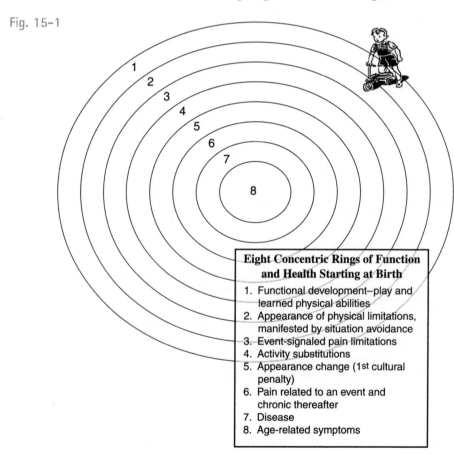

Eight Concentric Rings of Function and Health Starting at Birth

1. Functional development–play and learned physical abilities
2. Appearance of physical limitations, manifested by situation avoidance
3. Event-signaled pain limitations
4. Activity substitutions
5. Appearance change (1st cultural penalty)
6. Pain related to an event and chronic thereafter
7. Disease
8. Age-related symptoms

loskeletal system function. When you cross the border and enter new territory, you can immediately recognize where you are and what's happening. I've drawn you a picture (Figure 15–1).

Ring 1 encompasses the explosive functional development associated with childhood that comes about as the result of free-form play, exploration, and learned physical abilities. It establishes a rugged, long-lasting musculoskeletal foundation that can be maintained by way of a motion-rich environment and lifestyle. There's no reason we can't stay in this ring for decades. But whenever this period ends, "aging" begins. The primary characteristic of Ring 2 is what I call "situation avoidance." The individual, whether she's a young child or a middle-aged woman, no longer moves in a direct response to any and all stimuli. Instead, she chooses or edits her motion and activity according to her own criteria. Her choices are determined by likes, dislikes, opportunities, abilities, and—importantly—inabilities. She avoids certain situations that don't fit her requirements, and that avoidance creates ongoing physical limitations. In short, what she doesn't use, she loses.

Ring 3 reinforces limitations through an experience of pain that has been triggered by an event. For example, a runner gives up running after she twists a knee. Ring 4, activity substitution, follows when she switches from running to bike riding. With Ring 5, changes in her physical appearance set in. She may gain or lose weight, or she may undergo more subtle changes like slumping posture or skin problems. Since looking youthful is so highly valued, there's a cultural penalty associated with Ring 5 that makes it easy to mistake for a sign of aging. But looking old actually amounts to looking like you're an exile from Ring 1. Therefore the cultural penalty imposed on those who look old may reflect the more basic instinct to reward those who show the outward signs of musculoskeletal system function and the good health that comes with it. Unfortunately, cosmetics, plastic surgery, and the latest fashions can make someone look younger without moving him or her out of Ring 5.

Next is Ring 6, which occurs when an accident (event) causes recurring chronic pain, such as being in a fender bender that inflicts on the driver a sore neck from the whiplash. Ring 7 entails disease. Months or years may go by before the whiplash victim is diagnosed with arthritis in her neck and shoulders. Now we've arrived at Ring 8—age-related symptoms. The arthritis sufferer, if she happens to be fifty years old or older, is told she has an age-related disease.

Does it really make a difference whether chronic pain and disease are age-related or ring-related? It does because we can't do anything about the passage of time, except enjoy the ride. But by being aware of the rings and what they entail, we can take action that will bring us back toward Ring 1 or at least slow the movement away from it.

The Macro Forest, the Micro Tree

The body has so many components and structures, systems and subsystems, primary reactions and secondary phases, that it has convinced medical science to focus on the tiniest elements of human biology. Less is more. It's important work, but this emphasis deprives us of the vision to see what we're actually looking for in the first place—the sum of all the parts; the more that is the most.

The practitioners of microscience know this and escape from the dead end by shifting back to macroscience. We get sick and die, the hybrid micro-macro reasoning goes, for one of four reasons: bad luck, bad genes, bad bodies that are inherently prone to mistakes and breakdown, or age.

Bad genes will probably soon become the favorite explanation, but bad luck, bad bodies, and age all finish neck-and-neck. I think all four are losers. The sum of the parts that lead us to sicken and die prematurely is actually *metabolic deterioration*. Without it, opportunistic infection and disease (bad luck) does not get a foothold. Without it, all but the most deranged DNA encoding (bad genes) sorts itself out in the earliest stages of prenatal life. Without it, growth and strength preempt lost capability and decline (bad bodies and age).

Historically, humankind has not been prolific enough to endure runs of bad luck, bad genes, bad bodies, and age. For hundreds of thousands of years, the breeding stock was too small to tolerate the gene expression that undercut survival capability. Bad bodies didn't cross the Pacific in reed boats, and preliterate societies that didn't have the benefit of the practical experience and wisdom of their ancestors were not likely to remember the best route over the mountains and how to avoid the quicksand.

What we know in the twenty-first century that our primitive ancestors didn't is how extraordinarily complex the human body is. To us—children of the industrial age—that means high maintenance and frequent breakdowns. Machines Я Us. Our body machine is indeed complicated internally, but it's blessed with a nearly indestructible musculoskeletal system that responds to the stimulus of the environment. Partnered with the metabolic process, the musculoskeletal system ensures that aging is not governed by chronology; rather, chronology is sculpted, enriched, and enlivened by aging.

Ready or Not

Nature apparently does not intend for any living organism to be immortal. Metabolic efficiency amounts to an ongoing test to determine whether we will stay or go. It's a measure of our bodies' ability to perform useful physiological work. If we can't summon the energy to replace and rebuild our cells, then there's not much point in wasting food, water, and other resources on us. Mercifully, we have a built-in margin in case the body goes into temporary metabolic deficit as a result of accident or other circumstances beyond our control. The margin in most cases is quite substantial, but it is not limitless. There are many ingenious ways to crush one's metabolism. Getting run through by a dirty spear tip will do it. Our ancestor who didn't die of blood loss may have been killed by infection. Starvation, drought, exposure to the elements, and poor sanitation and hygiene did them in as well. But most premature deaths were probably infants, young children, and women in childbirth. Metabolism, in those cases, was either still well below peak or severely strained.

Because of the requirements of the development cycle, children are the most metabolically endangered until a few years after puberty. They need about fifteen years to get all their systems up to speed. During that period they are subject to a raft of diseases that target immature and weak systems that are not yet supported by fully functional metabolic processes. The metabolism is there, but not robust enough to withstand a full-scale invasion by pathogens.

Neither age nor gender was the key to survival, though. Once an individual had logged enough miles on the musculoskeletal system odometer, he or she lived for a long time. Their metabolisms were sturdy enough to handle most emergencies.

Graphically, the metabolic development cycle looks something like a bell curve that's had the top lopped off to form a plateau, as in Figure 15–2.

Roughly speaking, this bell curve represents the situation for the U.S. population in the first half of the twentieth century. As metabolic capacity increased through childhood and adolescence, the individual gained metabolic strength to fuel mental and physical development. As the pitch increased in the teen years, many childhood ailments were left behind. Strength and confidence rapidly accumulated. The vertical line at age eighteen marks the point when the individual arrived at peak metabolic strength and efficiency, where it leveled for several years until crossing the next vertical line, at age thirty-five. That's the point where metabolic deficit set in. The flat area between the vertical lines constitutes the zone of optimal health.

Since midcentury, motion has dwindled. What I believe is happening to the bell curve today (2001) looks like Figure 15–3.

The onset of full metabolic strength has shifted to the right, around age twenty. Deprived of motion, stimulus, and musculoskeletal system function, it's taking young people longer to get their metabolism up to speed, and they are staying longer in the danger zone of childhood disease and illness. Then musculoskeletal system dysfunction pulls metabolic capacity downward sooner than it did in the past, just before age thirty. Hence the zone of optimal health is shortening, to about ten years. For men the onset of metabolic decline occurs between thirty-five and forty and proceeds until the mid-seventies; for women it lasts until the early to mid-eighties. Aging in the classic sense is not involved: where you are positioned on the bell curve indicates your metabolic capacity, not your chronological age. But what these charts are telling us is that our metabolic capacity has been affected by our profile earlier in life. If you are now in your fifties, sixties, or seventies, your personal metabolic chart would likely resemble Figure 15–2, with its larger zone of optimal health and its more gradual metabolic decline. It sug-

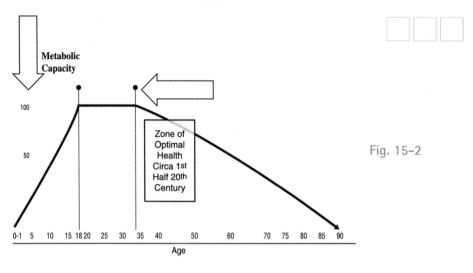

Fig. 15–2

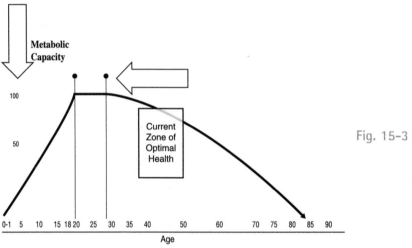

Fig. 15–3

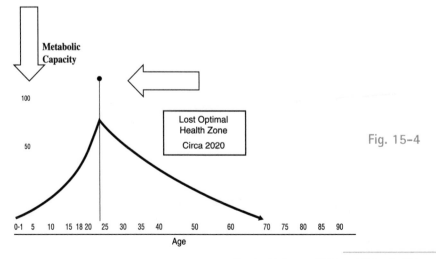

Fig. 15–4

gests a lifespan into the late eighties and early nineties, thanks to the metabolic strength developed early in life.

Within the next twenty years, the bell curve will start looking like Figure 15–4.

On the left, the slope's lower terrace leads to a steep ascent to the peak, around age twenty-five. The metabolic launch is slower and is spread over a longer span of childhood, which indicates prolonged developmental problems and potential illness. Adolescent emotional and physical maturation come more slowly. The plateau has disappeared altogether. Individuals will need approximately an extra ten years to get their metabolism cranked up; by which time they'll be in their mid-twenties. As soon as they reach it, however, metabolic decline will set in. They will never enter the zone of optimal health, or if they do, it will be a brief stay of only a few weeks or months. In general, when metabolism peaks, it will fall short of 100 percent.

In this worst-case scenario, the illness and disease of childhood metabolic insufficiency merge with the illness and disease of adult metabolic insufficiency. A metabolic surplus never exists, which increases the angle of descent toward illness and mortality on the right side. If the trend continues, the metabolic mountain will start to look like a molehill. It doesn't bode well for members of the middle– to late–baby boom generation, who'll enter their senior years at around 2025. Their optimal zone of metabolic health is much smaller and the line descends more precipitously and indicates a shorter lifespan.

Fig. 15-5

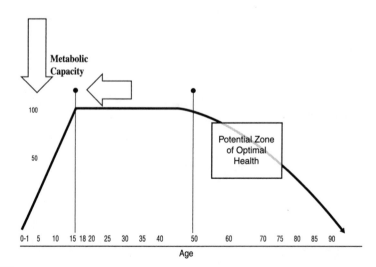

But that decline doesn't have to happen. Figure 15–5 displays the consequences of full musculoskeletal system function combined with a metabolism-enhancing lifestyle—one with proper diet, hydration, and rest, plus abstinence from tobacco, alcohol, and drugs.

Here the bell curve lifts off smartly, as young people more rapidly engage their functions in support of their metabolism. They achieve peak metabolic strength soon after puberty. With metabolic efficiency and power to spare, they enjoy a long plateau of optimal health, lasting well into late middle age. The descending curve is much more gradual.

In effect, years don't matter. The only two relevant points are the one that marks the realization of full metabolic strength and the one that marks the beginning of metabolic decline. Both points can be shifted, but not infinitely. The onset line cannot be pushed much farther to the left than puberty. The childhood development cycle needs time and stimulus to unfold. Likewise, the right vertical can shift under the proper conditions into the seventies, eighties, and nineties, but based on what we know about longevity, the mortality endpoint will probably continue to hover in the lower one hundreds.

The Elder Model

All living things die, but not all go through a prolonged period of extreme senescence or decrepitude. For most creatures the end appears to come quickly, without many outward signs of lost capability. Large mammals could be the exception, but many primates, especially chimpanzees, which share close similarities with humans, peak early, live for many years without signs of flagging, go into a quick nosedive, and then die.

"Dotage" may well be a product of culture and circumstance. With historically short lifespans prior to the twentieth century, those who survived famine, drought, poor diet, infection, accident, and violence probably gravitated to leadership, ceremonial, and teaching roles. They had important information to impart that was at least as valuable as hunting and gathering. Possessed of peak metabolism until that point, the change in stimulus provoked a slow metabolic decline and a gradual loss of physiological capability. Conceivably, if they had remained fully involved in hunting and gathering or other physically demanding activities, the top end of life expectancy could have extended to 125 or 130 years—or perhaps on the order of Methuselah's 969 years. Even as the general population started living longer (mostly by dint of avoiding death at birth and childhood diseases), this declining elder model stayed with us and turned a third or more of a lifetime into a slow-motion collapse.

Demographers and gerontologists are concerned that the upward trend in longevity that's been fostered to some extent by advanced medical technology may lead to the Western world becoming choked with many millions of enfeebled old women and men. That will indeed happen if the current elder model remains in place. Ironically, the *deceleration of mortality* after sixty-five, to use a term favored by experts, confirms that an efficient metabolism is the key to a longer, fully functional life. In terms of availability alone, health care is today more widely available than ever before. Powered by metabolism that was revved up by active, physically stimulating lifestyles as children, adolescents, and young adults, their downward glide-path is longer and more gradual.

Early baby boomers, born from 1946 to about 1956, had the benefit of the revolution in antibiotics in childhood. There's evidence that by avoiding major illnesses early in life, individuals may live longer, healthier lives in general. This is consistent with my belief that putting down a strong metabolic foundation is essential. But these early baby boomers may be the last to benefit fully from the antibiotic revolution because their metabolic systems were allowed to develop before the sedentary modern lifestyle totally engulfed American culture. They got in just under the wire.

Younger baby boomers and other upcoming generations may live longer than their parents and grandparents (though that's iffy), but the time gained may be in dysfunctional years characterized by increasing pain and physiological decline. Without engaged and strong musculoskeletal systems and with lifestyles that further undermine metabolic efficiency, the long-lived elderly of the not-too-distant future may be headed for more years of increasingly elaborate life support than they spent as healthy, independent, active beings.

Back to Burning and Churning

The E-cises in this section are designed to help get you over one of the biggest hurdles standing in the way of metabolic efficiency: a disengaged, dysfunctional musculoskeletal system. Any number of enzyme powders, mineral and nutritional supplements, diets, and exercise programs can bring about temporary spikes in your metabolism. But without the help of your musculoskeletal system, the natural baseline is insufficient to keep the metabolic process from sinking lower and lower after the spike wears off. The burning, the churning, and the chemical reactions that keep the cells fired up will dwindle.

Wouldn't the menus in earlier chapters work as well? No. They may appear similar and even share some of the same E-cises, but the arrangement of the menu is crafted to undo the misalignment and muscular disengagement often found in women over fifty.

By opening the door to efficient metabolism, these E-cises will probably whet your appetite for more physical activity. Go for it! There's no surer sign of increased metabolism than the desire to get moving. Remember, the more you move, the more you *can* move. Dormant, disengaged muscles cannot play a part in the supply-and-demand dynamic that's at the core of the metabolic process. Without demand from the major muscle groups, the metabolic supply (output) falls off.

If you have chronic musculoskeletal pain, you might want to consult my book *Pain Free* for advice on what to do about specific conditions. But use this menu as a warm-up first, then alternate between the two. As for acute illness, ask your doctor if he or she knows of any ailment that wouldn't benefit from improved metabolism. If there is one, I haven't heard of it.

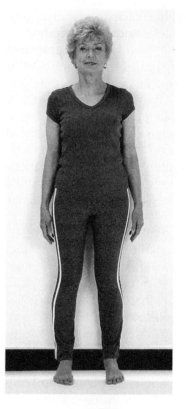

[Over-Fifty Restoration and Maintenance Menu]

**▶ STANDING at WALL
(Figure 15–6)**

PURPOSE This E-cise reminds the body what an upright and truly vertical posture feels like.

Stand with your heels, buttocks, upper back, and head against a wall. If you cannot get your head against the wall without straining too hard, then place it in a comfortable and relaxed position. Relax your stomach muscles and your arms. Let your body settle into this new position. Make sure that your feet remain pointed straight ahead for the entire E-cise and that your stomach is relaxed out. Hold this position for five minutes.

**✝▶ WALL STORK
(Figure 15–7)**

PURPOSE This E-cise levels the hips into a parallel position, under a load that's held in vertical alignment.

Stand against a wall with your feet pointed straight ahead. Your heels, hips, upper back, and head should be against the wall. Place your right foot on the seat of a chair positioned about twelve inches in front of you. Make sure this foot is pointed straight. Do not allow your left foot to twist or your left leg to bend. The right leg, on the chair, should be bent at about ninety degrees at the knee joint. Hold this position without allowing the left foot, leg, or hip to shift to the side or to roll away from the wall. Hold for three minutes. Switch legs and repeat.

▸ WALL PRESSES
(Figure 15–8 a, b, c, and d)

PURPOSE This E-cise repositions the shoulders to the correct posterior position.

Stand against a wall with your feet pointing straight ahead, about a hip-width apart. Your hips, upper back, and head should be against the wall. Place your hands with their backs against the wall, arms straight, and arrange them at the four and eight o'clock positions. *Set 1:* Your palms face out from the wall, and your head is level (a). Squeeze your shoulder blades together (back and down), and release. Don't *lift* your shoulders and squeeze—it's a *downward* squeeze and release. Do ten repetitions. *Set 2:* Keep your palms facing out, but lower your head till your chin rests on your chest (b). Squeeze and release your shoulder blades. Do ten repetitions. *Set 3:* Your palms face the wall, and your head is level (c). Do ten repetitions. *Set 4:* Your palms face the wall, and your head is lowered again (d). Do ten repetitions.

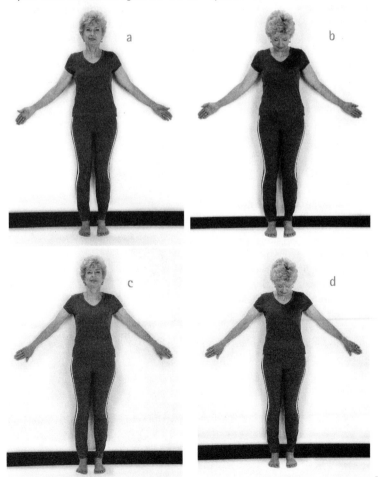

▶ STANDING ARM CIRCLES
(Figure 15–9)

PURPOSE This E-cise strengthens the muscles of the upper back that are involved with the shoulders' ball and socket function.

Stand facing a mirror with your feet parallel, about a hip-width apart, your arms at your sides. Curl your fingertips into the pads of each palm (the fleshy area at the base of the fingers), and point your thumbs straight out. This hand position, called the "golfer's grip," is imperative to the success of the E-cise. Squeeze your shoulder blades together, and bring your arms out to your sides at shoulder level, elbows straight. With your palms facing down, thumbs pointing forward, circle up and forward for forty repetitions. Now with your palms facing up, circle up and back for forty repetitions. Remember to keep your wrists and elbows straight and your shoulder blades squeezed together—the circles must come from the shoulders.

✾▶ STANDING FORWARD BEND
(Figure 15–10)

PURPOSE This E-cise strengthens the back and hips.

Stand with your feet facing straight ahead, a hip-width apart. Place your palms on your low back–upper buttocks area. Tilt your pelvis forward to put an exaggerated arch in your low back, pull your elbows and shoulder blades together, and hold. Your hips should initiate the bend, not your low back. Keep your back arched. Tighten your thighs, and allow your weight to shift forward onto the balls of your feet. Hold this position for one minute.

*
▸ CATS and DOGS
(Figure 15–11 a and b)
PURPOSE This E-cise works the hips, spine, shoulders, and neck in coordinated flexion and extension.

Get down on the floor on your hands and knees. Make a table by aligning your knees with your hips and your wrists with your shoulders. Your lower legs should be parallel with each other and with your hips. Your weight should be distributed evenly. For the Cat, smoothly round your back upward and let your head curl under to create a curve that runs from your buttocks to your neck—like a cat with an arched back (a). For the Dog, smoothly sway the back down while bringing the head up (b). Make these two moves flow continuously back and forth. Exhale as you move into the Cat position; inhale during the Dog. Do one set of ten repetitions.

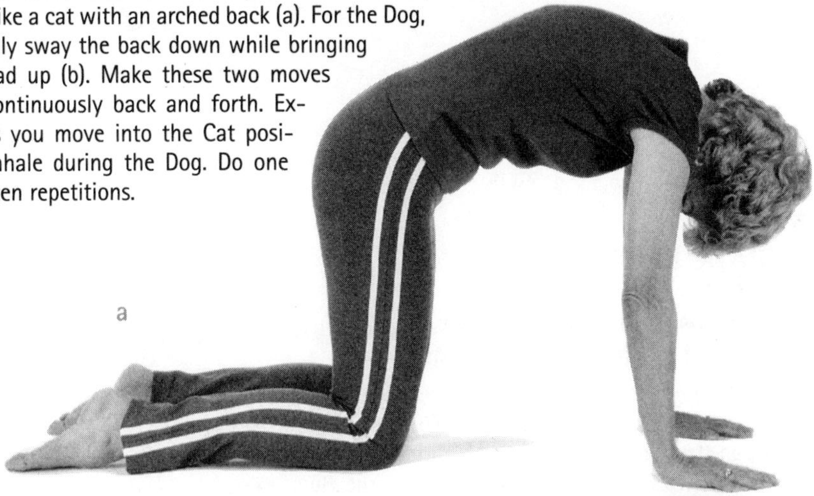

a

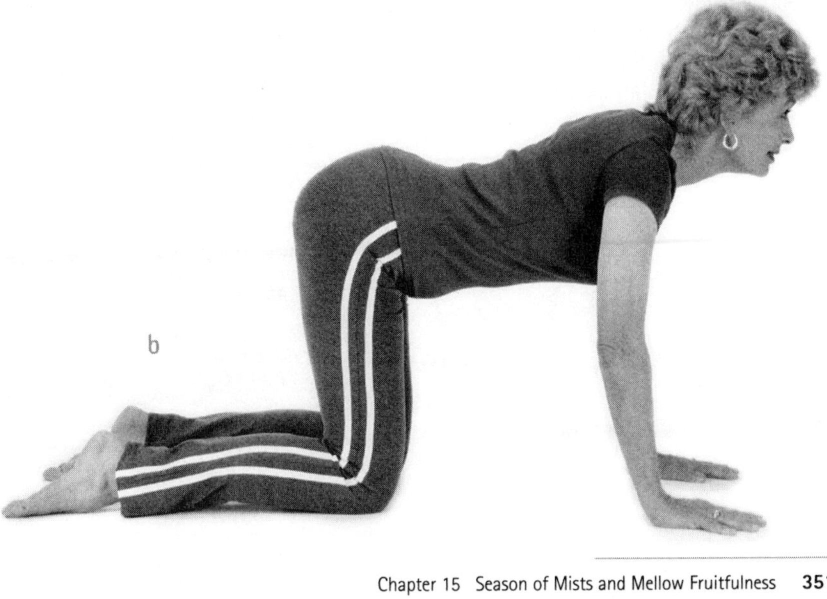

b

✱

▶ **STATIC BACK**
(Figure 15–12)

PURPOSE This E-cise uses gravity to flatten the back and put it in a neutral position.

Lie on your back, with both legs bent at right angles and resting on a chair, bench, or block. (The large blocks we use in the clinic are 20 inches high by 14 inches wide by 24 inches long.) Rest your hands on the floor, extended below shoulder level, with the palms up. Let your back settle into the floor. Breathe from your diaphragm, so your abdominal muscles rise as you inhale and fall as you exhale. Hold this position for five minutes.

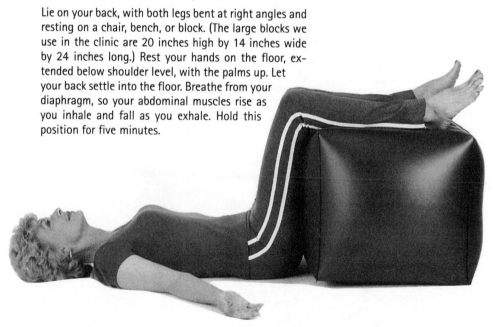

▶ STATIC BACK—PULLOVERS
(Figure 15–13 a and b)

PURPOSE This E-cise relaxes and strengthens the muscles of the thoracic back.

While in the Static Back position, clasp your hands together tightly, and extend your arms up toward the ceiling with your elbows straight (a). Now bring your arms back—keep them straight—to touch the floor behind your head (b). Return them to the starting position. Do three sets of ten repetitions each.

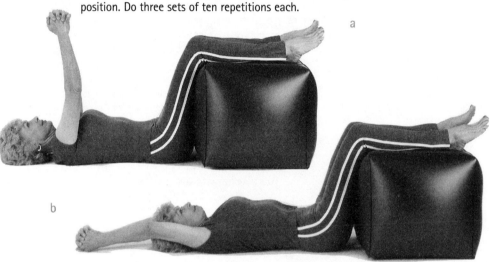

a

b

▶ STATIC BACK—PULLOVER PRESSES
(Figure 15–14)

PURPOSE This E-cise reminds the shoulders' ball and socket that it is not exclusively a hinge.

Stay in the Static Back position. Extend both arms straight back behind your head with the hands clasped, elbows locked. Press your clasped hands into a block or pillow, and release. Don't contract your abdominal muscles. Let your lower back muscles react. Keep your feet parallel to each other. Do three sets of ten repetitions each.

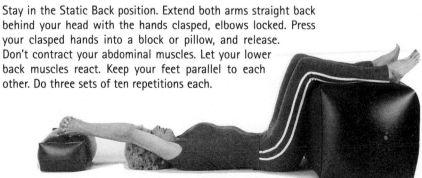

▸ FOOT CIRCLES and POINT/FLEXES
(Figure 15–15 a, b, and c)

PURPOSE This E-cise reminds the knees, ankles, and feet how to interact according to their designs.

Lie on your back with your left leg extended flat on the floor and your right leg bent toward your chest. For the Foot Circles, clasp your hands behind your bent knee to hold it in position while you circle your right foot clockwise (a). The Foot Circles emanate from the ankle, not from the knee. Keep your knee still, and try to make full circles. (You may tend to make half circles; it will help to slow down and concentrate.) Meanwhile, keep the left foot pointed straight up toward the ceiling, with the left thigh muscles tight. Do forty repetitions. Then reverse direction and circle your right foot counterclockwise. Repeat forty times. For the Point/Flexes, keep your legs in the same position. On the bent right leg, bring your toes back toward the shin to flex (b), then reverse the direction to point your toes (c). Do this forty times. Switch legs and do forty repetitions of both Foot Circles and Point/Flexes with the left foot.

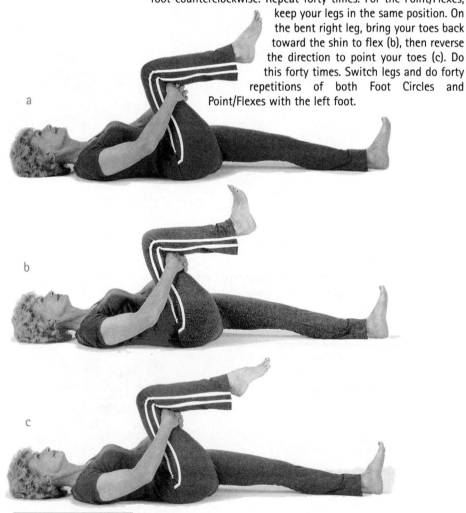

a

b

c

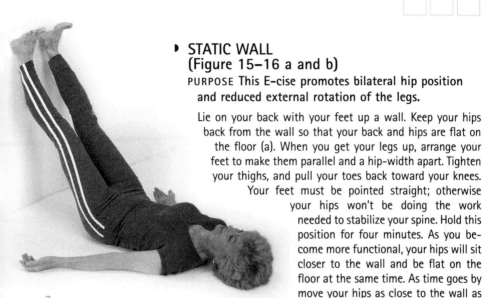

STATIC WALL
(Figure 15–16 a and b)

PURPOSE This E-cise promotes bilateral hip position and reduced external rotation of the legs.

Lie on your back with your feet up a wall. Keep your hips back from the wall so that your back and hips are flat on the floor (a). When you get your legs up, arrange your feet to make them parallel and a hip-width apart. Tighten your thighs, and pull your toes back toward your knees. Your feet must be pointed straight; otherwise your hips won't be doing the work needed to stabilize your spine. Hold this position for four minutes. As you become more functional, your hips will sit closer to the wall and be flat on the floor at the same time. As time goes by move your hips as close to the wall as you can and adjust your feet (b).

a

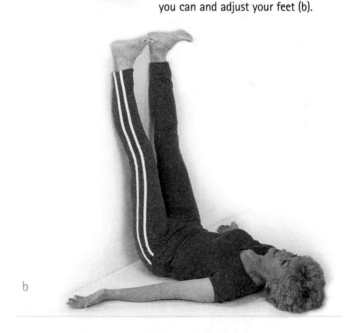

b

Will these E-cises get you back to a metabolic balance point where cell consumption equals cell construction? It's feasible but impossible to guarantee. The cellular deficit could be too steep to completely reverse. Even so, trying is better than not trying. Just slowing the trend of cellular deficit can be beneficial. Every uptick in the metabolic process can take us closer to the goal of optimal health, closer to being *ageless*.

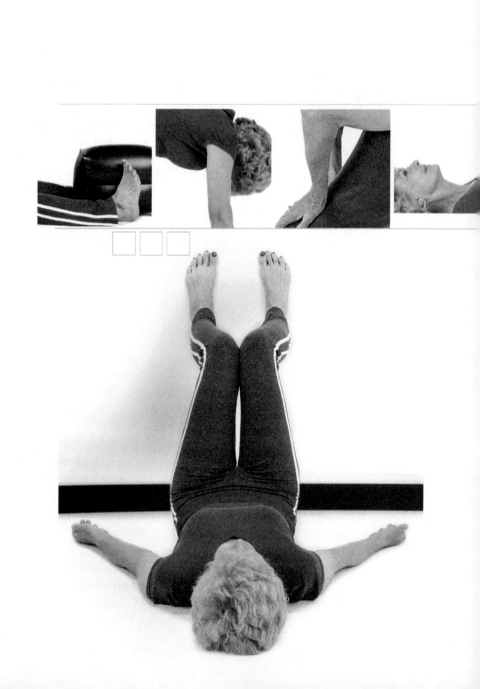

CHAPTER 16

balance: lost and found

As the end of this book comes into sight, it's time for me to write about a serial killer of women. He has no fancy scientific name. He's an old friend who's done no harm in the past other than perhaps cause a painful bump or bruise. You've known him since childhood as "tripping," "stumbling," "falling down"—alias "I don't know what happened. I just lost my balance."

The complications of hip fractures from falls hold a lifetime risk of death for women that is comparable to their rate of death from breast cancer. This extraordinary statistic is usually blamed on osteoporosis, but the real culprit is a dysfunctional musculoskeletal system that causes muscle and bone loss and deprives women of the strength and balance they need to stay on their feet.

It does not necessarily deprive *older* women of strength and balance. Injuries from falls are common in all age groups. In younger people they are rationalized as freak accidents; in older folks brittle bones and unsteady balance are blamed. But I believe that regardless of age, the key factor in the majority of cases is poor balance produced by skeletal misalignment and muscular disengagement. Musculoskeletal system dysfunctions are so pervasive that falling down is becoming more and more commonplace. And instead of bouncing back without damage, knees, wrists, and other joints are getting smashed up to the point that young children and teenagers regard braces and bandages as standard equipment for most sports and physical activities (including using a personal computer).

The mechanics of standing and moving on two feet is the same no matter what your age—and that's very good news.

Eyes and Ears

Compare the two women in Figures 16–1a and 16–1b. The one in 16–1b is fully functional from a musculoskeletal system standpoint. Her head and shoulders are back, her spine has an S-curve, her hips are square, and all her load-bearing joints are vertically aligned and parallel. The vertical dotted line shows her center of gravity. Check it out.

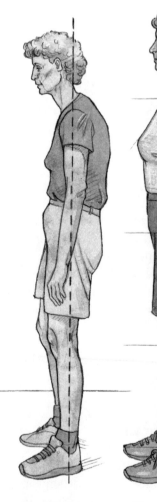

The other woman in 16–1a isn't so fortunate. She is severely misaligned. Yet she doesn't look unusual for someone her age, does she? Notice her head, shoulders, and back. Where's her center of gravity? Instead of being on a vertical axis that runs from her feet through her hips, spine, shoulders, and head, her center of gravity actually floats approximately where her head is, well forward of the rest of her body. The dotted vertical line shows what's happening to the equilibrium of her structure; it's essentially trying to topple forward. Most of her muscle strength and energy allocation are directed at preventing that from happening. She doesn't have much left over for anything else. That's why she tends to move slowly and stiffly.

Look at what happens when the two women descend stairs (Figures 16–2a and 16–2b). The aligned, fully functional woman in 16–2b is anchored to each tread by the force of gravity, which projects straight down through her head,

Fig. 16-1a   Fig. 16-1b

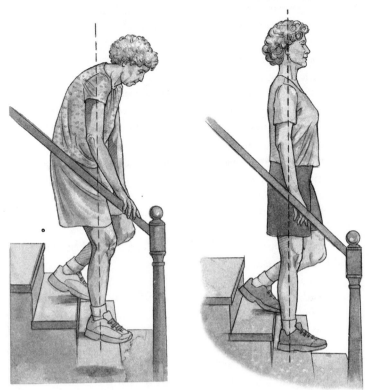

Fig. 16–2a

Fig. 16–2b

shoulders, spine, hips, and supporting leg. Her hips and legs are in the proper position to alternately flex and extend. She's in control and doesn't have a feeling that she is about to lurch off into space. Her aligned hips and head act as counterweights.

The woman in 16–2a, by contrast, is being pulled forward and down. The counterweight is gone. Her hips and head are actually trying to flip over and exchange places. To guard against such a disastrous somersault, she locks her hips—even more than they are already—and pops them from side to side to swing her legs clear of the front edge of the upper tread and down to the next. There's no way she can naturally flex and extend her hips, knees, and legs. She is in danger of falling with each step.

As you'll recall from Chapter 4, Figures 4–3 through 4–6 depicted another pair of functional and dysfunctional women on a staircase. In those illustrations I was showing you how misalignment undermines strength and stamina. Those models were in their late twenties or thirties. Imagine that forty years have elapsed: forty years of strength being undermined with every staircase climbed, forty years of gradually losing flexion and extension. Is it fair to blame the cumulative effects on age? While time has passed, the functional woman in Figure 16–2b is handling the stairs better than the dysfunctional younger woman. Function, not age, is the key.

On an irregular surface or where sudden shifts of weight are required—a rocky path, a cracked sidewalk, icy spots, and even especially thick carpeting—a dysfunctional woman's range of motion and response time are severely restricted. All of her resources are committed to dealing with the process of moving forward on a straight line. She can't cope with anything else. Even the slightest bump or wobble threatens to send her crashing to the ground.

To avoid a calamity, most people in this situation avoid stairs and every rough, unpredictable surface. It's one reason why shopping malls are now popular as exercise venues for the elderly. But the problem is our old "Use it or lose it" rule. The less we employ any given set of physical functions, the more inaccessible they become. In fairly short order, a little bit of trouble getting up and down stairs becomes a lot of trouble—and dangerous.

Many people blame their unsteadiness on impaired vision. They're partially correct, but it's not *what* you see that affects your balance, it's the *way* you see. In Figures 16–1 and 16–2, note the head positions of the two models. One reason the dysfunctional woman's head is sagging forward and down is that she is "reading" the ground. She is gathering information that her musculoskeletal system is designed to collect through other means but can't because it's dysfunctional. When they are functional, your feet, ankles, and knees are acutely sensitive to surface variations. Even encased in a hard-soled shoe, the lateral and transverse arches of the foot are the next best things to combination shock absorber–gyroscopes that send a constant stream of data to the central nervous system about whether the road is hard or soft, rough or smooth, wet or dry, flat or pitched. That information flow triggers a muscular response literally from head to foot.

But when feet are flat or averted, or knees are rotated, or you're wearing high heels or high-tech shoes, that doesn't happen. Your eyes are used as a substitute. They're not nearly as good at the job; they're cruder, slower, and have a tendency to over- and underreact. Furthermore, to examine the surface, we have to crane our necks forward and roll our head down, shifting the center of gravity in front of us even farther than it is already. Not only does this contribute to loss of balance, it actually impairs our vision all the more.

The optic nerve and muscles of the eye require oxygen—lots of it. In fact, the optic nerve uses more oxygen than any other single nerve in the body. But the back, shoulders, and neck muscles of a misaligned body gobble up a disproportionate share of that oxygen in order to fuel the muscle contractions needed to fight gravity, which drags the head forward and down. It's a constant tug-of-war. The resulting diversion of oxygen away from the eyes has the perverse effect of making it harder to see, and that in turn leads to more slumping, more eye strain, and more lost vision.

But the body doesn't give up. It goes to its back-up guidance system—the inner ear. Both ears have fluid-filled, U-shaped canals that act much like carpenters' levels. Each canal is lined with tiny filaments that react to the fluid as it sloshes back and forth in response to the body's traversing terrain. The system is designed to keep the torso on a rough vertical axis to the surface of the earth. Without it we would be immobilized at night and whenever the horizon is obscured even momentarily. It's pure genius. But there's a hitch.

The inner ear doesn't know that we've lost musculoskeletal alignment. It reads a head that is in the forward position as an indication of descending terrain. If the head is also tipped to the right or left, it interprets that information as signaling an irregular surface. And we may be standing stock-still! When we start to move, it gets even more confusing. The eye overrides the ear, but as vision is impaired, the ear becomes more assertive; the two systems come into conflict. One says zig and the other says zag. Occasionally they both shrug and say, "Beats the hell out of me."

In the meantime, we feel like hell. We may have evolved out of the sea, but enough time has elapsed that our inner ear is more suited to terrestrial navigation. It can handle quick turns and changes in elevation, but it has difficulty with slow, persistent side-to-side rocking. That's why many of us tend to get seasick when we're out on the water. I contend that many older people feel lousy in part because they are operationally seasick. Their gait-patterns are such that they walk swaying from side to side. The head rocks and rolls along, and fluid in the inner ear sloshes left-right-right-left-left-right. . . . Consequently, walking is no pleasure because it's making us queasy.

On Balance

Joint restrictions also lead to poor balance. You might want to turn back to Chapter 1 to reacquaint yourself with the body's basic grid design. Whenever the body loses the vertical and horizontal alignment of its principal load-bearing joints, those joints—ankles, knees, hips, and shoulders—are no longer able to open and close without extra friction. It takes more muscular effort; in some cases there's nerve impingement, and often the joint's articulating surfaces grind, bind, and grate.

Combine this situation with the additional gravitational burden of skeletal misalignment, and unsteadiness is inevitable. Okay, you may say, but times are changing—high-tech medicine will come to the rescue, won't it? Sorry. Joint-replacement surgery is no miracle cure. While it may alleviate the pain—living tissue is being replaced by cold, dead hardware, after all—the misalignment remains and still puts continued stress on the other load-joints. That's why one artificial hip tends to lead to another, and to artificial knees as well.

Nor does this surgery guarantee total pain abatement. There's still plenty of wear and tear on muscles, tendons, ligaments, and supporting joints. When the skeleton starts rearranging itself, there are only so many places the bones can go before they start rubbing up against nerves.

"Incurable" Arthritis

According to the U.S. Public Health Service, 40 million Americans are affected by arthritis and other rheumatic diseases. Some experts believe that figure is too conservative and that, in fact, nearly everyone older than sixty is afflicted by the condition to some degree or another.

I don't agree. Based on my experience in the clinic, those numbers are wildly exaggerated. I would estimate that roughly half the people who come in thinking they have arthritis pain, based either on a physician's cursory diagnosis or on their own opinion, are mistaken. Now,

I'm not a medical doctor, and so the mysteries of arthritis pathology may be eluding my grasp, but joint and muscle pain that is present when skeletal misalignment is apparent and absent when that misalignment is corrected seems to be telling us in a straightforward way that arthritis isn't happening.

Arthritis is a real disease, however. In its nastiest forms it attacks and destroys bone and cartilage with relentless ferocity by inflaming and deforming joints and in some cases damaging muscles, skin, blood vessels, and other internal systems. But musculoskeletal system dysfunction and misalignment also destroy bone and cartilage and inflame joints. This similarity has led to confusion, misdiagnosis, drastically inappropriate treatment, and needless suffering. And it's no wonder—such is the logical consequence of treating the wrong disease.

For decades researchers have been baffled by arthritis's tendency to go into and out of remission and by its apparent incurability. These characteristics are also shared—or so it seems—by musculoskeletal system dysfunction. This is where the confusion arises. Suppose a remission in arthritis pain comes out of the blue. One day the pain is horrible, the next it's gone. A remission in chronic musculoskeletal pain and swelling comes out of the blue too, since it usually follows a change in lifestyle or a demand that can be almost unnoticeable and apparently unrelated. That's why doctors often suggest bed rest for sore backs. Left on their own to figure it out, if people can make a link between pain and a given activity, they usually modify or drop the activity. They don't give it much thought. If it hurts their back to bend over to tie their shoes, they buy a pair of loafers. Within a few days or weeks, the pain abates. In other words, it goes into *remission*. "Amazing! I'm cured."

But that really doesn't fix the problem—the posture of musculoskeletal system dysfunction is still causing friction and stress elsewhere. So pain usually recurs at some point. It may come and go several times, but it always returns and keeps getting worse. In other words, the pain is *incurable*. Therefore remissions plus renewed pain and incurability equal arthritis. Just as easily, the math could add up to chronic musculoskeletal pain, and when the individual is under fifty years old, it generally does. By popular definition, incorrect as it is, age and disease travel together. Once we pass the magic number of fifty, it's time for the Big A. Only in many cases, it's the Big MSD—musculoskeletal dysfunction.

As a result, drugs and surgery are brought to bear on a condition that is indeed truly incurable by that treatment protocol. Chronic musculoskeletal pain laughs off most drugs and surgery. This means that the "disease" spreads, the pain intensifies, and the drug and surgical wars escalate. And everyone sits back and marvels at how intractable and resistant arthritis seems to be, how no one seems immune, and how it's beginning to strike younger and younger people.

For just this once, let's assume the best rather than the worst. Maybe there's a good reason that there's no cure for arthritis after all these years and billions of dollars in research. What if joint inflammation, pain, and even overt cartilage and bone loss mean that the individual's musculoskeletal system is not under attack by a disease but is simply dysfunctional? Forget about arthritis. Let's try a simple explanation. One of the marvelous things about the human body is, it lends itself to simple self-restoration and self-maintenance. In a rough-and-ready world where the nearest hospital is in the next millennium or the next galaxy, do-it-yourself has to be simple. We got along fine for a couple of million years without oncologists, radiologists, and surgeons. Self-restoration and self-maintenance happened as our ancestors interacted with their physically stimulating environment. We can do the same. By deliberately and systematically stimulating musculoskeletal system functions in accordance with our design and motion requirements, we can eliminate friction and stress that cause joint inflammation and damage. Let's cure arthritis by not curing arthritis.

If simple doesn't work, we can try something more complicated. But you know what? Even if arthritis is also present, a reduction in friction and stress will ease the crisis for the afflicted joint. Consequently, a less drastic drug or surgical intervention might work just as well or better. That's precisely why several recent research studies have found that light to moderate exercise can help relieve arthritis pain and make it easier to move. Light to moderate exercise would have even more benefits once the body has been restored to musculoskeletal function.

Osteoarthritis and rheumatoid arthritis are both

classified as autoimmune diseases. The immune system goes bonkers and attacks cartilage and bone. But I believe a motion trigger and a metabolic trigger set off this event. The body isn't bonkers at all—it is its usual rational self. A hot, disengaged, functionally motionless joint is neither being kept supplied with oxygen and nutrients nor being flushed of toxins and other waste products. Under the body's strict "Use it or lose it" rule, the joint and its supporting mechanism are, in effect, dying. The immune system senses this and mobilizes to dispose of the corpse. It treats the joint the way it would any invading virus or antigen: with an all-out counterattack of potent biological weaponry. It makes perfect sense: dead and decayed tissue will poison the rest of the body—get rid of it! Autoimmune diseases aren't mistakes, they're self-defense.

The other trigger, metabolism, is equally important. Without adequate musculoskeletal system function, the metabolic process is unable to supply enough cellular material to maintain healthy cartilage and bone. As they deteriorate, joints become more disengaged, less viable, and ever-riper targets for immune system counterattacks. In addition, the immune system loses its ability to discriminate between appropriate and inappropriate levels of response. Like an overworked, tired, and frustrated person who lashes out in anger at minor irritations, the stressed immune system becomes very cranky indeed.

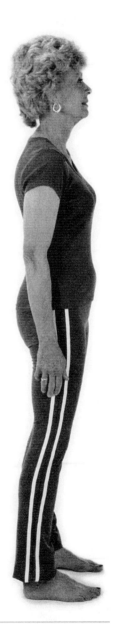

A May 2000 study found that lupus, another rheumatic disease related to arthritis, may be caused by the failure of a key enzyme to clean up waste products. The body's enzyme "factory" makes Intel, the world's number-one computer chip maker, look like a mom-and-pop store. Its incredible output is fueled by metabolism.

In important ways, the disease we know as arthritis is a symptom of motion starvation and the profound musculoskeletal system dysfunction that it creates.

Parkinson's and Alzheimer's: Unsteady as She Goes

Metabolic weakness is a common thread in Parkinson's and Alzheimer's diseases as well. Both neurological disorders display symptoms of a musculoskeletal nature. Parkinson's is characterized by muscular tremors, loss of motor control, rigidity of movement, and a drooping posture. A deficiency in the neurotransmitter dopamine is believed to be responsible.

This disease tends to get progressively worse over time. The rate varies from individual to individual depending on a host of factors and the course of treatment with synthetic dopamine and other drugs. In the Egoscue Method Clinic, we handle people with Parkinson's as if they were solely afflicted with a posture-related musculoskeletal system disorder. I believe Parkinson's symptoms can only worsen if the musculoskeletal system is allowed to weaken and spiral into dysfunction. By strengthening muscles, engaging joints, and restoring alignment, the often-startling rapidity of the disease can be slowed. Otherwise, as with *any* dysfunctional person, the less a Parkinson's victim moves according to the body's inherent design, the less she is capable of moving.

In addition, the dopamine deficiency is very likely caused or aggravated by a failure of the motion-driven metabolic process to provide the wherewithal to create sufficient dopamine and other neurotransmitters to smoothly carry out muscular contraction and other musculoskeletal system requirements.

Once again it's a case of supply and demand—and its mirror image, demand and supply. The metabolic process is not being asked to make available the energy necessary to fire up basic biochemical reactions and cell building. Everything is scarce, including dopamine and all the other neurotransmitters. When the volume of a substance is small to begin with—as is the case with neurotransmitters and hormones—tiny fluctuations have major impact.

I've found that many Parkinson's sufferers are intense, type-A personalities. Without a vigorous metabolism supported by strong, engaged muscles, they may be spending many years driving with the needle of the dopamine gauge hovering around empty until the tank finally runs dry. The usual pattern is that something stressful or demanding happens to use up metabolic resources. It could be the death of a loved one or the prospect of retirement, a high fever, or chronic dehydration. Shortly thereafter a Parkinson's-triggering event occurs. In the case of Alicia, a client who had undergone a traumatic divorce, it was a tennis lesson conducted on a particularly hot day. Immediately afterward she noticed her hands were trembling. She figured it was just the result of a hard workout. When the trembling persisted for several days, Alicia went to a doctor, who told her it was Parkinson's.

Typically, Parkinson's sufferers curtail their physical activity. But this reduces metabolic demand all the more and curbs the supply of fuel, further limiting the dopamine supply. Therefore the tremors and other symptoms get worse. On top of that, muscles are losing strength and disengaging, the joints are becoming restricted, and skeletal misalignment is setting in because the body is no longer being adequately stimulated. It's getting harder to move from a mechanical standpoint, just as the brain's dopamine supply is dwindling.

A recent study suggests that Parkinson's victims benefit from drinking coffee. This finding doesn't surprise me. The caffeine is goosing the body's metabolism. It provides a temporary jolt that either stimulates an uptick in the available amount of neurotransmitters or stretches the limited amount enough to suppress the musculoskeletal symptoms.

But caffeine and other drugs don't address the underlying and ongoing metabolic weakness. When the buzz or dosage wears off, the metabolism slumps again, and the symptoms are likely to recur. Likewise, medication for Alzheimer's disease has limited success due to the body's inability to supply the fuel necessary to carry out proper brain cell replication and maintenance. The lesions and plaque deposits found in the brains of Alzheimer's patients may be the result of improper bonding between glucose molecules and proteins that form a gloppy mass that prevents the proteins from going about their rightful business. Without strong metabolic activity to make them behave themselves, the protein and glucose are like a couple of teenagers who have nothing better to do than get into trouble. That's one possible explanation. Another is that the body is attempting to work around the metabolic weakness by improvising cell replication in the brain as best it can. In effect, it skips a few steps by not completely processing the glucose according to the standard recipe because it doesn't have the metabolic energy to do it properly. The stove isn't hot enough, and as in cooking, the chef may either get away with it or end up with a blob. Alzheimer's is the blob. Perhaps the body can tolerate a few of them from time to time, but years of metabolic insufficiency and years of serving up glucose/protein blobs may take a terrible toll.

A third possibility that may explain the brain lesions harkens back to my conviction that the body is rarely confused or mistaken. Confident that strong and efficient metabolism will be restored sooner rather than later, the body may simply be stockpiling valuable protein and glucose molecules on the principle of "Waste not, want not." It's conceivable that a metabolically driven mechanism for decoupling the gloppy glucose and protein combination is never activated due to the lack of metabolic activity. Eventually, the blob becomes a real-life horror story.

Cancer: Self-Defense or Self-Destruction?

The same perspective may provide insights into the puzzling nature of cancer. If the body is rarely confused or mistaken, why does it allow deviant cells to massively divide and multiply to the point that they launch a potentially deadly helter-skelter invasion of surrounding tissue? Surely, that's a mistake.

Or is it? Could it be a form of self-defense that, through our actions and lifestyle, we both provoke and ultimately undermine, so instead of working to save us, it may ultimately mean our destruction?

A popular theory on the origins of cancer is that one or more genes in a cell accidentally mutate. The accident disrupts the essential function of the cell, which when it divides creates other deviant cells with the same shortcoming. Since some internal organ systems are more cancer prone than others—like the colon, the stomach, the lymph system, and the lungs—and since they tend to be composed of tissue that does more cell replication than, say, the heart muscle or the brain, the assumption is that, by the law of averages, these mutations will randomly occur wherever there is a lot of cell building going on.

It sounds plausible—if you believe the body is accident prone, which I don't. We may be accident prone by way of our actions and behavior patterns, but the body works hard to avoid the accidents that we create for ourselves. The metabolic accident is a primary example. By suppressing our metabolism, we make it difficult for the body to build new cells. The fuel isn't available to do the job properly. But the body doesn't close up shop. It does what it can with the available resources. It may be that deviant cells are the products of having to scrimp and improvise cell building when there isn't enough of the right material on hand. The body leaves out certain features, figuring that when full metabolism is restored, the immune system will get rid of the shoddy cells. But metabolism is never fully restored, so the improvisation continues, the deviant cells keep dividing and multiplying, and the compromised immune system cannot cope.

Another way to explain cancer as a rational response to metabolic deficiency is on the level of the operation of the individual organs. Digestion, for instance, uses enormous amounts of energy. Without adequate fuel and without the aid of an active musculoskeletal system, the transit time of waste moving through the colon increases. This exposes the lining of the colon to toxins, killing cells off or polluting them. The body tries to turn up the rate of cell replication but runs into the problem that it cannot produce all the right ingredients. Here again it does the best it can with what it has to work with. The object is to protect the body from toxins. Colon cancer is an accident all right, and when we look into the mirror and observe the posture of musculoskeletal system dysfunction, we can see it waiting to happen.

Better Balance and Breathing

The E-cises in this menu will help you regain what you may not even know you've lost—balance and proper breathing. Without them, there's no way you can rev up your metabolism. With them, it's a done deal.

[Balance and Breathing Menu]

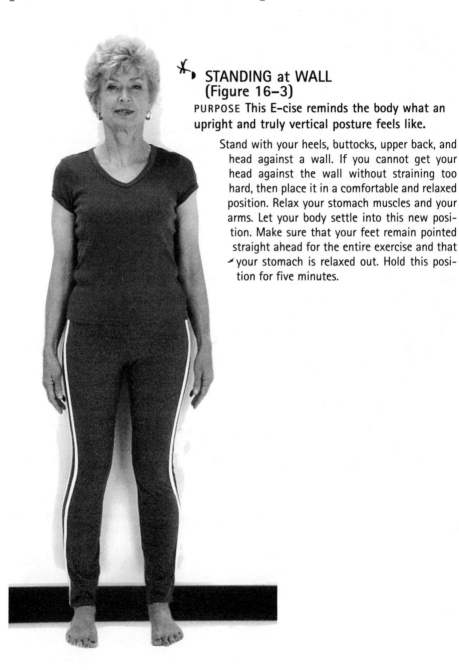

**STANDING at WALL
(Figure 16–3)**

PURPOSE This E-cise reminds the body what an upright and truly vertical posture feels like.

Stand with your heels, buttocks, upper back, and head against a wall. If you cannot get your head against the wall without straining too hard, then place it in a comfortable and relaxed position. Relax your stomach muscles and your arms. Let your body settle into this new position. Make sure that your feet remain pointed straight ahead for the entire exercise and that your stomach is relaxed out. Hold this position for five minutes.

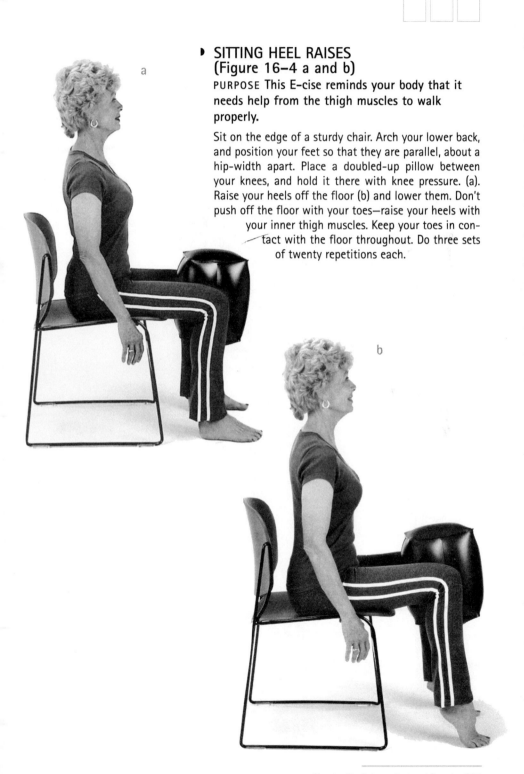

▶ SITTING HEEL RAISES
(Figure 16–4 a and b)

PURPOSE This E-cise reminds your body that it needs help from the thigh muscles to walk properly.

Sit on the edge of a sturdy chair. Arch your lower back, and position your feet so that they are parallel, about a hip-width apart. Place a doubled-up pillow between your knees, and hold it there with knee pressure. (a). Raise your heels off the floor (b) and lower them. Don't push off the floor with your toes—raise your heels with your inner thigh muscles. Keep your toes in contact with the floor throughout. Do three sets of twenty repetitions each.

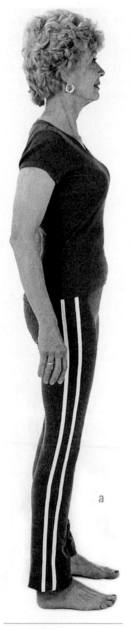

▶ STANDING SHOULDER SHRUGS
(Figure 16–5 a and b)

PURPOSE This E-cise unlocks your shoulder blades.

Stand with your back against a wall, feet parallel, about a hip-width apart. Your hips, upper back, and head should be in contact with the wall. Let your arms hang at your sides. Squeeze your shoulder blades together (a) and hold while you shrug your shoulders up (b) and down. You should hear your shoulder blades gliding up and down the wall. Do three sets of ten repetitions.

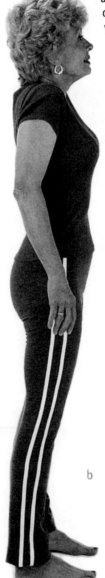

a

b

▸ STANDING SHOULDER ROLLS
(Figure 16–6 a, b, c, and d)

PURPOSE This E-cise strengthens the shoulders' ball and socket function.

Stand with your hips, upper back, and head against a wall. Let your arms hang at your sides with your elbows straight. Keep your head back and shoulders square (a). Circle your shoulders by pulling them up (b), forward, and down. After ten repetitions, reverse by pulling them up, back (c), and down (d) for ten more circles in that direction. Do three sets of ten each way.

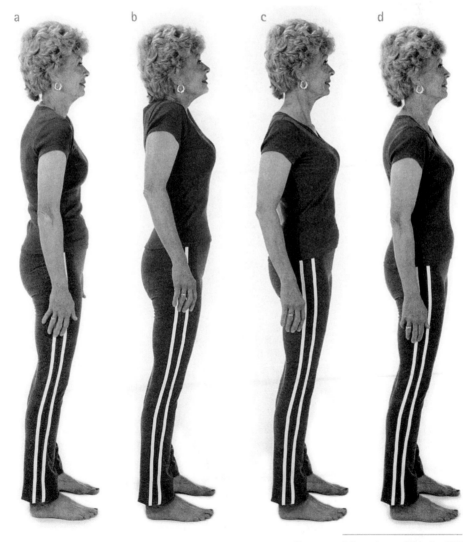

a   b   c   d

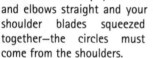

✦ STANDING ARM CIRCLES
(Figure 16–7)

PURPOSE This E-cise strengthens the muscles of the upper back that are involved with the shoulders' ball and socket function.

Stand facing a mirror with your feet parallel, about a hip-width apart, your arms at your sides. Curl your fingertips into the pads of each palm (the fleshy area at the base of the fingers), and point your thumbs straight out. This hand position, called the "golfer's grip," is imperative to the success of the E-cise. Squeeze your shoulder blades together, and bring your arms out to your sides at shoulder level, elbows straight. With your palms facing down, thumbs pointing forward, circle up and forward for forty repetitions. Now with your palms facing up, circle up and back for forty repetitions. Remember to keep your wrists and elbows straight and your shoulder blades squeezed together—the circles must come from the shoulders.

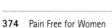

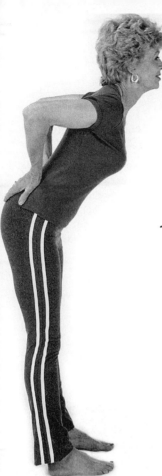

✻ ▸ **STANDING FORWARD BEND**
(Figure 16–8)

PURPOSE This E-cise strengthens your hips and low back.

Stand with your feet facing straight ahead, a hip-width apart. Place your palms on your low back–upper buttocks area. Tilt your pelvis forward to put an exaggerated arch in your low back, pull your elbows and shoulder blades together, and hold. Your hips should initiate the bend, not your low back. Keep your back arched. Tighten your thighs, and allow your weight to shift forward onto the balls of your feet. Hold this position for one minute.

✻

▸ **STATIC BACK (Figure 16–9)**

PURPOSE This E-cise uses gravity to flatten the back and put it in a neutral position.

Lie on your back, with both legs bent at right angles and resting on a chair, bench, or block. (The large blocks we use in the clinic are 20 inches high by 14 inches wide by 24 inches long.) Rest your hands on the floor, extended below shoulder level, with the palms up. Let your back settle into the floor. Breathe from your diaphragm, so your abdominal muscles rise as you inhale and fall as you exhale. Hold this position for five minutes.

STATIC BACK FOOT CIRCLES and POINT/FLEXES (Figure 16–10 a, b, c, and d)

PURPOSE This E-cise gives your foot and ankle functions a workout.

Stay in the Static Back position. For the Foot Circles, circle your right foot in a clockwise direction for twenty repetitions (a). Then circle the same foot in a counterclockwise direction for twenty repetitions (b). Switch to the left foot, and repeat. For the Point/Flexes, point the toes of your right foot straight ahead by flexing the ankle forward (c), then pull the toes back toward the knee (d). Repeat for twenty repetitions. Switch to the left foot, and repeat.

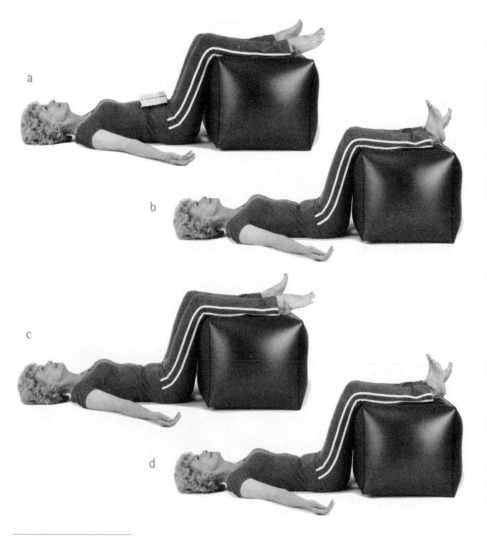

a

b

c

d

▶ ABDUCTION–ADDUCTION (feet close) (Figure 16–11 a and b)

PURPOSE This E-cise engages the muscles on the inside and outside of the thighs, which often interfere with the muscle function on the front and rear of the thighs.

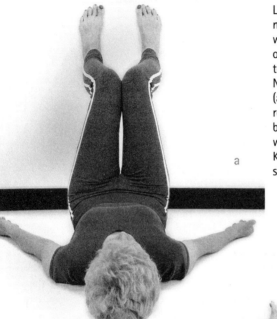

Lie on your back with your knees bent at ninety degrees and your feet on the wall. Set your feet parallel to each other on the wall, about ten inches apart, with toes pointing up toward the ceiling. Now bring your knees together slowly (a), then move them apart so your feet roll laterally (b). As your feet roll, the bottoms of your feet will leave the wall while the outside edges remain on it. Keep your upper body relaxed. Do three sets of ten repetitions each.

a

b

▶ LYING SUPINE (with a pillow) (Figure 16–12)

PURPOSE This E-cise links the foot and ankle flexors to the extensor functions of the thighs, knees, and legs.

Lie on your back with your knees and feet a hip-width apart, holding a pillow lightly between your ankles. Your arms are extended at your sides on the floor at a forty-five-degree angle, with your palms up. Relax your upper torso, and keep your knees and feet pointed straight up toward the ceiling. While in this position, use the quadriceps muscles of the thighs (on the front of the thighs) to pull your toes straight back. Relax your stomach, and breathe. Hold this position for ten minutes.

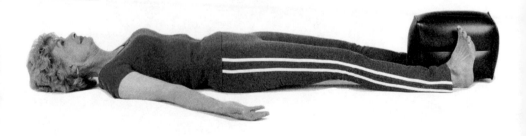

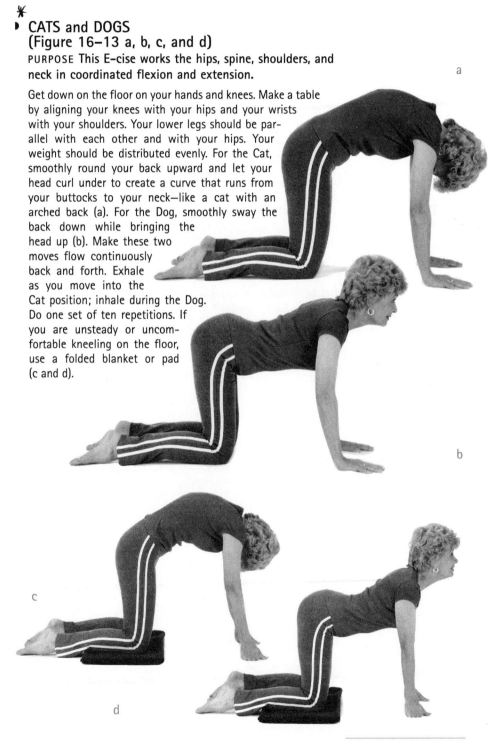

✱
▶ CATS and DOGS
(Figure 16–13 a, b, c, and d)

PURPOSE This E-cise works the hips, spine, shoulders, and neck in coordinated flexion and extension.

Get down on the floor on your hands and knees. Make a table by aligning your knees with your hips and your wrists with your shoulders. Your lower legs should be parallel with each other and with your hips. Your weight should be distributed evenly. For the Cat, smoothly round your back upward and let your head curl under to create a curve that runs from your buttocks to your neck—like a cat with an arched back (a). For the Dog, smoothly sway the back down while bringing the head up (b). Make these two moves flow continuously back and forth. Exhale as you move into the Cat position; inhale during the Dog. Do one set of ten repetitions. If you are unsteady or uncomfortable kneeling on the floor, use a folded blanket or pad (c and d).

a

b

c

d

Why is there no E-cise menu to fight arthritis, cancer, Parkinson's, or Alzheimer's? There is such a menu—turn back to Chapter 15, where you'll find the Over-Fifty Restoration and Maintenance Menu. A fully functional musculoskeletal system is both your best defense and your best offense.

Message in a Body

Former president Ronald Reagan was called the Great Communicator, and he was pretty good at it. But the greatest communicator of all is the human body. It always tells us what we need to know, when we need to know it.

It seems to me that one advantage of being a woman of a certain age is that you're aware of that fact already. You don't need the message to wash up on a beach inside a bottle. You've lived long enough to know firsthand that the body keeps its promise of health, happiness, and achievement if we keep faith in this splendid birthright of ours—a priceless legacy of flesh and bone, muscle and blood that, in words from Shakespeare's *Tempest*, "doth suffer a sea change into something rich and strange."

How can I be so sure? My mother told me; so did Shakespeare's—and so did yours. Pass it on.

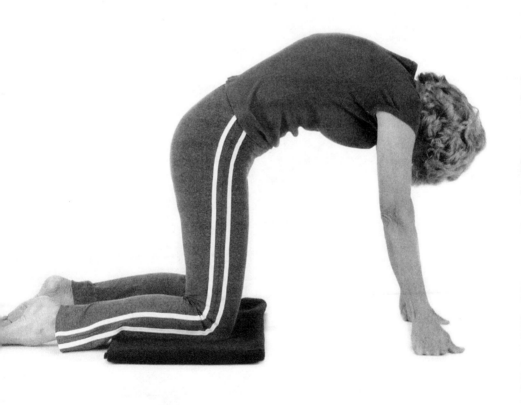

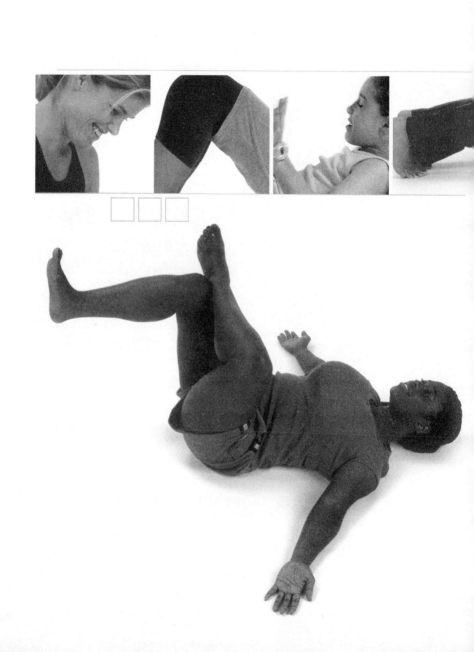

women's wisdom

It's time to round up the usual suspects—readers of all ages, in this case—for one last meeting on common ground. Age, as I've said more than once, is irrelevant.

What is relevant is the musculoskeletal system. All of us have one, and it's always based on the exact same design. The assembly line has been cranking along for three million years, and it's likely to keep at it for a while longer. But you know that, so let's end by circling back to the beginning to let Little Gramma walk us home.

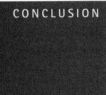

One of the things that I enjoyed about writing this book is that it gave me a chance to share her biography with you—her musculoskeletal biography. The babies, toddlers, young children, teenagers, young adults, and the adults in prime time and those in a season of "mists and mild fruitfulness" are Little Gramma come again.

Yes, *come again*. That old country-bred expression for re-birth catches the magic of generation after generation of embodied strength, beauty, and wisdom on the move, leading the human procession deeper into time's farthest reaches. This awesome long march of Little Grammas is a feat of self-replication and self-renewal that depends ultimately on willpower. The will is our master muscle. The others serve and wait to be commanded into motion.

No matter whether our ruling impulse is hope or fear, love or hate, a desire for riches or fame, or restless curiosity, we put ourselves into motion—or we weaken and die. The will to move is so central to our existence that if we lose it, we lose ourselves.

As medical science and modern technology conquer disease, there is a grave risk that other technology will subdue motion. Technology is ready to move for us in almost every way. It will work for us, play for us, even raise our children and do our healing for us. If we let it, it will bring the march of the Little Grammas to a halt. Motionless internal systems are dying systems. Healthy muscles and bones offer life support of the most fundamental kind. For too many of us— young and old alike—our muscles and bones have lost the ability to provide this support, and we urgently need to find it again.

I'm worried, very worried. The pressure to relinquish motion is enormous and seductive. But I don't think that's going to happen. The will to move is safe because it's guarded not by strong men but by wise women. I can't say conclusively why this is, but I'll take a perhaps overly romantic stab at it:

The moon sets these things in motion, and women keep them going. As that gleaming barren rock glides across the sky, women are drawn toward a fertile moment and are imbued with a deeper knowledge of the forces of nature. Men move because they have to. Women, struck by moonlight and gravity, move because they want to. They feel the enchantment and promise of motion deep within.

Now as never before, women are being wooed away from motion. They're offered quicker and easier ways to get stronger, smarter, and sexier. Based on past performance, I predict their answer will be "No thanks"— thanks to all our Little Grammas.

My fondest hope is that this book has energized your will to move and given you valuable tools to do so every day for the rest of your life. By sharing them with friends and family, you'll be helping them remember something they didn't know they knew—the secret of good health and a long life.

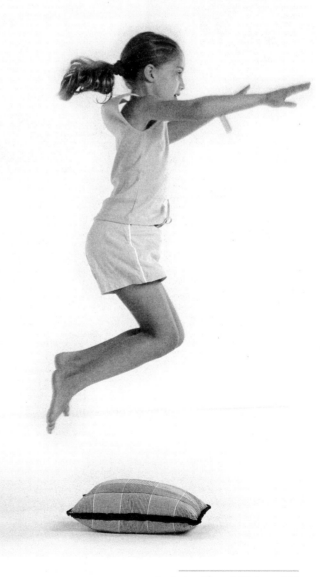

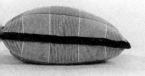

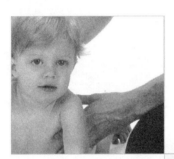

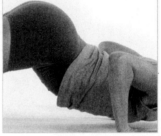

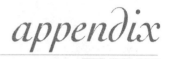

appendix

For easy reference, I've grouped E-cise menus for early childhood (infants and toddlers), middle childhood, and adolescence here in the Appendix.

Babies

Babies are too young to walk, but they're not too young to move. In the pretoddler stage (as in the rest of life), unstructured, spontaneous movement is the best way to go. Encourage your baby to reach and grasp by dangling colorful soft objects. Encourage her to move her head and engage her neck muscles with tickles and touches. Keep it simple with a variety of small, inexpensive toys, including that old standby, a ball that can be tossed and chased after (when she's ready for creeping and crawling). Forget about formal baby calisthenics or workouts unless your pediatrician recommends them to treat a specific condition.

You can supplement free, spontaneous play with the following four baby E-cises. You don't have to worry about overdoing them. Repeat them until the child loses interest. She'll tell you when she's had enough.

[Babies Menu]

▶ **CROSS-CRAWLING**
(Figure A-1 a and b)
PURPOSE This E-cise helps engage the creeping and crawling muscles.

Have your baby lie on her back. Dangle a piece of jewelry, some keys, or a toy (something to catch her eye) off the floor by about six inches above her head so she tries to grab the object with one hand. Simultaneously, bend the baby's opposite knee toward her chest, trying to keep the other leg straight in an extended position (a). Switch sides (b).

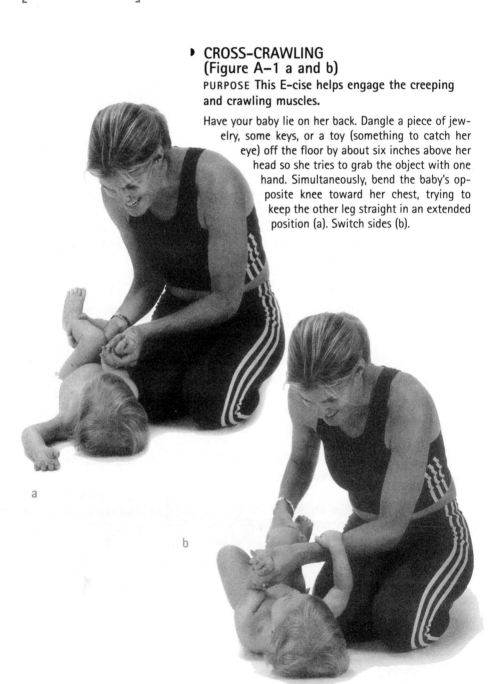

a

b

▶ COBRA
(Figure A–2)

PURPOSE This E-cise engages the shoulders, neck, and spine.

Lay your baby on his stomach, and dangle an object in front of him, about one foot up from the floor. If he is in the precrawling stage, he will go right into this Cobra position by trying to raise his head and chest off the floor.

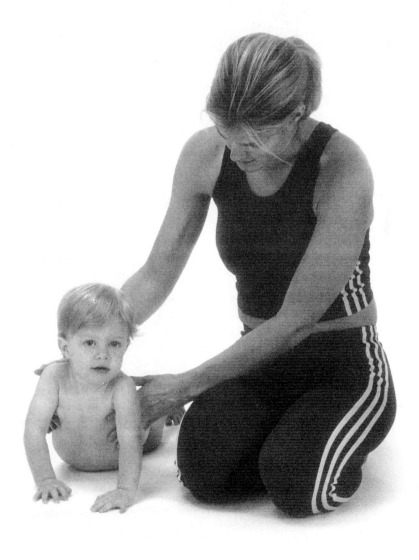

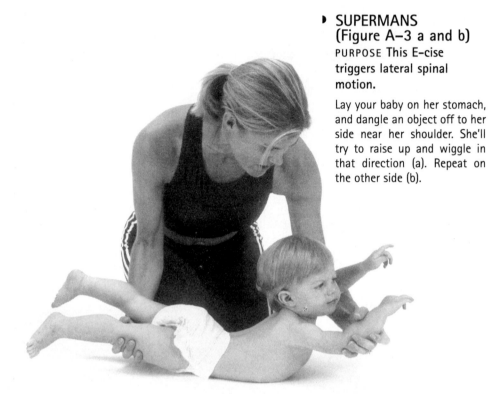

▸ SUPERMANS
(Figure A–3 a and b)

PURPOSE This E-cise triggers lateral spinal motion.

Lay your baby on her stomach, and dangle an object off to her side near her shoulder. She'll try to raise up and wiggle in that direction (a). Repeat on the other side (b).

a

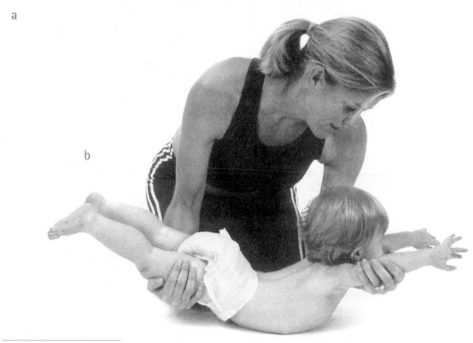

b

▶ SITTING CORE AB-DOMINALS
(Figure A–4 a and b)

PURPOSE This E-cise strengthens the core abdominal muscles. The stronger the core abdominals, the more stable he will be.

When your baby is able to sit on his own, gently apply pressure against his torso with the palm of your hand (a). This will stimulate his reactions to work the muscles required to maintain this position. Apply pressure to the front, sides, and back (b).

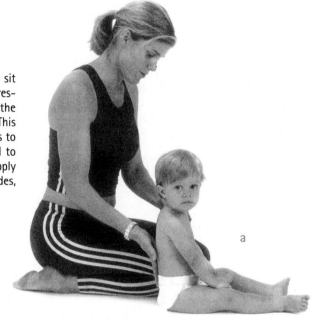

a

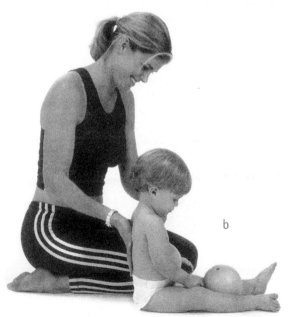

b

Toddlers

Toddlers slurp down the "motion potion" big-time. Learning games and activities are fine, but don't overdo them. There's nothing wrong—and everything right—about motion for the sake of motion. Select an idea or two from the menu below. It's not necessary to do them all or to follow any particular order.

[Toddlers Menu]

▶ CHAIR CRAWL
Set up a maze or fun fort-area where your child will have to crawl under things (chairs are perfect) to get to you.

▶ TUPPERWARE TWO-STEP
Place Tupperware (or other unbreakable soft-edged objects) on the floor and have your toddler side-step over them. Do this in both directions.

▶ REACH for the STARS
In a standing position, ask your child to reach for the stars. It might help to dangle ribbons from a doorway that are just beyond reach.

▶ TOOTSIE TOUCHES
From a standing position, have your child reach down and touch her toes and hold while you count. (It doesn't matter how long they hold it.)

▶ CRAWLING AROUND the HOUSE
Play follow the leader as your toddler crawls around the house on his hands and knees. (Mom, this is great for you too!) If you have stairs and your child is strong enough, have him go up the stairs too.

▶ SOMERSAULTS
Teach your toddler to do somersaults. This works best when you physically show your toddler what to do, because she'll think it's funny to see Mom or Dad going head over heels.

▶ SUPERMANS
Have your child lie on his stomach and lift his arms and legs off the floor and fly like Superman (or Superwoman!).

The idea is to engage as many musculoskeletal system functions as possible, from head to toe. You'll know you are succeeding if your child's legs are straight, his knees point straight ahead and over his feet, and his feet are slightly pigeon-toed. The illustration in Figure A–5 is an example.

Middle Childhood

Like infants and toddlers, children in middle childhood are still too young to be put through a regimen of structured exercises.

They hate them. Even a twelve-year-old who seems to take to a sports drill or workout program is probably doing it more to please her parents and other adult authority figures. If she's functional, that's okay, as long as she continues to stay functional by getting enough varied, unstructured movement as well. But dysfunctional older children are engaged in a consolidation process at the expense of exploration that can build and maintain overall musculoskeletal system functions.

This age group, however, isn't too old for games that are crossed with E-cises. Try some from this menu:

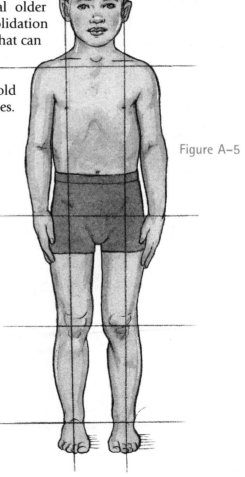

Figure A–5

[Middle Childhood Menu]

▶ CRAB WALKS
(Figure A–6)

PURPOSE This E-cise builds extensor muscle strength.

Your child raises himself with his legs bent, the soles of his feet flat on the floor, his arms behind his back, and his hands on the floor, with his fingers pointing in the opposite direction from his feet. Your child should lift his bottom as high as he can off the floor and "walk" using his hands and feet. Move forward ten steps and back ten. Repeat.

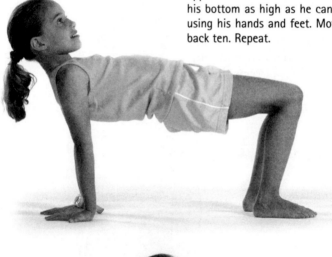

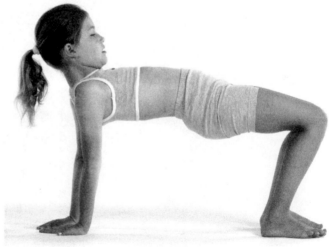

▶ CATS and DOGS
(Figure A–7 a and b)

PURPOSE This E-cise works the hips, spine, shoulders, and neck in coordinated flexion and extension.

Have your child get on her hands and knees. For the Cat, she should round her back upward by rolling her hips under and tucking her chin in toward her chest (a). For the Dog, she should roll her hips forward to put an arch in her back and pull her head up and back to look at the ceiling (b). In this position, she should let her shoulders collapse together.
Repeat six times.

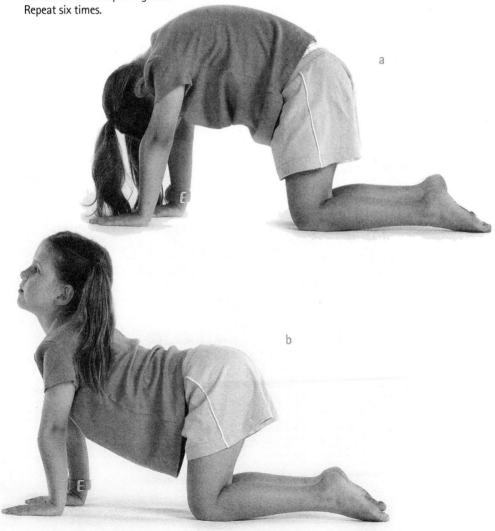

a

b

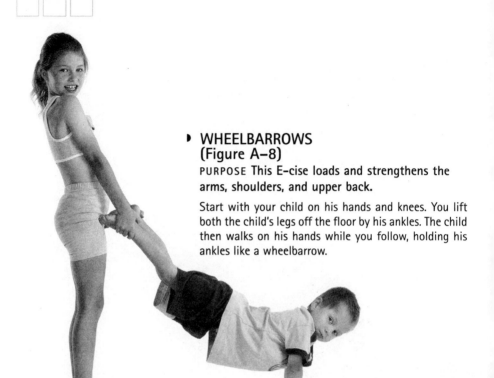

▶ WHEELBARROWS
(Figure A–8)

PURPOSE This E-cise loads and strengthens the arms, shoulders, and upper back.

Start with your child on his hands and knees. You lift both the child's legs off the floor by his ankles. The child then walks on his hands while you follow, holding his ankles like a wheelbarrow.

▶ STORK WALKS
(Figure A–9)

PURPOSE This E-cise engages the hips, thighs, and knees in coordinated action.

With her hands behind her head (or alternately straight out as shown in the photo, if she has trouble keeping her balance), your child walks slowly forward with an exaggerated high lift of each knee. Encourage her to keep her head and shoulders back, her hips level, and her feet pointed straight ahead. This works well in a game of follow-the-leader.

▸ BEAR CRAWLS
(Figure A–10)

PURPOSE This E-cise induces muscular engagement all the way from the feet through the neck, shoulders, arms, wrists, and hands.

Have your child get down on the floor or lawn in a crawling position on his hands and feet (instead of the knees). His feet should be straight, and his knees shouldn't flare out to the sides in a waddle. Crawl on!

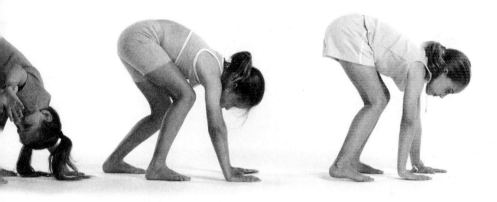

▸ LEAP FROG
(Figure A–11)

PURPOSE This E-cise strengthens hip and thigh functions.

Two or more children alternate squatting and hopping over each other.

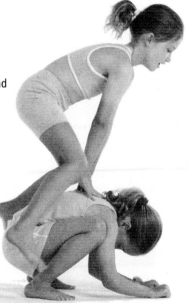
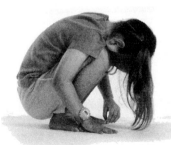

▸ CRAWL UNDERS (two variations) (Figure A–12 a and b)

PURPOSE This crawling E-cise strengthens core posture muscles and enhances agility.

Variation 1: Line the kids up. The child at the head of the line ducks around and under to crawl between the legs of the others (a). When she gets to the end, she rejoins the line for another turn.

Variation 2: Arrange an obstacle course of ladders, tables, and chairs for the kids to crawl under (b).

a

b

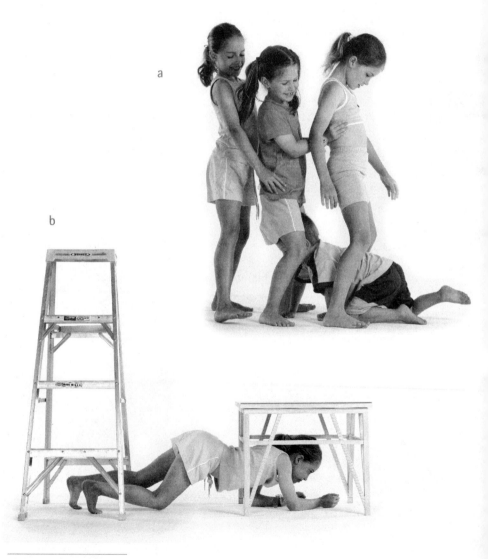

▶ SUMMER SALTS
(Figure A–13 a, b, and c)
PURPOSE This E-cise builds hip and spine strength and flexibility.

It's a fun way to spell somersaults. Shoes off, heads down, and over they go (a, b, c).

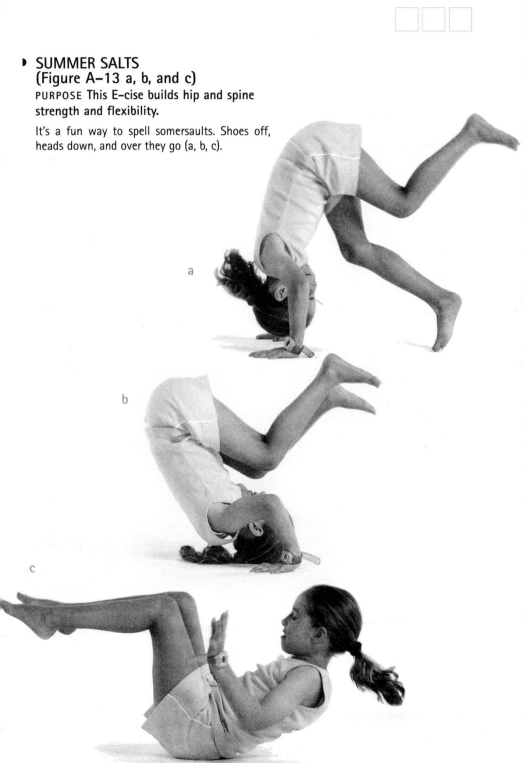

a

b

c

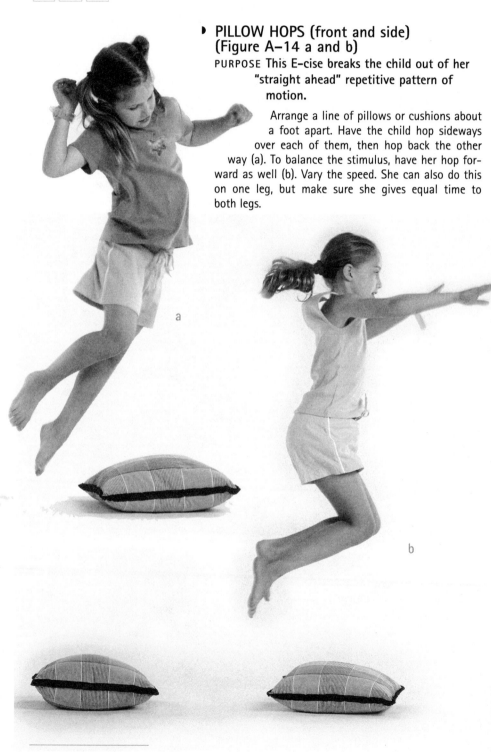

▶ PILLOW HOPS (front and side) (Figure A–14 a and b)

PURPOSE This E-cise breaks the child out of her "straight ahead" repetitive pattern of motion.

Arrange a line of pillows or cushions about a foot apart. Have the child hop sideways over each of them, then hop back the other way (a). To balance the stimulus, have her hop forward as well (b). Vary the speed. She can also do this on one leg, but make sure she gives equal time to both legs.

a

b

Teens

This section contains three menus for teenagers. They should do the first menu daily for at least four months or until it becomes relatively undemanding. Then switch to the second menu for about the same length of time, and finally move on to the third menu. Follow the sequence as presented, and don't skip any E-cise unless it causes pain. It will be easier to obtain cooperation if the teenager is interested in sports; explain that these E-cises will enhance her performance. If sports are not her thing, you'll have to fall back on the art, science, and voodoo of parental leadership.

$$[\text{Teens Menu I}]$$

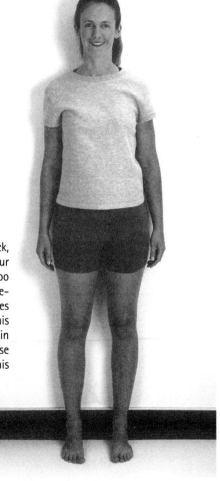

› STANDING at WALL (Figure A–15)

PURPOSE This E-cise reminds the body what an upright and truly vertical posture feels like.

Stand with your heels, buttocks, upper back, and head against a wall. If you cannot get your head against the wall without straining too hard, then place it in a comfortable and relaxed position. Relax your stomach muscles and your arms. Let your body settle into this new position. Make sure that your feet remain pointed straight ahead for the entire E-cise and that your stomach is relaxed out. Hold this position for five minutes.

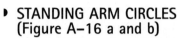

▶ STANDING ARM CIRCLES
(Figure A–16 a and b)

PURPOSE This E-cise strengthens the muscles of the upper back that are involved with the shoulders' ball and socket function.

Stand facing a mirror with your feet parallel, about a hip-width apart, your arms at your sides. Curl your fingertips into the pads of each palm (the fleshy area at the base of the fingers), and point your thumbs straight out. This hand position, called the "golfer's grip," is imperative to the success of the E-cise. Squeeze your shoulder blades together, and bring your arms out to your sides at shoulder level, elbows straight. With your palms facing down, thumbs pointing forward, circle up and forward for forty repetitions (a). Now with your palms facing up, circle up and back for forty repetitions (b). Remember to keep your wrists and elbows straight and your shoulder blades squeezed together—the circles must come from the shoulders.

a

b

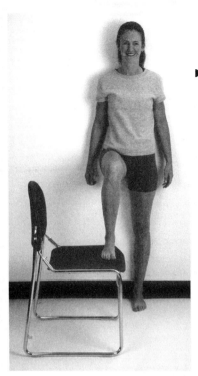

▶ **WALL STORK**
(Figure A–17)
PURPOSE This E-cise levels the hips into a parallel position, under a load that's held in vertical alignment.

Stand against a wall with your feet pointed straight ahead. Your heels, hips, upper back, and head should be against the wall. Place your right foot on the seat of a chair positioned about twelve inches in front of you. Make sure this foot is pointed straight. Do not allow your left foot to twist or your left leg to bend. The right leg, on the chair, should be bent at about ninety degrees at the knee joint. Hold this position without allowing the left foot, leg, or hip to shift to the side or to roll away from the wall. Hold for three minutes. Switch legs, and repeat.

▶ **STANDING ELBOW CURLS**
(Figure A–18 a and b)
PURPOSE This E-cise reminds the shoulder's "hinge" what full flexion and extension feel like.

Stand with your heels, buttocks, upper back, and head against a wall. Your feet, pointed straight ahead, are about a hip-width apart. Raise your hands in the "golfer's grip" (see Standing Arm Circles), placing your knuckles along your temples, thumbs extended down your cheeks (a). Bring your elbows together to meet in front (b). Make sure your elbows meet in the middle of your body (and are not skewed to the left or right, which would mean that one shoulder is flexing more than the other).
Then pull your elbows back even with your shoulders to touch the wall. Your head should remain still, and your knuckles should not lift off your temples. Do one set of twenty-five repetitions.

▶ CATS and DOGS
(Figure A–19 a and b)

PURPOSE This E-cise works the hips, spine, shoulders, and neck in coordinated flexion and extension.

Get down on the floor on your hands and knees. Make a table by aligning your knees with your hips and your wrists with your shoulders. Your lower legs should be parallel with each other and with your hips. Your weight should be distributed evenly. For the Cat, smoothly round your back upward and let your head curl under, to create a curve that runs from your buttocks to your neck—like a cat with an arched back (a). For the Dog, smoothly sway the back down while bringing your head up (b). Make these two moves flow continuously back and forth. Exhale as you move into the Cat position; inhale during the Dog. Do one set of ten repetitions.

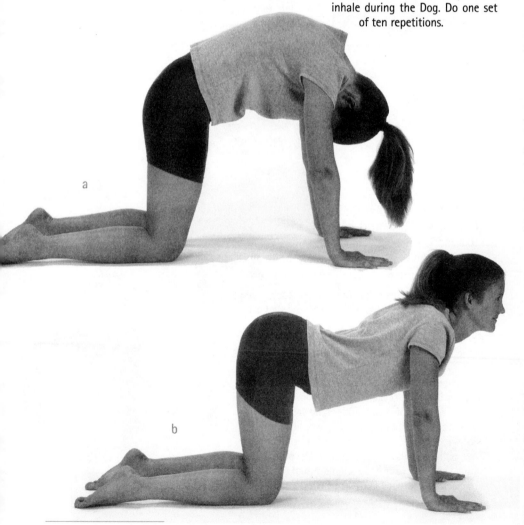

▶ STATIC EXTENSION
(Figure A-20)

PURPOSE This E-cise tackles hip rotation. Hips that "rotate" are actually twisting to the right or left and disrupt knee and ankle function. If you look closely in the mirror, one hip will appear to be a little nearer to the mirror than the other.

Kneel on a large block (approximately three feet square) with your hands on the floor ahead of you. Keep your elbows straight and locked while you ease your hips in front of your knees. (Please refer to the photograph.) You don't want your knees and hips to align one atop the other, or for your hips to be behind your knees. The idea is to let the pelvis swing free and engage with the upper torso. Allow your low back to arch, with the movement coming from the tilt of your pelvis. Your shoulder blades should collapse together and form a distinct valley. Keep your elbows straight. Drop your head, and hold the position. If your low back begins to hurt, back your hips up toward your knees a bit. This will also make it easier on your arms. Hold this position for three minutes.

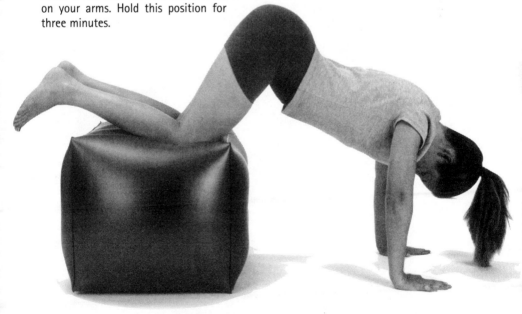

▶ ABDUCTION–ADDUCTION
(Figure A–21 a and b)

PURPOSE This E-cise engages the muscles on the inside and outside of the thighs, which often interfere with muscle function on the front and rear of the thighs.

Lie on your back with your knees bent at ninety degrees and your feet on the wall. Set your feet parallel to each other on the wall, three or four inches wider than your hips, with your toes pointing up toward the ceiling. Now bring your knees together slowly (a), then move them apart so that your feet roll laterally (b). As your feet roll, the bottom of your feet will leave the wall while the outside edges remain on it. Keep your upper body relaxed. Do three sets of ten repetitions each.

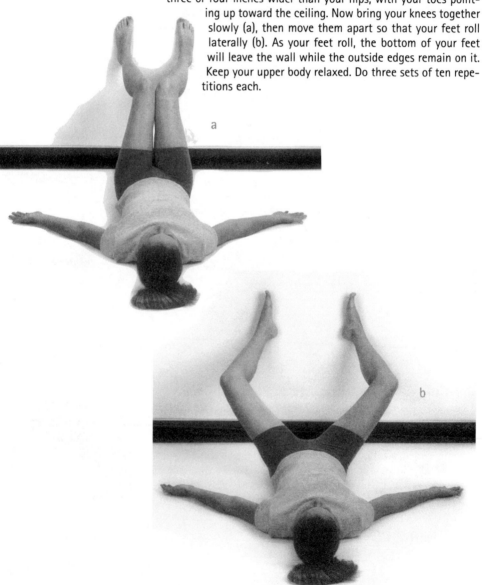

a

b

▶ ABDOMINAL CRUNCHES
(Figure A–22 a and b)

PURPOSE This E-cise forces the abdominal muscles to do the lifting, rather than the hip flexors or thoracic back muscles.

Lie on your back with your knees bent and your feet on the wall pointed straight up, parallel to each other. Interlace your fingers, and place them behind your head (a). Looking up at the ceiling and keeping your elbows back and level, use your abdominal muscles to "sit up" about two inches off the floor (b). Your back, shoulders, neck, and head should lift as a unit. Don't yank your neck and head forward; keep looking at the ceiling. Repeat, and do not allow your knees to spread apart from their original position. Do two sets of twenty-five repetitions each.

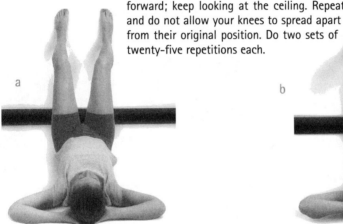
a

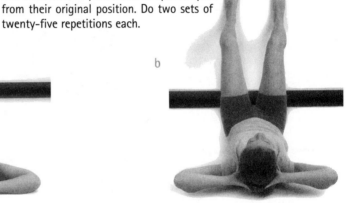
b

▶ COBRA on ELBOWS
(Figure A–23)

PURPOSE This E-cise isolates the upper and lower torsos, to allow design flexion and extension to take place.

Lie on your stomach propped on your elbows. Keeping your toes together, allow your heels to drop away to the side. Move your hands away from each other, thumbs extended upward, fingers lightly curled, pivoting on your elbows. Put tension on your arms, as though you were trying to pull them apart. Allow your shoulder blades to collapse inward to create a furrow between them. Look straight ahead. Remember to relax your buttock muscles. Hold this position for one minute.

▶ CATS and DOGS
(Figure A–24 a and b)

Follow the instructions for this E-cise earlier in this menu. We're repeating this one now that you've loosened up. You'll achieve better flexion and extension.

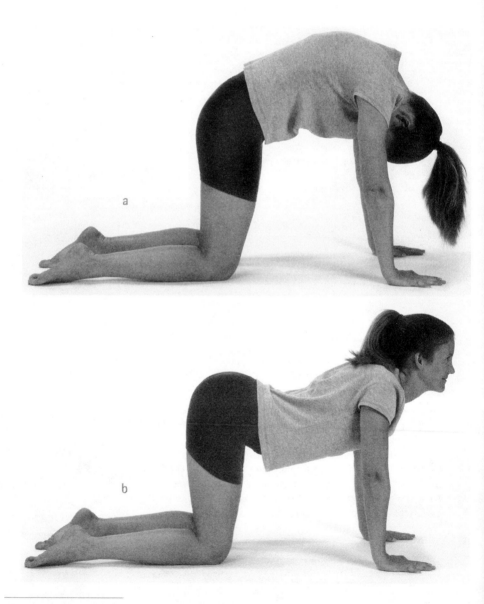

a

b

At first, dysfunctional teenagers won't be happy about doing these E-cises. They'll need parental encouragement and supervision. For them, motion is no longer a pleasure, and they'll have trouble remembering the last time it was. But that memory will return fairly quickly. Exactly how long it takes will depend on the extent of the motion deprivation that the teenager has suffered. You should probably brace yourself for about a month of hassles and complaints. Motionlessness is a habit and an illness. But habits can be broken and illnesses cured.

Gradually, the grumbling will subside as motion becomes more pleasurable. The E-cises will jump-start an increase in physical activity levels. The more a teen moves, the more she can move—and will want to move. You may also see a reversion to a more "childish" rambunctiousness such as wrestling matches with younger siblings, chasing the dog, and other high-jinks. Don't let it bother you. A rediscovery process is under way. Your teen could show a heretofore uncharacteristic interest in athletic competition. Often younger children and teenagers who show no interest or aptitude for sports have been discouraged by their musculoskeletal system dysfunctions and are rationalizing it behind a facade of indifference.

Teens Menu II

If the teenager has been doing Teen Menu I for four months and the entire routine has become relatively undemanding, she should switch at this point to Teen Menu II and do it for another four months.

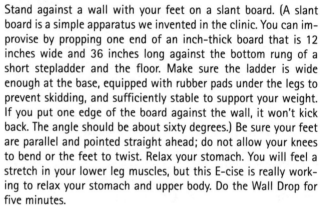

[Teens Menu II]

▶ **WALL DROP**
(Figure A–25)

PURPOSE This E-cise allows the hips to be properly repositioned while keeping the knees and feet functionally aligned.

Stand against a wall with your feet on a slant board. (A slant board is a simple apparatus we invented in the clinic. You can improvise by propping one end of an inch-thick board that is 12 inches wide and 36 inches long against the bottom rung of a short stepladder and the floor. Make sure the ladder is wide enough at the base, equipped with rubber pads under the legs to prevent skidding, and sufficiently stable to support your weight. If you put one edge of the board against the wall, it won't kick back. The angle should be about sixty degrees.) Be sure your feet are parallel and pointed straight ahead; do not allow your knees to bend or the feet to twist. Relax your stomach. You will feel a stretch in your lower leg muscles, but this E-cise is really working to relax your stomach and upper body. Do the Wall Drop for five minutes.

▶ WALL DROP—WALL GLIDES
(Figure A–26 a and b)

PURPOSE This E-cise gives the shoulder blades a workout in a vertically aligned position.

Stand on the slant board with your feet pointed straight and parallel. Put your arms and hands against the wall in the "stick 'em up!" position, with the elbows roughly on the same level as the shoulders and the palms facing out (a). Keep the arms and backs of the hands in contact with the wall. Glide them up the wall, and bring them together over your head (b). You'll be making a semicircle. Your stomach should stay relaxed; your arms and hands remain in contact with the wall through the entire range of motion. Return to the starting position and repeat. Do four sets of ten repetitions each.

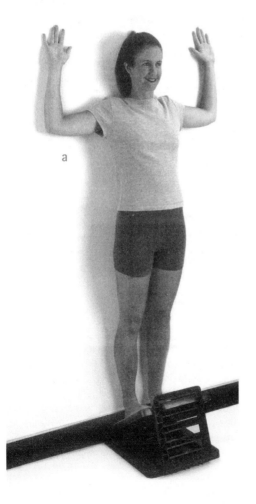

a

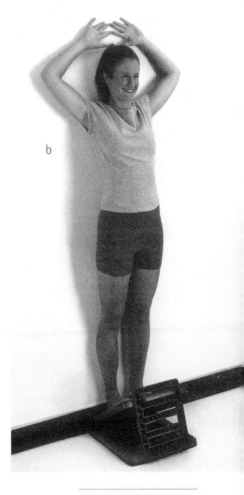

b

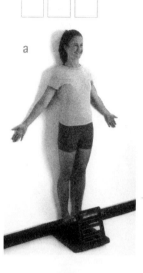

a

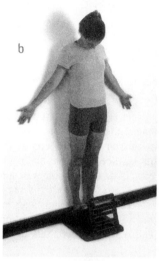

b

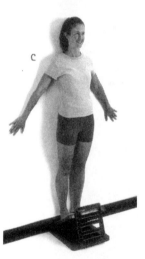

c

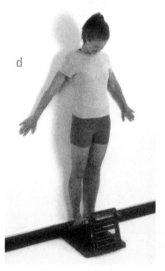

d

▶ WALL DROP—WALL PRESSES (Figure A-27 a, b, c, and d)

PURPOSE This E-cise runs the shoulders through a range of motion that they're not asked to do very often, but they need the function to keep the head and shoulders from rounding forward.

Stand on the slant board with your feet pointed straight ahead and parallel. Relax your stomach. Place your hands with their backs against the wall, arms straight, and arrange them at the four and eight o'clock positions. You'll do four sets of this E-cise. In each set squeeze your shoulder blades together (back and down) and release. Don't lift your shoulders and squeeze—it's a *downward* squeeze and release. *Set 1:* Your palms face out from the wall, and your head is level (a). *Set 2:* Your palms remain face out, but your head is lowered, looking down at your feet (b). *Set 3:* Your palms face the wall, and your head is level (c). *Set 4:* Your palms remain facing the wall, but your head again looks down at your feet (d). Do ten repetitions in each set.

▶ WALL DROP—GLUTEAL CONTRACTIONS (not illustrated)

Stand against a wall with your feet on the slant board and pointed straight ahead. Relax your stomach, do not allow your knees to bend or your feet to twist laterally, and keep your upper body relaxed. Contract and release your left and right buttock muscles at the same time. Do not tighten your stomach muscles or thighs. This E-cise gets your buttock muscles working in unison. You'll probably find that one side is stronger—it contracts more deeply—than the other. We want to equalize them. Do three sets of twenty repetitions each.

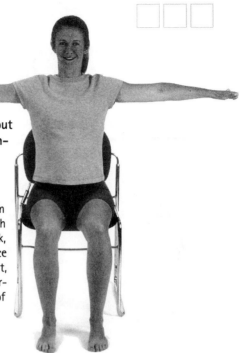

▸ SITTING ARM CIRCLES (Figure A–28)

PURPOSE This E-cise makes sure the shoulders and hips are in alignment without help from the thighs, knees, lower legs, ankles, or feet. It puts the shoulders' ball and socket joints through a full range of motion.

Follow the basic instructions for Standing Arm Circles, but sit on the edge of a chair or bench that's not going to move or tip. Arch your back, and pull your head and shoulders back. Place your feet on the floor about a hip-width apart, point them straight ahead, and keep them parallel. Do two sets (one forward, one back) of forty repetitions each.

a   b

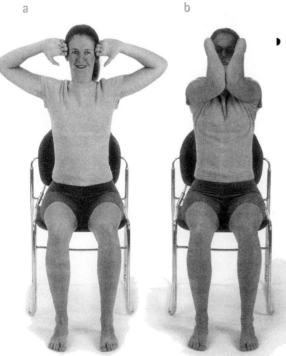

▸ SITTING ELBOW CURLS (Figure A–29 a and b)

PURPOSE This E-cise helps the shoulder's "hinge" joint relearn its proper function without nondesign help from the thighs, knees, lower legs, ankles, or feet.

Follow the basic instructions for Standing Elbow Curls, but sit on the edge of a chair or bench. Arch your back, and pull your head and shoulders back. Place your feet on the floor about a hip-width apart, pointed straight ahead, and parallel. Raise your hands in the "golfer's grip," placing your knuckles along your temples, thumbs extended down your cheeks (a). Bring your elbows to meet in front (b). Then pull your elbows back even with your shoulders. Do forty repetitions.

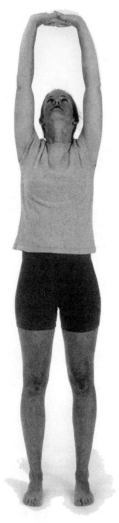

▶ OVERHEAD EXTENSION—STANDING (Figure A–30)

PURPOSE This E-cise opens up the thoracic back (upper back and neck) and the abdominal cavity, increases oxygen flow, and strengthens the extensor muscles of the back.

Stand with your feet pointed straight ahead, a hip-width apart. Interlace your fingers together, raise your hands and arms over your head, and roll your hands palm up. Look up at the backs of your hands. Your arms should be straight, holding on a line even with your ears, with elbows locked. Don't lean back; reach straight up. Keep your hands directly over your head, not in front of your head. Relax your stomach muscles, and remember to breathe. Hold this position for one minute.

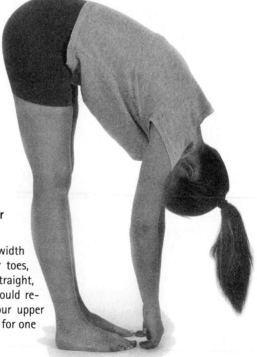

▶ HANGING (Figure A–31)

PURPOSE This E-cise works on your back's flexor muscles.

Stand with your feet parallel, a hip-width apart. Bend over till you touch your toes, and just hang there. Keep your knees straight, drop your head (the neck muscles should relax), and concentrate on relaxing your upper back. Don't bounce. Hold this position for one minute.

CATS and DOGS
(Figure A-32 a and b)

PURPOSE This E-cise works the hips, spine, shoulders, and neck in coordinated flexion and extension.

Get down on the floor on your hands and knees. Make a table by aligning your knees with your hips and your wrists with your shoulders. The lower legs should be parallel with each other and with the hips. Your weight should be distributed evenly. For the Cat, smoothly round your back upward and let your head curl under, to create a curve that runs from your buttocks to your neck—like a cat with an arched back (a). For the Dog, smoothly sway your back down while bringing your head up (b). Make these two moves flow continuously back and forth. Exhale as you move into the Cat position; inhale during the Dog. Do one set of ten repetitions.

a

b

▸ STATIC BACK
(Figure A–33)

PURPOSE This E-cise uses gravity to flatten the back and put it in a neutral position.

Lie on your back, with both legs bent at right angles and resting on a chair, bench, or block. (The large blocks we use in the clinic are 20 inches high by 14 inches wide by 24 inches long.) Rest your hands on the floor, extended below shoulder level, with the palms up. Let your back settle into the floor. Breathe from your diaphragm, so your abdominal muscles rise as you inhale and fall as you exhale. Hold this position for five minutes.

▸ LYING SUPINE (with a pillow)
(Figure A–34)

PURPOSE This E-cise links the foot and ankle flexors to the extensor functions of the thighs, knees, and legs.

Lie on your back with your knees and feet a hip-width apart, holding a pillow lightly between your ankles. Your arms are extended at your sides on the floor at a forty-five-degree angle with the palms up. Keeping your upper torso relaxed and your knees and feet pointing straight up toward the ceiling, pull your toes straight back. The quadriceps muscles of the thighs (on the front of the thighs) are relaxed. Relax your stomach, and breathe. Hold this position for ten minutes.

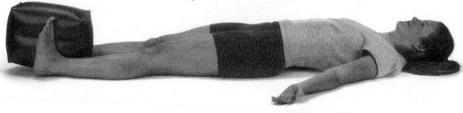

▶ CATS and DOGS
(Figure A–35 a and b)
Follow the instructions for this E-cise earlier in this menu.

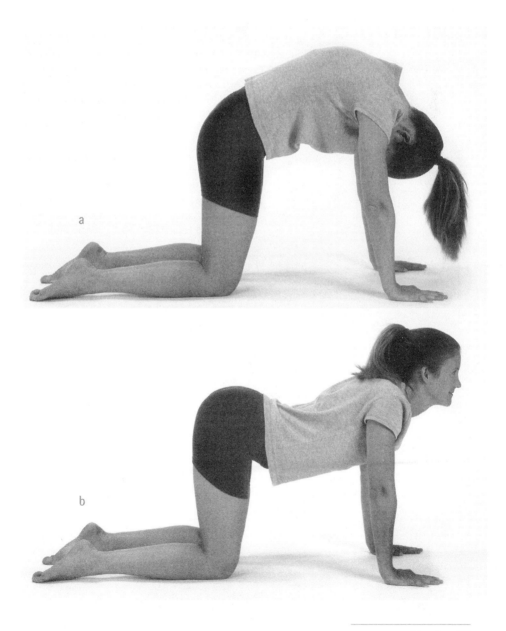

a

b

▶ **FOOT CIRCLES and POINT/FLEXES
(Figure A–36 a, b, and c)**

PURPOSE This E-cise reminds your knees, ankles, and feet how to interact according to their designs.

Lie on your back with your left leg extended flat on the floor and your right leg bent toward your chest. For the Foot Circles, clasp your hands behind your bent knee to hold it in position while you circle your right foot clockwise (a). The Foot Circles emanate from the ankle, not from the knee. Keep your knee still, and try to make full circles. (You may tend to make half circles; it will help to slow down and concentrate.) Meanwhile, keep the left foot pointed straight up toward the ceiling, with the left thigh muscles tight. Do forty repetitions. Then reverse direction and circle your right foot counterclockwise. Repeat forty times. For the Point/Flexes, keep your legs in the same position. On the bent right leg, bring your toes back toward the shin to flex (b), then reverse the direction to point your toes (c). Switch legs, and do forty repetitions of both Foot Circles and Point/Flexes with the left foot.

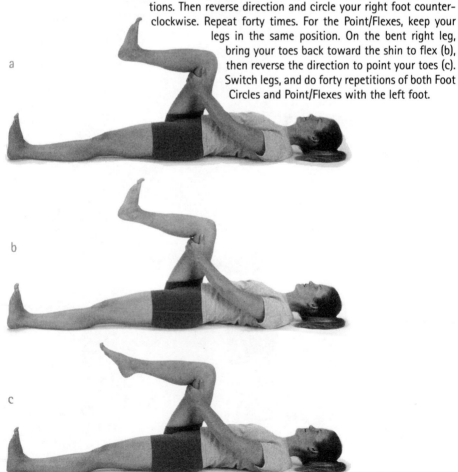

a

b

c

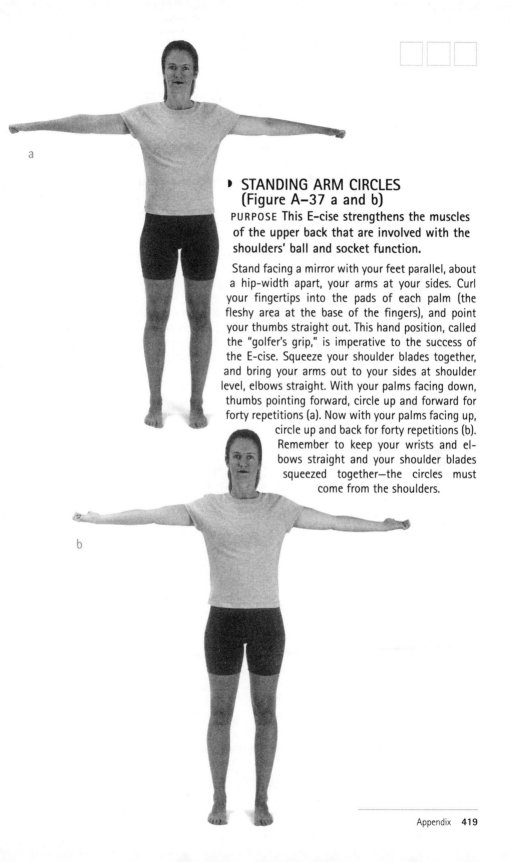

▶ STANDING ARM CIRCLES
(Figure A–37 a and b)

PURPOSE This E-cise strengthens the muscles of the upper back that are involved with the shoulders' ball and socket function.

Stand facing a mirror with your feet parallel, about a hip-width apart, your arms at your sides. Curl your fingertips into the pads of each palm (the fleshy area at the base of the fingers), and point your thumbs straight out. This hand position, called the "golfer's grip," is imperative to the success of the E-cise. Squeeze your shoulder blades together, and bring your arms out to your sides at shoulder level, elbows straight. With your palms facing down, thumbs pointing forward, circle up and forward for forty repetitions (a). Now with your palms facing up, circle up and back for forty repetitions (b). Remember to keep your wrists and elbows straight and your shoulder blades squeezed together—the circles must come from the shoulders.

a

b

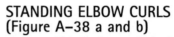

STANDING ELBOW CURLS
(Figure A-38 a and b)

PURPOSE This E-cise reminds the shoulder's "hinge" what full flexion and extension feel like.

Stand with your heels, buttocks, upper back, and head against a wall. Your feet, pointed straight ahead, are about a hip-width apart. Raise your hands in the "golfer's grip" (see Standing Arm Circles), placing your knuckles along your temples, thumbs extended down your cheeks (a). Bring your elbows together to meet in front (b). Make sure your elbows are meeting in the middle of your body (and are not skewed to the left or right, which would mean that one shoulder is flexing more than the other). Then pull your elbows back even with your shoulders to touch the wall. Your head should remain still, and your knuckles should not lift off your temples. Do one set of twenty-five repetitions.

a

b

▶ KNEELING GROIN STRETCH
(Figure A-39)

PURPOSE This E-cise works to rebalance your hips and shoulders.

From a kneeling position, place one foot out in front of the other with the knee bent. Place your interlaced hands on the top-front of the forward knee. Lunge forward, but don't let the knee go forward of the ankle. You should feel this in the groin. Keep an arch in your back and your head up and back. Your forward foot must point straight, and the toes and top of the rear foot need to be on the floor pointing straight back. Hold this position for one minute, then switch legs.

▶ CATS and DOGS
(Figure A–40 a and b)

PURPOSE This E-cise works the hips, spine, shoulders, and neck in coordinated flexion and extension.

Get down on the floor on your hands and knees. Make a table by aligning your knees with your hips and your wrists with your shoulders. Your lower legs should be parallel with each other and with your hips. Your weight should be distributed evenly. For the Cat, smoothly round your back upward and let your head curl under, to create a curve that runs from your buttocks to your neck—like a cat with an arched back (a). For the Dog, smoothly sway your back down while bringing your head up (b). Make these two moves flow continuously back and forth. Exhale while moving into the Cat position; inhale during the Dog. Do one set of ten repetitions.

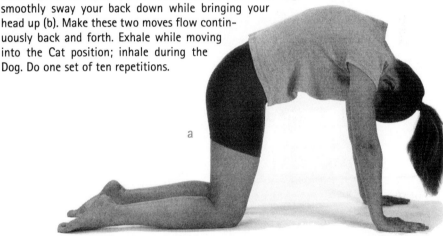

a

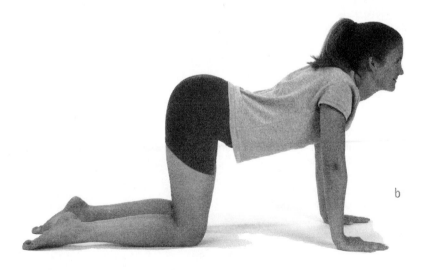

b

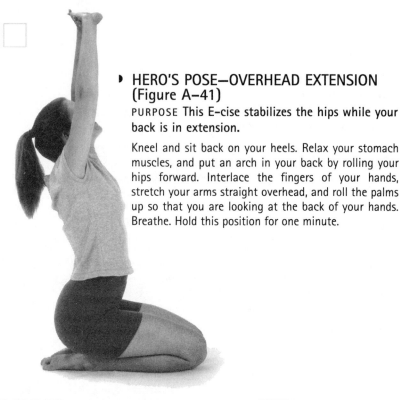

‣ HERO'S POSE—OVERHEAD EXTENSION (Figure A–41)

PURPOSE This E-cise stabilizes the hips while your back is in extension.

Kneel and sit back on your heels. Relax your stomach muscles, and put an arch in your back by rolling your hips forward. Interlace the fingers of your hands, stretch your arms straight overhead, and roll the palms up so that you are looking at the back of your hands. Breathe. Hold this position for one minute.

‣ HERO'S SQUATS (Figure A–42 a and b)

PURPOSE This E-cise strengthens the quadriceps.

Kneel and sit back on your heels. Interlace your hands and place them behind your head. Keep your elbows back and even on both sides (a). To begin the movement, roll your pelvis forward to put an arch in your back. Hold this arch. Next, lift your hips off your feet by using your thigh muscles on the front (top) of the thighs (b). Don't lean forward or twist; come straight up. At first it will be tough, and you may not be able to lift yourself at all. But make the effort for the required number of repetitions. In due time you'll make the lift, and it will get stronger and stronger. Do three sets of fifteen each.

a

b

▶ DOWNWARD DOG
(Figure A–43)

PURPOSE This E-cise reestablishes linkage from the wrists to the feet.

Assume the Cats and Dogs position. Curl your toes under, and push with your legs to raise your torso until you are off your knees and your weight is resting on your hands and feet. Keep pushing until your hips are higher than your shoulders and have formed a tight, stable triangle with the floor. Your knees should be straight, your calves and thighs tight. Don't let your feet flare outward; keep them pointing straight ahead in line with your hands, which need to stay in place—no creeping forward! Your back should be flat, not bowed, as your hips push up and back into the heels. Breathe. If you cannot bring your heels flat onto the floor, get them as close as possible. Don't force them. It may take several sessions before they go all the way down. Hold this position for one minute.

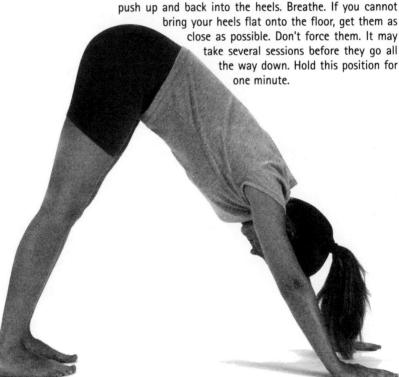

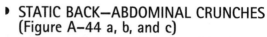

▸ STATIC BACK—ABDOMINAL CRUNCHES (Figure A–44 a, b, and c)

PURPOSE This E-cise allows your abdominals to work without help from your legs.

Lie on your back on the floor, with both legs bent at right angles and resting on a large block, bench, or chair (about four feet high) (a). Interlace your hands behind your head (b). Keep your shoulders and elbows back. Use your abdominal/stomach muscles to pull your upper body off the floor by about two inches (c), then lower it to the floor. Don't let the head come forward; concentrate on looking straight up at the ceiling. Do two sets of thirty repetitions each.

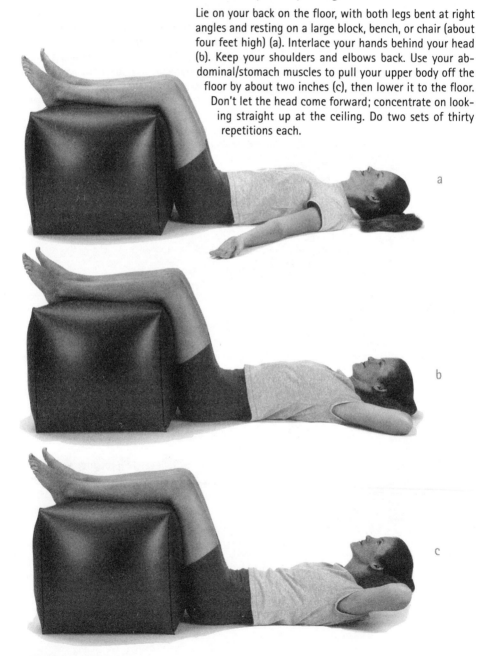

a

b

c

▶ SUPINE GROIN STRETCHES
(Figure A–45)

PURPOSE This E-cise disengages your groin muscles and those along the outside of your thighs.

Lie on your back on the floor, with one leg bent at a right angle and resting on a large block, bench, or chair. The other leg is extended straight out on the floor, with the foot propped on the outside to keep it pointing straight up. Extend your arms out to your sides at forty-five-degree angles (resting on the floor). Relax your upper body, knees, and feet. The longer you are in this position, the more your back settles into the floor. Breathe from your diaphragm. Hold for fifteen minutes. Switch sides, and repeat. Don't skip this! Do two sets, one on each side.

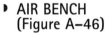

▶ AIR BENCH
(Figure A–46)

PURPOSE This E-cise promotes lower leg, thigh, and hip strength, and it relaxes the muscles of the torso.

Stand against a wall with your feet pointing straight ahead, parallel, a hip-width apart. Walk your feet away from the wall approximately 2 to 2½ feet, as you bend your knees and slide your back down the wall. Stop sliding and walking when your thighs and hips form approximately a ninety-degree angle. Your knees should be over your ankles, not your toes. If you feel pain in your kneecaps, raise your body up the wall to relieve the pressure. Keep your weight on your heels. Hold this position for two minutes.

Your teenager can do this menu daily or every other day for . . . forever. There's no reason to stop once she gets started. She can incorporate the menu into whatever fitness routine or sport catches her interest.

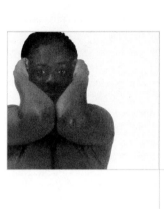

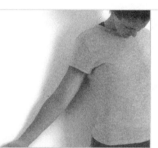

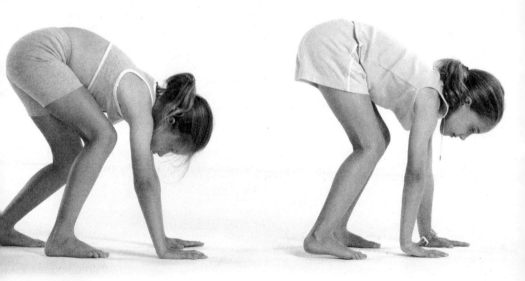

notes

Chapter 1

Page 2: Henry Gray, F.R.S., *Anatomy Descriptive and Surgical*, 1901 ed. (Philadelphia: Courage Books/Running Press, 1974).

Page 4: Colin Tudge, *The Time Before History: Five Million Years of Human Impact* (New York: Simon & Schuster, 1996), pp. 186–87.

Chapter 3

Page 32: "Brain May Grow New Cells Daily," *New York Times*, October 15, 1999.

Page 34: Andrew Weil, M.D., *Spontaneous Healing* (New York: Alfred A. Knopf, 1995), pp. 81–82.

Page 38: Sherwin B. Nuland, *The Wisdom of the Body* (New York: Alfred A. Knopf, 1997), p. 182.

Chapter 4

Page 56: "Preventing Fatal Medical Errors," *New York Times*, December 1, 1999.

Page 58: Natalie Angier, *Woman: An Intimate Geography* (New York: Houghton Mifflin, 1999), p. 290.

Chapter 5

Page 65: Benjamin Spock, M.D., and Steven J. Parker, M.D., *Dr. Spock's Baby and Child Care*, 7th ed. (New York: Pocket Books, 1998), p. 77.

Page 69: Ibid., p. 250.

Chapter 6

Page 81: Michael Cole and Sheila R. Cole, *The Development of Children*, 3rd ed. (New York: W. H. Freeman, 1996).

Page 87: "Behavioral Drug Use in Children Up Sharply," *Washington Post*, February 23, 2000.

Chapter 7

Page 108: Cole and Cole, *Development*, pp. 485–88, 282. I have relied heavily on the authors' discussion of the work of psychologist Jean Piaget.

Page 117: *Lancet*'s figures on the historic trend in puberty onset are quoted in James Pinkerton, "Today's Puberty Is Too Fast for Society," *Newsday*, April 2, 1998.

Page 120: Tavris, *Mismeasure*, pp. 135–36.

Page 122: "The Face of Teenage Sex Grows Younger," *New York Times*, April 2, 2000.

Chapter 9

Page 138: The statistics on average U.S. height come from Barry Bogin, "The Tall and Short of It," *Discover*, February 1998. It's also an informative essay on what Bogin terms human "plasticity."

Page 141: The soft drink demographic and consumption data are drawn from Michael F. Jacobson, Ph.D., "Liquid Candy: How Soft Drinks Are Harming Americans' Health," Center for Science in the Public Interest, http://cspinet.org/sodapop/liquid_candy.htm.

Chapter 10

Page 184: Eldra Pearle Solomon, Richard R. Schmidt, and Peter James Andragna, *Human Anatomy and Physiology*, 2nd ed. (New York: Saunders College Publishing, 1990), pp. 1075–76.

Page 185: Nuland, *Wisdom*, pp. 188–89.

Page 186: "Premature Births Up Among White Women, Down For Minorities," Associated Press, March 12, 1999.

Chapter 11

Page 219: The figures on muscle loss are drawn from Miriam E. Nelson, Ph.D., with Sarah Wernick, Ph.D., *Strong Women Stay Young* (New York: Bantam Books, 1998), p. 22.

Page 220: Angier, *Woman*, p. 292.

Page 221: The photos of bone and muscle loss are in ibid., p. 23.

Page 221: Miriam E. Nelson, Ph.D., with Sarah Wernick, Ph.D., *Strong Women Stay Slim* (New York: Bantam Books, 1998).

Chapter 12

Page 250: "Fat," *Frontline* (WGBH/PBS), aired November 3, 1998.

Page 252: Barry Sears, Ph.D., with Bill Lawren, *The Zone: A Dietary Road Map* (New York: HarperCollins, 1995).

Page 254: Nelson with Wernick, *Strong Women Stay Slim*, p. 6.

Chapter 13

Page 306: Angier, *Woman*, p. 94.

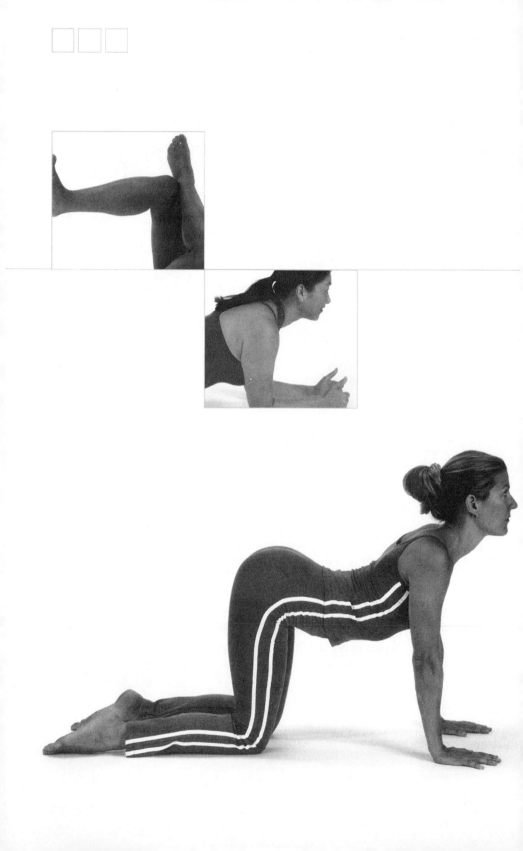

about the authors

Pete Egoscue, an anatomical physiologist since 1978, operates the Egoscue Method Clinic in San Diego. His exercise therapy program is acclaimed worldwide for treating chronic musculoskeletal pain attributed to workplace and sports injuries, accidents, aging, and other conditions. He is also author with Roger Gittines of *Pain Free: A Revolutionary Method for Stopping Chronic Pain* and *The Egoscue Method of Health Through Motion.*

Roger Gittines is a writer living in Washington, D.C.

For more information on the Egoscue Method Clinic, please call 1-800-995-8434 or visit www.egoscue.com

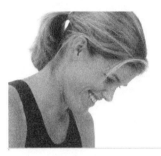

index

Note: Page numbers in *italics* refer to illustrations. See list of illustrations on pages xi-xvii. Capitalized entries refer to specific exercises.

A

Abdominal Crunches, 407, *407*, 424, *424*
Abduction-Adduction, 151, *151*, 170, *170*, 191, *191*, 377, *377*, 406, *406*
abductor muscles, 23–24
abortion, spontaneous, 183
abstract thinking, 108
Active Bridges, 169, *169*
adaptiveness, 53
ADD (attention deficit disorder), 86–91
adductor muscles, 23–24
ADHD (attention deficit hyperactivity disorder), 86–91
adipose tissue, 57
adolescents, *see* teenagers
adrenal glands, 140
adrenaline, 120, 123
adulthood, 219–47
  aging and, *see* aging
  E-cise menus, 224, 226–47
  muscle and bone loss in, 219–21
  strength in, 221–24
  weight in, *see* weight management
  young, *see* young adulthood

aging, 333–55
  Alzheimer's disease, 365, 367–68
  anti-aging, 290–91
  arthritis in, 362–65
  and balance, *see* balance
  Balance and Breathing Menu, 370–79
  and cancer, 368–69
  cosmetic signs of, 260–61
  as deceleration of mortality, 346
  and degeneration, 34–35, 336
  and disease, 333–34, 338–40
  E-cises for, 346–47, 348–55, 370–79
  elder model, 345–46
  eyes and ears in, 358–62
  and hip fractures, 357
  and injury, 357–58
  metabolic deterioration in, 340–41
  muscle and bone loss in, 219–21
  and negative capability, 336–38
  Over-Fifty Restoration and Maintenance Menu, 348–55
  Parkinson's disease and, 365–68
  and pregnancy, 187–88
  ring-related symptoms in, 338–40
  and stiffness, 30, 40
Air Bench, 278, *278*, 285, *285*, 320, *320*, *323*, 425, *425*
alcohol abuse, 122
alignment, checking for, 7–9

educational reform for, 89–90
eye-hand coordination of, 75
first years of, *see* babies
free play for, 91–93
games for, 98–99
gender differentiation of, 90–91
good behavior of, 82–84
hyperactive, 75, 85–91, 95
imagination and, 97–99
learning mechanisms of, 81–84, 100
locomotor skills of, 75
Middle Childhood Menu, 393–400
movement patterns of, 81–82, 85, 100
movement restrictions on, 80, 83–84, 92
musculoskeletal system dysfunctions of, 82, 85, 93–97, *93*, *94*, 99–100
obesity of, 138
outcome-oriented, 98
perception of, 81
posture of, 75, *99*
reading readiness of, 89, 99
size increases in, 118
sleep patterns of, 92, 96, 100
socialization of, 83
as "straight-ahead kids," 97
structured lives of, 92, 93
symptoms of, 94–96
television watched by, 93
Toddlers Menu, 392
vulnerability of, 341
weight-to-muscle ratio of, 118
chromosomal abnormalities, 182
chronic pain, 9–11, 18, 20
circulatory system, and water, 144
Cobra, 389, *389*
Cobra on Elbows, 407, *407*
communication systems, 177–79, 380
compensating motion, 20–21, 22–23
computer use, 93, 106–7, *107*
Core Abdominals, 155, *155*, 167, *167*, 239, *239*, 269, *269*
Counter Stretch, 204, *204*
Coyle, Joseph T., 87
Crab Walks, 394, *394*
crawling, babies and, 69–70, 72

Crawling Around the House, 392
Crawl Unders, 398, *398*
Cross-Crawling, 388, *388*

D

dehydration, 144, 145
depression, 124–25
Diagnosis and Nonsurgical Treatment Menu, 315–22
diet, *see* nutrition
digestion, and water, 144
digestive system, 180
dopamine deficiency, 366
dotage, use of term, 345
Downward Dog, 173, *173*, 205, *205*, 233, *233*, 246, *246*, 423, *423*
Dr. Spock's Baby and Child Care (Spock and Parker), 65
drug abuse, 122

E

ears, and balance, 361–62
eating disorders, 122–23, 140
E-cises (Egoscue-cises), 30, 129–35
   Abdominal Crunches, 407, *407*, 424, *424*
   Abduction-Adduction, 151, *151*, 170, *170*, 191, *191*, 377, *377*, 406, *406*
   Active Bridges, 169, *169*
   for adults, 224, 226–47
   aging and, 346–47, 348–55, 370–79
   Air Bench, 278, *278*, 285, *285*, 320, *320*, *323*, 425, *425*
   for babies, 387–91
   balance and, 130, 369, 370–79
   Bear Crawls, 397, *397*
   Bench Hops, 277, *277*
   benchmarks for, 132–33, 134
   Bicep Curls, 288, *288*
   Cats and Dogs, *see* Cats and Dogs
   Chair Crawl, 392
   in childhood, 393–400
   Cobra, 389, *389*, 407, *407*
   Core Abdominals, 155, *155*, 167, *167*, 239, *239*, 269, *269*
   Counter Stretch, 204, *204*
   Crab Walks, 394, *394*

Z